Multicultural Health

Lois A. Ritter, EdD, MS, MA

Assistant Professor, Nursing and Health Sciences Department
California State University, East Bay

Nancy A. Hoffman, JD, BSN

Assistant Professor, Nursing and Health Sciences Department
California State University, East Bay

JONES AND BARTLETT PUBLISHERS

Sudbury, Massachusetts

BOSTON   TORONTO   LONDON   SINGAPORE

World Headquarters
Jones and Bartlett Publishers
40 Tall Pine Drive
Sudbury, MA 01776
978-443-5000
info@jbpub.com
www.jbpub.com

Jones and Bartlett's books and products are available through most bookstores and online booksellers. To contact Jones and Bartlett Publishers directly, call 800-832-0034, fax 978-443-8000, or visit our website www.jbpub.com.

Substantial discounts on bulk quantities of Jones and Bartlett's publications are available to corporations, professional associations, and other qualified organizations. For details and specific discount information, contact the special sales department at Jones and Bartlett via the above contact information or send an email to specialsales@jbpub.com.

Production Credits

Acquisitions Editor: Shoshanna Goldberg
Senior Associate Editor: Amy L. Bloom
Production Assistant: Jill Morton
Associate Marketing Manager: Jody Sullivan
V.P., Manufacturing and Inventory Control: Therese Connell
Composition: International Typesetting and Composition
Cover Design: Kristin E. Parker
Assistant Photo Researcher: Bridget Kane
Cover and Title Page Images: See
  Photography Credits page
Printing and Binding: Edwards Brothers Malloy
Cover Printing: Edwards Brothers Malloy

Library of Congress Cataloging-in-Publication Data

Ritter, Lois A.
    Multicultural health / by Lois A. Ritter and Nancy A. Hoffman.
      p. ; cm.
    Includes bibliographical references and index.
    ISBN-13: 978-0-7637-5742-7
    ISBN-10: 0-7637-5742-X
    1. Transcultural medical care—United States. I. Hoffman, Nancy A. II. Title.
    [DNLM: 1. Cultural Competency—United States. 2. Cross-Cultural Comparison—United States. 3. Delivery of Health
    Care—United States. 4. Ethnic Groups—United States. W 21 R614m 2010]
    RA418.5.T73R58 2010
    362.1089—dc22
                                    2009007713
6048

Printed in the United States of America
18 17 16 15 14   10 9 8 7 6 5

To Juls and Sammie, my unselfish friends who never desert me and provide unbounded and limitless love and joy. —LR

CONTENTS

PREFACE

Your mind is like a parachute . . . it functions only when open.

—Author unknown

Health care professionals are increasingly aware of the importance of working in a diverse society and the challenges this can present. As a result, there is a need and demand for these professionals to move toward becoming culturally competent. Knowing about every culture is not a possible task. *Multicultural Health* provides an introduction and overview to some of the major cultural differences related to health. Through this text, those engaged in health care can acquire the skills necessary to improve their effectiveness when working with diverse groups, regardless of the culture of the community in which they live or work. The content is useful to working in the field on both individual and community levels. This text serves as a guide to the concepts and theories related to cultural issues in health and as a primer on health issues and practices specific to certain cultures and ethnic groups.

Multicultural Health is divided into three units. Unit I, "The Foundations," includes Chapters 1 through 6 and focuses on the context of culture, cultural beliefs regarding health and illness, health disparities, law and ethics, models for cross-cultural health and communication, and approaches to culturally-appropriate health promotion programs and evaluation. Unit II, "Specific Cultural Groups," includes Chapters 7 through 12 and focuses on specific cultural and ethnic groups and various issues related to their health concerns. Unit III, "Looking Ahead," outlines priority areas in health disparities and strategies to eliminate health disparities.

Chapter 1, "Introduction to Multicultural Health," discusses the reasons for becoming knowledgeable about the cultural impact of health practices. It defines terminology and key concepts that set the foundation for the remainder of the text. The chapter addresses diversity in the United States and the racial makeup of the country, health disparities and their causes among cultures, and issues related to medical care in the context of culture.

Chapter 2, "Cross-Cultural Concepts of Health and Illness," addresses different cultural theories regarding the occurrence of illness and its treatment. It discusses the concept of worldview on illness and treatment, and it explores cultural influences on communication. Terms and theoretical models related to cultural competence are provided.

Chapter 3, "Complementary and Alternative Medicine," provides an introduction to folk, complementary, and alternative medicine and health practices. It explores the major non-Western medicine modalities of care, including ayurvedic medicine, traditional Chinese medicine, herbal medicine, holistic and naturopathic medicine, and chiropractic. The history, theories, and beliefs regarding the source of illness and treatment modalities are described.

Chapter 4, "Religion, Rituals, and Health," explores the role of religion and spiritual beliefs in health and health behavior. The similarities and differences between religion and rituals are described. The chapter also includes an overview of the prevalent religious beliefs in the United States and their impact on health decisions and outcomes.

Chapter 5, "Multicultural Health: Legal and Ethical Impacts," provides a review of the various laws that impact cultural health practices in the United States. The chapter explains the laws and regulations that limit and protect those practices and the various policies designed to further culturally competent health care. Finally, the basic ethical tenets that apply to health care are explored and discussed in relation to cultural issues.

Chapter 6, "Health Promotion in Diverse Societies," includes information about community program planning, implementation, and evaluation. The content is tailored toward special considerations for working with diverse populations. Social marketing and tailoring your message are highlighted in this chapter.

Unit II addresses the history of specific cultural groups in the United States, beliefs regarding the causes of health and illness, healing traditions and practices, common health problems, and health promotion and program planning for the various cultural groups. These points are applied to specific cultural groups as follows:

Chapter 7, "Hispanic and Latino American Populations"
Chapter 8, "American Indian and Alaska Native Populations"
Chapter 9, "African American Populations"
Chapter 10, "Asian American and Pacific Islander Populations"
Chapter 11, "Caucasian American Populations"
Chapter 12, "Nonethnic Populations: Lesbian, Gay, Bisexual, and Transgender (LGBT) Individuals; Migrant Farmworkers"

Unit III contains Chapter 13, "Closing the Gap: Strategies for Eliminating Health Disparities," which explores the implications of the growth of diversity in the United States in relation to future disease prevention and treatment. It further addresses diversity in the health care workforce and its impact on care, as well as the need for ongoing education in cultural competence for health care practitioners.

Each chapter includes chapter review questions and a case study with topics to consider. The chapters in Unit II also include discussions of model programs that are directed toward the group discussed in that particular chapter.

We hope that the information contained in *Multicultural Health* will introduce students to the rich and fascinating cultural landscape in the United States and the diverse health practices and beliefs of various cultural groups. This book is not intended to be an end point; rather, it is a starting place in the journey to becoming culturally competent in health care.

ANCILLARIES

The Web site that accompanies this text, http://health.jbpub.com/multicultural, includes study tools for students, including Chapter Outlines and Web Links. Online instructor resources, including PowerPoint presentations, Instructor's Manual, and TestBank questions are also available. Contact your sales representative or visit www.jbpub.com for access.

ACKNOWLEDGMENTS

We would like to express our gratitude to the many dedicated people whose contributions made this book possible. We extend a special thanks to those who provided us with permission to reprint their work in this textbook. We also are grateful to the Jones and Bartlett Publishers team who assisted with the writing, editing, design, and marketing of this book. We would like to particularly acknowledge Jacqueline Geraci, Shoshanna Goldberg, Amy Bloom, and Jill Morton at Jones and Bartlett for their efforts. Two students at California State University, East Bay, are to be acknowledged for their assistance with the research conducted for this publication: Cherilyn Aranzamendez and Jessica Ross, we appreciate your tireless efforts to locate research and case studies on the topic of multicultural health. We are also indebted to the reviewers for their thoughtful and valuable suggestions:

Patricia Coleman Burns, PhD, University of Michigan
Mary Hysell Lynd, PhD, Wright State University
Maureen J. Dunn, RN, Pennsylvania State University, Shenango Campus
Sharon B. McLaughlin, MS, ATC, CSCS, Mesa Community College
Melba I. Ovalle, MD, Nova Southeastern University

Our families, friends, and colleagues are probably the most difficult people to express our gratitude to because they provided continued encouragement, support, and recognition throughout the process. Of course, we also want to thank our dogs for sitting by our sides and keeping us company while we spent an uncountable number of hours in our home offices writing this text.

ABOUT THE AUTHORS

Dr. Lois A. Ritter has earned a doctorate in education and master's degrees in health science and anthropology. She is an assistant professor in the nursing and health sciences department at California State University, East Bay, where she teaches community health and evaluation. Dr. Ritter also is a consultant specializing in program planning and evaluation in the public health field.

Nancy A. Hoffman is a registered nurse and attorney practicing in health law. She is an assistant professor of nursing and health sciences at California State University, East Bay.

UNIT I: The Foundations

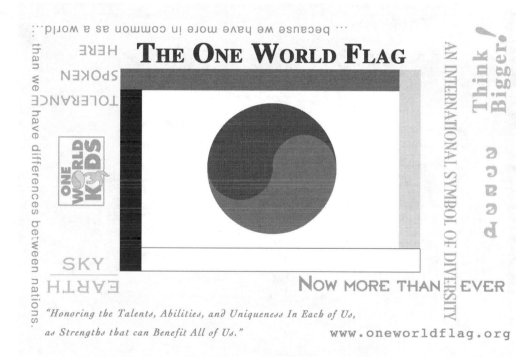

THE ONE WORLD FLAG

AN INTERNATIONAL SYMBOL OF DIVERSITY

Think Bigger!

...because we have more in common as a world...

HERE

SPOKEN

TOLERANCE

...than we have differences between nations.

SKY

EARTH

NOW MORE THAN EVER

"Honoring the Talents, Abilities, and Uniqueness In Each of Us, as Strengths that can Benefit All of Us."

www.oneworldflag.org

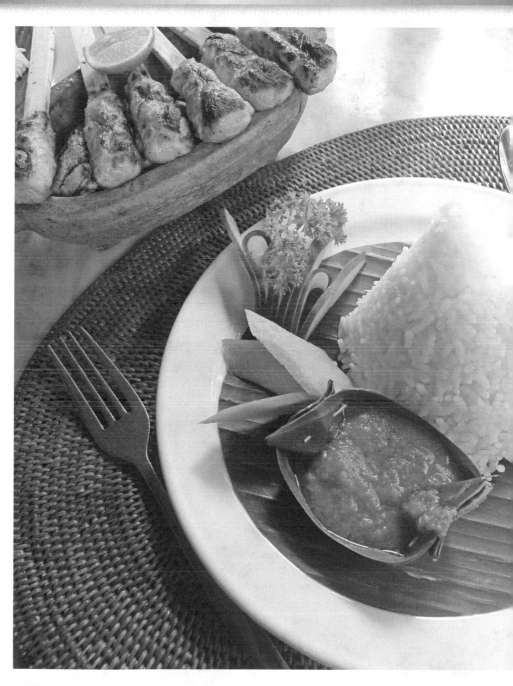

CHAPTER 1

Introduction to Multicultural Health

We have become not a melting pot but a beautiful mosaic. Different people, different beliefs, different yearnings, different hopes, different dreams.

—Author unknown

One day our descendants will think it incredible that we paid so much attention to things like the amount of melanin in our skin or the shape of our eyes or our gender instead of the unique identities of each of us as complex human beings.

—Author unknown

KEY CONCEPTS

- Multicultural health
- Culture
- Cultural competency
- Race
- Acculturation
- Ethnicity
- Ethnocentricity
- Cultural relativism
- Racism

- Discrimination
- Minority
- Cultural adaptation
- Dominant culture
- Assimilation
- Heritage consistency
- Health disparities
- *Healthy People 2010*

CHAPTER OBJECTIVES

1. Explain why cultural considerations are important in health care.
2. Describe the processes of acculturation and assimilation.
3. Define race, culture, ethnicity, ethnocentricity, and cultural relativism.
4. Explain what cultural adaptation is and why it is important in health care.
5. Explain what health disparities are and their related causes.
6. List the five elements of the determinants of health and describe how they relate to health disparities.

Why do we need to study **multicultural health**? Why is **culture** important if we all have the same basic biological make-up? Isn't health all about science? Shouldn't people from different cultural backgrounds just adapt to the way that we provide health care in the United States if they are in this country?

For decades, the role that culture plays in health was virtually ignored, but the links have now become more apparent. As a result, the focus on the need to educate health care professionals about the important role that culture plays in health has escalated. Health is influenced by factors such as genetics, the environment, and socioeconomic status, as well as cultural and social forces. Culture impacts people's perception of health and illness, how they pursue and adhere to treatment, their health behaviors, beliefs about why people become ill, how symptoms and concerns about the problem are expressed, what is considered to be a health problem, and ways to maintain and restore health. This is why recognizing cultural similarities and differences is an essential component to delivering effective health care services. To provide quality care, health care professionals need to provide services within a cultural context, which is the focus of multicultural health.

Multicultural health is the phrase used to reflect the need to provide health care services in a sensitive, knowledgeable, and nonjudgmental manner with respect for people's health beliefs and practices when they are different than your own. It entails challenging your own assumptions, asking the right questions, and working with the patient and/or community in a manner that takes into consideration their lifestyle and approach to maintaining health and treating illness. Multicultural health integrates different approaches to care and incorporates the culture and belief system of the health care recipient while providing care within the legal, ethical, and medically sound practices of the practitioner's medical system.

Knowing the health practices and cultures of all groups is not possible, but becoming familiar with various groups' general health beliefs and variances can be very beneficial and improve the effectiveness of health care services. In this book, we make generalizations about cultural groups, but it is important to realize that many sub-cultures exist within those cultures, and people vary in the degree to which they identify with the beliefs and practices of their culture of origin. Awareness of general differences can help health care professionals provide services within a cultural context, but it is important to distinguish between stereotyping (the mistaken assumption that everyone in a given culture is alike) and generalizations (awareness of cultural norms) (Juckett, 2005). Generalizations can serve as a starting point and do not preclude factoring in individual characteristics, such as education, nationality, faith, and level of cultural adaptation. Stereotypes and assumptions can be problematic and can lead to errors and ineffective care. Remember, every person is unique, but understanding the generalizations can be beneficial, because it moves people in the direction of becoming culturally competent.

Cultural competency refers to possessing knowledge, awareness, and respect for other cultures (Juckett, 2005). Cultural competence occurs on a continuum, and this is the first chapter of a book that is geared to help you progress along the cultural competency scale. There are many key terms used that are related to multicultural health, such as **race** and **acculturation**, that need to be clarified, so we begin this chapter by defining and describing these terms. Then we move into a discussion about types and degrees of cultural adaptation, how the demographic landscape of the population in the United States is changing, and why it is important to take those demographic changes into consideration when delivering health care services.

KEY CONCEPTS AND TERMS

Some of the terminology related to multicultural health can be confusing, because the differences are difficult to distinguish. This section is designed to clarify the terminology. The terms described here are culture, race, **ethnicity**, **ethnocentricity**, and **cultural relativism**.

Culture

There are countless definitions of culture. The short explanation is that culture is everything that makes us who we are. E. B. Tylor, who is considered to be the founder of cultural anthropology, provided the classical definition of culture. Tylor stated in 1871, "Culture, or civilization, taken in its broad, ethnographic sense, is that complex whole which includes knowledge, belief, art, morals, law, custom, and any other capabilities and habits acquired by man as a member of society" (Tylor, 1924/1871, p. 1). Tylor's definition is still widely cited today. A more current definition is, "The thoughts, communications, actions, customs, beliefs, values, and institutions of racial, ethnic, religious, or social groups" (Office of Minority Health, 2001, p. 131).

Culture is learned, changes over time, and is passed on from generation to generation. It is a very complex system, and many subcultures exist within the dominant culture. For example, universities, businesses, neighborhoods, age groups, homosexuals, athletic teams, and musicians are sub-cultures of the American dominant culture. People simultaneously belong to numerous sub-cultures, because we can be students at a university, fathers or mothers, and employees at the same time.

Race and Ethnicity

Race refers to a person's physical characteristics and/or genetic or biological makeup, but the reality is that race is not a scientific construct; it is a social construct. Race was developed so that people can be categorized, and it is based on the notion that some races are superior to others. Many professionals in the fields of biology, sociology, and anthropology have determined that race is a social construct and not a biological one because not one characteristic, trait, or gene distinguishes all the members of one so-called race from all the members of another so-called race. "There is more genetic variation within races than between them, and racial categories do not capture biological distinctiveness" (Williams, Lavizzo-Mourey, & Warren, 1994). So why is race important if it does not really exist? Race is important because society makes it important. Race shapes social, cultural, political, ideological, and legal functions in society. The result is that race is an institutionalized concept that has had devastating consequences. Race has been the basis for deaths from wars and murders and suffering caused by discrimination, violence, torture, and hate crimes. The ideology of race has been the root of suffering and death for centuries even though it has no scientific merit.

In the 2000 U.S. census, the question of race was asked differently than in previous years. Respondents were given the option of selecting one or more race categories to indicate their racial identities. The race categories and their related definitions were:

White: a person having origins in any of the original peoples of Europe, the Middle East, or North Africa

Black or African American: a person having origins in any of the black racial groups of Africa

American Indian or Alaska Native: a person having origins in any of the originals peoples of North and South America (including Central America) and who maintain tribal affiliation or community attachment

Asian: a person having origins in any of the original peoples of the Far East, Southeast Asia, or the Indian subcontinent, including, for example, China, India, and the Philippine Islands

Native Hawaiian or other Pacific Islander: a person having origins in any of the original peoples of Hawaii, Guam, Samoa, or other Pacific Islands

The United States government declared that Hispanics and Latinos are an ethnicity and not a race, which is correct, and the rationale is explained in Chapter 7. The government defines Hispanic or Latino as a person of Cuban, Mexican, Puerto Rican, South or Central American, or other Spanish culture or origin regardless of race.

PLEASE DO NOT FILL OUT THIS FORM.
This is not an official census form. It is for informational purposes only.

United States
Census 2000

U.S. Department of Commerce • Bureau of the Census

This is the official form for all the people at this address. It is quick and easy, and your answers are protected by law. Complete the Census and help your community get what it needs — today and in the future!

Start Here

Please use a black or blue pen.

1. How many people were living or staying in this house, apartment, or mobile home on April 1, 2000?

Number of people

INCLUDE in this number:
- foster children, roomers, or housemates
- people staying here on April 1, 2000 who have no other permanent place to stay
- people living here most of the time while working, even if they have another place to live

DO NOT INCLUDE in this number:
- college students living away while attending college
- people in a correctional facility, nursing home, or mental hospital on April 1, 2000
- Armed Forces personnel living somewhere else
- people who live or stay at another place most of the time

2. Is this house, apartment, or mobile home — *Mark* ☒ *ONE box.*
- ☐ Owned by you or someone in this household with a mortgage or loan?
- ☐ Owned by you or someone in this household free and clear (without a mortgage or loan)?
- ☐ Rented for cash rent?
- ☐ Occupied without payment of cash rent?

3. Please answer the following questions for each person living in this house, apartment, or mobile home. Start with the name of one of the people living here who owns, is buying, or rents this house, apartment, or mobile home. If there is no such person, start with any adult living or staying here. We will refer to this person as Person 1.

What is this person's name? *Print name below.*

Last Name

First Name   MI

4. What is Person 1's telephone number? *We may call this person if we don't understand an answer.*

Area Code + Number

5. What is Person 1's sex? *Mark* ☒ *ONE box.*
- ☐ Male   ☐ Female

6. What is Person 1's age and what is Person 1's date of birth?
Age on April 1, 2000

Print numbers in boxes.
Month   Day   Year of birth

→ **NOTE: Please answer BOTH Questions 7 and 8.**

7. Is Person 1 Spanish/Hispanic/Latino? *Mark* ☒ *the "No" box if not Spanish/Hispanic/Latino.*
- ☐ **No,** not Spanish/Hispanic/Latino   ☐ Yes, Puerto Rican
- ☐ Yes, Mexican, Mexican Am., Chicano   ☐ Yes, Cuban
- ☐ Yes, other Spanish/Hispanic/Latino — *Print group.* ↗

8. What is Person 1's race? *Mark* ☒ *one or more races* to indicate what this person considers himself/herself to be.
- ☐ White
- ☐ Black, African Am., or Negro
- ☐ American Indian or Alaska Native — *Print name of enrolled or principal tribe.* ↗

- ☐ Asian Indian   ☐ Japanese   ☐ Native Hawaiian
- ☐ Chinese   ☐ Korean   ☐ Guamanian or Chamorro
- ☐ Filipino   ☐ Vietnamese   ☐ Samoan
- ☐ Other Asian — *Print race.* ↗   ☐ Other Pacific Islander — *Print race.* ↗

- ☐ Some other race — *Print race.* ↗

OMB No. 0607-0856: Approval Expires 12/31/2000

Form **D-61A**

→ **If more people live here, continue with Person 2.**

Source: U.S. Census Bureau, Public Information Office, http://www.census.gov/dmd/www/2000quest.html.

It is important to note that there is great variation within each of the government's racial and ethnic categories, and in this book we address the basic foundation of each group. It is rare to identify all of the themes in any individual due to differences in the level of their acculturation. Also, within each racial and ethnic category is great variation. For example, the Asian category includes Chinese and Indians, who have variations between them. Therefore, it is essential to be aware of the differences that occur within these groups and to not stereotype people.

Stereotyping people by their race and ethnicity may lead to **racism**. Racism is the belief that some races are superior to others by nature and can result in discrimination. **Discrimination** occurs when people act on a belief, and differences in treatment transpire as a result. Discrimination can occur because of beliefs related to factors such as race, sexual orientation, dialect, religion, or gender.

Ethnicity is "the characteristic of a group of people who share a common and distinctive racial, national, religious, linguistic, or cultural heritage" (Office of Minority Health, 2001, p. 131). Ethnicity is made up of the following characteristics:

- Geographic origins
- Family patterns
- Language
- Values and symbols
- Cultural norms
- Religion
- Literature
- Music
- Dietary patterns
- Gender roles
- Employment patterns

So how is ethnicity different from culture? One can belong to a culture without having ancestral roots to that culture. For example, a person can belong to the hip–hop culture, but he or she is not born into the culture.

Cultural Ethnocentricity and Cultural Relativism

Cultural ethnocentricity refers to when a person believes that his or her culture is superior to another one. This can cause problems in the health care field if a professional believes that his or her way is the better way to prevent or treat a health problem and disrespects or ignores the patient's or client's cultural beliefs and values. The health care professional may not take into consideration that the listener may have different views than the provider. This can lead to ineffective communication and treatment and leave the listener feeling unimportant, frustrated, disrespected, or confused about how to prevent or treat the health issue, and he or she might view the professional as uneducated, uncooperative, unapproachable, or closed-minded. To be effective, one needs to see and appreciate the value of different cultures; this is referred to as cultural relativism.

Cultural relativism came about in an attempt to refute the idea of cultural ethnocentricity. The phrase was derived in the field of anthropology, and it is an approach that posits that all cultures are of equal value and need to be studied from a neutral point of view. It rejects value judgments on cultures and holds the belief that no culture is superior. Cultural relativism takes an objective view of cultures and incorporates the idea that if a society's moral code believes that something is right (or wrong), then it is right (or wrong) for members of that society.

DIVERSITY WITHIN THE UNITED STATES

A great strength of the United States is the diversity of the people. Historically, waves of immigrants have come to the United States to start their lives in the land of opportunity in pursuit of a better quality of life. The immigrants brought with them their traditions, languages, and cultures to create a country with a very diverse landscape. Some of the diverse landscape occurred for other reasons, such as Africans being forced to come to the United States and the American Indians who originated here. An unfortunate outcome of this diversity is that it has contributed to the history of racial and cultural clashes along with imbalances in equality and opportunities that continue today. These positive and adverse consequences of diversity must be considered in our health care approaches, particularly because the demographics are continuing to change and the inequalities persist. The delivery of health care to individuals, families, and communities must meet the needs of the wide variety of people who reside in and visit the United States.

The percentage of the United States population characterized as white is decreasing (see Figure 1.1). The term **minority** is becoming outdated because the minority population grew 11 times as rapidly as the white, non-Hispanic population between 1980 and 2000 (Hobbs & Stoops, 2002), and it is projected that by 2050 nearly one-half of the United States population will be composed of non-whites (McKenzie, Pinger, & Kotecki, 2005). This is an important consideration for health care providers, because ethnic minorities experience poorer health status. These disparities in health are discussed later in this chapter.

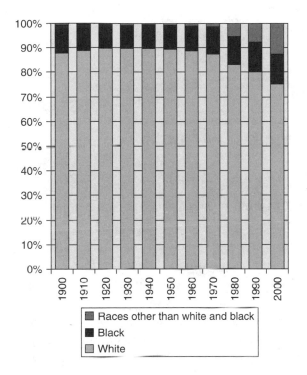

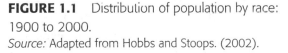

FIGURE 1.1 Distribution of population by race:
1900 to 2000.
Source: Adapted from Hobbs and Stoops. (2002).

CULTURAL ADAPTATION

With this changing landscape in the United States, professionals are encouraged to consider the degree of cultural adaptation that the person has experienced. **Cultural adaptation** refers to the degree to which a person or community has adapted to the **dominant culture** and retained their traditional practices. Generally, a first-generation individual will identify more with his or her culture of origin than a third-generation person. Therefore, when working with the first-generation person, the health care professional will need to be more sensitive to issues such as language barriers, distrust, lack of understanding of the American medical system, and the person's ties to his or her traditional beliefs. Acculturation and **assimilation** are terms that relate to the degree of adaptation that has taken place.

Acculturation refers to a process in which members of one cultural group adopt the beliefs and behaviors of another group. Essentially, members of one cultural

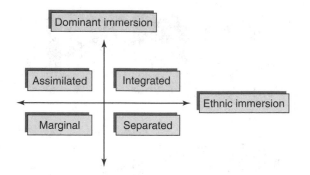

FIGURE 1.2   Acculturation framework.

group acquire a second culture. Usually the minority culture takes up many of the dominant culture's traits. People can experience different levels of acculturation as illustrated in Berry and colleagues' acculturation framework, which is illustrated in Figure 1.2.

An assimilated individual demonstrates high dominant and low ethnic society immersion. This entails moving away from one's ethnic society and immersing fully in the dominant society (Stephenson, 2000). An individual who rejects his or her country of origin would fall into this category. An integrated person has high dominant and ethnic immersion. Integration entails immersion in both ethnic and dominant societies (Stephenson, 2000). An example of an integrated person is a French American who socializes with the dominant group but chooses to speak French at home and marries a person who is French. Separated individuals have low dominant immersion and high ethnic immersion. A separated individual withdraws from the dominant society and completely immerges in the ethnic society (Stephenson, 2000). An example is a person who lives in ethnic communities such as Little Italy or Chinatown. A marginalized individual has low dominant and ethnic immersion and does not identify with any particular culture or belief system.

The marginalized people tend to have the most psychological problems and highest stress levels. These individuals often lack social support systems and are not accepted by the dominant society or their culture of origin. A person in the separated mode is accepted in his or her ethnic society but may not be accepted by the dominant culture, leaving the person feeling alienated. The integrated and assimilated modes are considered to be the most psychologically healthy adaptation styles, although some individuals benefit more from one than from the other. Western Europeans and individuals whose families have been in the United States for a number of generations (and are not discriminated against) are most likely to adopt an assimilated mode because they have many beliefs and attributes of the dominant society. Individuals who retain value structures from their country of origin and encounter discrimination benefit more from an integrated (bicultural) mode. To be bicultural one must be knowledgeable about both cultures and see the positive attributes of both of them.

Assimilation is the process that occurs when individuals or groups of different cultures are absorbed into the dominant society. As a result there is a disappearance of a minority group through the loss of particular identifying physical or socio-cultural characteristics. This usually occurs when people immigrate into a new geographic region, and through their contact with the dominant groups and their desire to be a part of the mainstream they give up most of their culture traits of origin and take on a new cultural identity, which is the one of the dominant culture. The reality is that many people do not fully assimilate because they tend to keep some of their cultural beliefs from the origin.

The degree to which people identify with their culture of origin is sometimes referred to as **heritage consistency**. Some indicators that can help professionals assess the level of cultural adaptation are inquiring about how long the person has been in the country, how often the person returns to his or her culture of origin, what holidays the person celebrates, what language the person speaks at home, and how much knowledge the person has of his or her culture of origin.

Are people who have higher levels of cultural adaptation healthier? Despite increasing research on the relationships between acculturation and health, the answer is not clearly defined. The influence of acculturation on health in the literature indicates contradictory results because the variables are complex. The answer also is dependent upon what health habits are incorporated into one's lifestyle and what ones are lost. For example, acculturation can have detrimental effects on one's dietary patterns if a person is from a culture where eating fruits and vegetables is common and the person incorporates the habit of eating at fast food restaurants, which is common in the United States. On the other hand, if someone moves from a culture where smoking is common to a culture where it is frowned upon, the person may stop smoking.

As noted, acculturation can have both negative and positive affects on health. Zambrana, Scrimshaw, Collins, and Dunkel-Schetter (1997) found that Mexican American women who are undergoing the process of immersion in the mainstream culture "experience a decrease in culture-specific protective factors that are integrally related to the quality of the community environment in which they live" (Zambrana, et al., 1997, p. 1025). In the study conducted by Zambrana and colleagues (1997), risky health behaviors, stress levels, and medical risks all seemed to increase with greater acculturation and decrease in protective factors, such as social support, in the Hispanic community. Lack of fluency in English may adversely affect health as the prevalence of risks for chronic disease and injury among certain racial and ethnic groups increases. Some immigrants are highly educated and have high incomes (Council of Economic Advisors for the President's Initiative on Race, 1998), but their lack of familiarity with the United States public and private health care systems, different cultural attitudes about the use of traditional and United States conventional medicine (Centers for Disease Control and Prevention [CDC], 1991), and lack of fluency in English may pose barriers to obtaining appropriate health care (CDC, 1997). Poverty also is associated with lower levels of acculturation, which affects immigrants' health as well.

On the contrary, acculturation can have a favorable impact on immigrants' health. For example, people with higher acculturation levels learn how to navigate the health care system in the United States and may have language skills that enable them to communicate more effectively. Tran, Fitzpatrick, Berg, and Wright (1996) wrote that the level of acculturation has a significant affect upon health status. Less acculturated respondents experienced higher rates of self-reported health problems than people with higher levels of acculturation. Fewer language skills and less education are factors that are related to the avoidance of obtaining health-care services (Tran, et al., 1996).

HEALTH DISPARITIES

Health disparities are differences in the incidence, prevalence, mortality, burden of diseases, and other adverse health conditions or outcomes that exist among specific population groups in the United States. The specific population groups can be based on gender, age, ethnicity, socioeconomic status, geography, sexual orientation, disability, or special health care needs. Health disparities occur among groups who have persistently experienced historic trauma, social disadvantage, or discrimination. They are widespread in the United States as demonstrated by the fact that many minority groups in the United States have a higher incidence of chronic diseases, higher mortality, and poorer health outcomes when compared to whites (Goldberg, Hayes, & Huntley, 2004).

Eliminating health disparities is an important goal for our nation as indicated by the fact that it is the second major goal of *Healthy People 2010*. Some ways to eliminate health inequalities include changing policy, increasing access to care, and creating a culturally competent health-care system. Examples of health disparities are addressed throughout this book, but the following sections describe a few revealing statistics.

African Americans

In 2003, the death rate for African Americans was higher than that for whites for heart diseases, stroke, cancer, asthma, influenza and pneumonia, diabetes, human immunodeficiency virus (HIV)–acquired immunodeficiency syndrome (AIDS), and homicide.

The following statistics were compiled by the Office of Minority Health (n.d.):

- In 2003, African American men were 1.4 times as likely to have new cases of lung and prostate cancer compared to non-Hispanic white men.
- African American men were twice as likely to have new cases of stomach cancer as non-Hispanic white men.
- In 2003, diabetic African Americans were 1.8 times as likely as diabetic whites to be hospitalized.
- In 2004, African Americans were 2.2 times as likely as non-Hispanic whites to die from diabetes.
- In 2004, African American men were 30% more likely to die from heart disease compared to non-Hispanic white men.
- African Americans were 1.5 times as likely as non-Hispanic whites to have high blood pressure.
- African American women were 1.7 times as likely as non-Hispanic white women to be obese.
- Although African Americans make up only 13% of the total United States population, they accounted for 47% of HIV–AIDS cases in 2005.
- African American males had more than eight times the AIDS rate of non-Hispanic white males.
- African American females had more than 23 times the AIDS rate of non-Hispanic white females.
- In 2005, African Americans aged 65 years and older were 40% less likely to have received an influenza (flu) shot in the past 12 months compared to non-Hispanic whites of the same age group.
- In 2005, African American adults aged 65 years and older were 30% less likely to have ever received a pneumonia shot compared to non-Hispanic white adults of the same age group.
- African American infants were almost four times as likely to die from causes related to low birth-weight compared to non-Hispanic white infants.
- African Americans had 2.1 times the sudden infant death syndrome mortality rate as non-Hispanic whites.

- African American mothers were 2.6 times as likely as non-Hispanic white mothers to begin prenatal care in the third trimester or not receive prenatal care at all.
- African American adults were 50% more likely than their white adult counterparts to have a stroke.

American Indians and Alaska Natives

Some of the leading diseases and causes of death among American Indians and Alaska Natives are heart disease, cancer, unintentional injuries (accidents), diabetes, and stroke (Office of Minority Health, n.d.). American Indians and Alaska Natives also have a high prevalence and greater risk factors for mental health problems and suicide, obesity, substance abuse, sudden infant death syndrome (SIDS), teenage pregnancy, and liver disease. American Indians and Alaska Natives have an infant death rate almost double the rate for Caucasians and are twice as likely to have diabetes as Caucasians. American Indians and Alaska Natives also have disproportionately high death rates from unintentional injuries and suicide.

The following statistics were compiled by the Office of Minority Health (n.d.):

- American Indian and Alaska Native men were twice as likely to be diagnosed with stomach and liver cancers as white men.
- American Indian women were 20% more likely to die from cervical cancer compared to white women.
- American Indian and Alaska Native adults were 2.3 times as likely as white adults to be diagnosed with diabetes.
- American Indian and Alaska Natives were twice as likely as non-Hispanic whites to die from diabetes in 2003.
- American Indian and Alaska Native adults were 1.3 times as likely as white adults to have high blood pressure.
- American Indian and Alaska Native adults were 1.2 times as likely as white adults to have heart disease.
- American Indian and Alaska Native adults were 1.4 times as likely as white adults to be current cigarette smokers.
- American Indian and Alaska Native adults were 1.6 times as likely as white adults to be obese.
- American Indian and Alaska Native adults were 1.3 times as likely as white adults to have high blood pressure.

- American Indians and Alaska Natives had a 40% higher AIDS rate than their non-Hispanic white counterparts.
- American Indian and Alaska Native babies were 2.2 times as likely as non-Hispanic white babies to die from sudden infant death syndrome (SIDS).
- American Indian and Alaska Native infants were 3.6 times as likely as non-Hispanic white infants to have mothers who began prenatal care in the third trimester or did not receive prenatal care at all.
- American Indian and Alaska Native adults were 60% more likely to have a stroke than their white adult counterparts.

Asian Americans

Asian American women have the highest life expectancy (85.8 years) of any other ethnic group in the United States (Office of Minority Health, n.d.). Life expectancy varies among Asian subgroups: Filipino (81.5 years), Japanese (84.5 years), and Chinese women (86.1 years). However, Asian Americans contend with numerous factors that may threaten their health. Some negative factors are infrequent medical visits due to issues such as the fear of deportation, language and cultural barriers, and the lack of health insurance. Asian Americans are most at risk for cancer, heart disease, stroke, unintentional injuries (accidents), and diabetes. Asian Americans also have a high prevalence of chronic obstructive pulmonary disease, hepatitis B, HIV–AIDS, smoking, tuberculosis, and liver disease.

The following statistics were compiled by the Office of Minority Health (n.d.):

- In 2006, tuberculosis was 10 times more common among Asian Americans and five times more common among Native Hawaiians and Pacific Islanders compared to the white population.
- In 2003, Asian American and Pacific Islander women were 1.2 times as likely to have cervical cancer compared to non-Hispanic white women.
- Asian American and Pacific Islander men and women had higher incidence and mortality rates for stomach and liver cancer.
- Asian Americans were 20% less likely than non-Hispanic whites to die from diabetes.
- Overall, Asian American and Pacific Islander adults were less likely than white adults to have heart disease, and they were less likely to die from heart disease.
- Asian Americans and Pacific Islanders were 40% less likely to die from heart disease compared to non-Hispanic whites.

- Asian Americans and Pacific Islanders had lower AIDS rates than non-Hispanic white counterparts, and they were less likely to die of HIV–AIDS.
- One Asian American–Pacific Islander child was diagnosed with AIDS in 2006.
- In 2005, Asian American and Pacific Islander adults aged 65 years and older were 40% less likely to have ever received a pneumonia shot compared to non-Hispanic white adults of the same age group.
- Asian American and Pacific Islander adults were less likely to die from a stroke.
- Asian American and Pacific Islander adults had lower rates of being overweight or obese, lower rates of hypertension, and they were less likely to be current cigarette smokers compared to white adults.

Hispanics and Latin Americans

Hispanics' health is often shaped by factors such as language and cultural barriers, lack of access to preventive care, and the lack of health insurance. The Centers for Disease Control and Prevention has cited some of the leading causes of illness and death among Hispanics, which include heart disease, cancer, unintentional injuries (accidents), stroke, and diabetes. Some other health conditions and risk factors that significantly affect Hispanics are asthma, chronic obstructive pulmonary disease, HIV–AIDS, obesity, suicide, and liver disease. Hispanics have higher rates of obesity than non-Hispanic Caucasians. There also are disparities among Hispanic subgroups. For example, although the rate of low birth-weight infants is lower for the total Hispanic population in comparison to non-Hispanic Caucasians, Puerto Ricans have a low birth-weight rate that is 50% higher than the rate for non-Hispanic Caucasians (Office of Minority Health, n.d.). Puerto Ricans also suffer disproportionately from asthma, HIV–AIDS, and infant mortality. Mexican-Americans suffer disproportionately from diabetes.

The following statistics were compiled by the Office of Minority Health (n.d.):

- Mexican American adults were two times more likely than non-Hispanic white adults to have been diagnosed with diabetes by a physician.
- In 2002, Hispanics were 1.5 times as likely to start treatment for end-stage renal disease related to diabetes compared to non-Hispanic white men.
- In 2004, Hispanics were 1.5 times as likely as non-Hispanic whites to die from diabetes.
- Mexican American women were 1.3 times more likely than non-Hispanic white women to be obese.
- Hispanic males had over three times the AIDS rate as non-Hispanic white males.

- Hispanic females had over five times the AIDS rate as non-Hispanic white females.
- In 2005, Hispanic adults aged 65 years and older were 50% less likely to have ever received a pneumonia shot compared to non-Hispanic white adults of the same age group.
- In 2004, infant mortality rates for Hispanic subpopulations ranged from 4.6 per 1,000 live births to 7.8 per 1,000 live births compared to the non-Hispanic white infant mortality rate of 5.7 per 1,000 live births.
- Puerto Rican infants were twice as likely to die from causes related to low birthweight compared to non-Hispanic white infants.
- Mexican American mothers were 2.5 times as likely as non-Hispanic white mothers to begin prenatal care in the third trimester or not receive prenatal care at all.

Gays, Lesbians, and Bisexuals

Gays, lesbians, and bisexuals also encounter disparate health concerns. For example, major health issues for gay men are HIV–AIDS and other sexually transmitted diseases, substance abuse, depression, and suicide. Some evidence suggests that lesbians have higher rates of smoking, being overweight, alcohol abuse, and stress than heterosexual women (CDC, 2007a). The issues surrounding personal, family, and social acceptance of sexual orientation can place a significant burden on mental health and personal safety (CDC, 2007a).

CAUSES OF HEALTH DISPARITIES

The causes of health disparities are due to both voluntary and involuntary factors. Voluntary factors are related to health behaviors, such as smoking and diet, and can be avoided. Factors such as genetics, living and working in unhealthy conditions, limited or no access to health care, language barriers, limited financial resources, and low health literacy skills are often viewed as being involuntary and unfair, because they are not within that person's control.

The Lalonde report was produced in Canada in 1974 and was titled *A New Perspective on the Health of Canadians*. This report probably was the first acknowledgment by a major industrialized country that health is determined by more than biological factors. The report led to the development of the health field concept, which identified four health fields that were interdependently responsible for individual health.

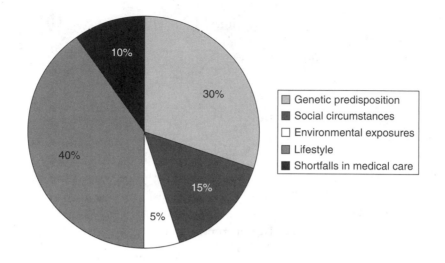

FIGURE 1.3   Domains and their percentage of contributions to early death.
Source: Data from: McGinnis, Williams-Russo, and Knickman. (2002).

1. *Environment.* All matters related to health external to the human body and over which the individual has little or no control. Includes the physical and social environment.
2. *Human biology.* All aspects of health, physical and mental, developed within the human body as a result of organic make-up.
3. *Lifestyle.* The aggregation of personal decisions over which the individual has control. Self-imposed risks created by unhealthy lifestyle choices can be said to contribute to, or cause, illness or death.
4. *Health care organization.* The quantity, quality, arrangement, nature, and relationships of people and resources in the provision of health care.

These four domains were later changed to five intersecting domains, which are environmental exposures, genetics, behavior (lifestyle) choices, social circumstances, and medical care (Institute of Medicine [IOM], 2001). A rough estimate of the impact of each domain on early deaths is illustrated in Figure 1.3.

We discuss each one of the five domains in more detail, but it is important to note that all of the domains are integrated and affected by one another. For example, people who have more education usually have higher incomes, are more likely to have healthcare coverage, and live in neighborhoods with fewer environmental health risks.

TABLE 1.1   Segregation of Ethnic Minorities Compared with Whites, United States, 1980 to 2000

	1980	1990	2000
American Indians	37.3	36.8	33.3
African Americans	72.7	67.8	64.0
Asian Americans and Pacific Islanders	40.5	41.2	41.1
Hispanics	50.2	50.0	50.9

Segregation was determined using the index of dissimilarity, which measures the evenness of groups over space and can be interpreted as the percentage of a particular group who would have to move to integrate the two groups over the region as a whole. For example, in 2000, 64% of all African Americans (or whites) would have to move to another census tract to integrate all metropolitan areas nationwide.

Data source: Gee and Payne-Sturges. (2004).

Environmental Exposures

Environmental conditions are believed to play an important role in producing and maintaining health disparities (Lee, 2002; Yen & Syme, 1999). The environment influences our health in many ways, including through exposures to physical, chemical, and biological risk factors and through related changes in our behavior in response to those factors. In general, whites and minorities do not have the same exposure to environmental health threats, because they live in different neighborhoods. Residential segregation still exists.

Segregation, the spatial separation of the residences of racial groups from one another, has persisted for many decades (Iceland, Weinberg, & Steinmetz, 2002; Massey, 2001; Massey & Denton, 1993). Table 1.1 shows the segregation of African Americans, Hispanics, American Indians, and Asian Americans–Pacific Islanders compared with whites from 1980 to 2000 for metropolitan areas, as measured with the index of dissimilarity (Logan, 2003; US Census Bureau, 2003). Scored from 0 to 100, a given value of the index indicates the percentage of that group who would have to move to integrate the metropolitan area. Segregation from whites is highest for African Americans, followed by Hispanics, Asian Americans and Pacific Islanders, and American Indians.

Although a common argument is that segregation is harmful to the health of minorities, there is some indication that segregation may have a counterbalancing effect by concentrating social resources, such as black political power (LaVeist, 1993). Others have reported that the clustering of ethnic groups may build a sense of collective identity that helps mitigate trauma (Mazumdar, Mazumdar, Docuyanan, & McLaughlin, 2000). Thus, supportive social relationships within minority communities may help promote health and ameliorate the effects of community risks. Segregation concentrates both risks and resources.

Minority Neighborhoods

Ethnicity is highly correlated with residential location, and minority neighborhoods experience greater exposure to environmental health risks. These two links lead to the idea that health disparities are, in part, caused by the difference in exposure levels to environmental hazards. Minority neighborhoods tend to have higher rates of mortality, morbidity, and health risk factors compared with white neighborhoods, even after accounting for economic and other characteristics (Cubbin, Hadden, & Winkleby, 2001; Deaton & Lubotsky, 2003; Geronimus, Bound, Waidmann, Colen, & Steffick, 2001).

A contributing factor is greater exposure to environmental toxicants, such as air pollution, pesticides, and lead, which can lead to health problems such as asthma, cancer, and chemical poisoning. Low socioeconomic neighborhoods are more likely than middle or higher socioeconomic neighborhoods to be situated near toxic waste sites and other potential environmental hazards (Mohai & Bryant, 1992).

People who live in poor neighborhoods might not have access to nutritious foods, safe places to exercise, and other resources that improve health. Poor and minority neighborhoods tend to have fewer grocery stores with healthy foods (Morland, Wing, Diez-Roux, & Poole, 2002) and fewer pharmacies with needed medications (Morrison, Wallenstein, Natale, Senzel, & Huang, 2000). Other research indicates that healthy foods are not only less abundant, they also are more costly in low-income neighborhoods. Poor nutrition can increase susceptibility to environmental pollutants by compromising immune function (Beck & Weinstock 1988; Rios, Poje, & Detels, 1993). Additionally, disadvantaged neighborhoods also are exposed to greater health hazards, including tobacco and alcohol advertisements, toxic waste incinerators, and air pollution (Morello-Frosch, Pastor, Porras, & Sadd, 2002). Finally, economic stress within a community may exacerbate tensions between social groups, magnify workplace stressors, induce maladaptive coping behaviors, such as smoking and alcohol use (Brenner, 1995), and translate into individual stress, which makes individuals more vulnerable to illness when they are exposed to environmental hazards. Tobacco and alcohol use can increase susceptibility to environmental toxicants that are normally metabolized by impairing host defense (Rios, et al., 1993).

Neighborhood physical conditions also may contribute to health disparities (Cohen, et al., 2003). Minorities are more likely to live in areas with building code violations and neighborhoods with deteriorated housing (Perera, et al., 2002). In 1999, 3.4% of blacks, 3.8% of Hispanics, and 1.7% of Asian Americans and Pacific Islanders reported living in housing units with severe problems with heating, plumbing, electricity, public areas, or maintenance, compared with 1.5% of whites (US Census Bureau, 2000). Substandard housing may contribute to a variety of problems, including exposure to toxicants, increased risk of injuries from falls and fires, and illness due to ineffective waste disposal and presence of disease vectors (Bashir, 2002; Jacobs, et al., 2002; Northridge, Stover, Rosenthal, & Sherard, 2003).

Factors associated with living in poor neighborhoods, such as crime and physical deterioration, can cause stress, which can lead to health problems. Stress is a state of activation of physical and psychological readiness to act, which helps an organism survive external threats. Stressors are the factors that produce stress and include such phenomena as crime, domestic violence, and noise (Babisch, Fromme, Beyer, & Ising, 2001; Ouis, 2001), traffic (Gee & Takeuchi, 2004), litter, density, and residential crowding (Fleming, Baum, & Weiss, 1987; Evans & Lepore, 1993). Stress has effects on the physical and psychological state of humans and as a result can lead to health problems such as high blood pressure or depression (Gee & Payne-Sturges, 2004).

Genetics

Genetics have been linked to many diseases, including diabetes, cancer, sickle-cell anemia, obesity, cystic fibrosis, hemophilia, Tay-Sachs disease, schizophrenia, and Down syndrome. Currently, about 4,000 genetic disorders are known. Some genetic disorders are a result of a single mutated gene, and other disorders are complex, multifactorial or polygenic mutations. Multifactorial means that the disease or disorder is likely to be associated with the effects of multiple genes in combination with lifestyle and environmental factors. Examples of multifactorial disorders are cancer, heart disease, and diabetes. Although there have been numerous studies that link genetics to health, social and cultural factors play a role as well. For example, smoking may trigger a genetic predisposition to lung cancer, but that gene may not have been expressed if the person did not smoke.

There are concerns about relating genetics and health disparities because race is not truly biologically determined, so the relationship between genetics and race is not clear cut. There are more genetic differences within races than among them, and racial categories do not capture biological distinctiveness (Williams, et al., 1994). Another problem with linking genetics to race is that many people have a mixed gene pool due to inter-racial marriages and partnerships. Also, it is difficult at times to determine which diseases are related to genetics and which are related to other factors, such as lifestyle and the environment. Sometimes disease is caused by a combination of factors. For example, African-Americans have been shown to have higher rates of hypertension than whites (Williams, et al., 1994), but is that difference due to genetics? African-Americans tend to consume less potassium than whites and have stress related to discrimination, which, instead of genetics, could be the cause of their higher rates of hypertension. Health disparities also can be related to the level of exposure to environmental hazards, such as toxins and carcinogens, that exist among racial groups. Therefore, it is difficult to link health disparities to genetics, because they could be a result of a variety of factors, but that does not mean that genetics do not play a role in health because some clear links have been made.

Lifestyle

Behavior patterns are factors that the individual has more control over. Many of the diseases of the twenty-first century are caused by personal modifiable factors, such as smoking, poor diet, and physical inactivity. So how does lifestyle relate to ethnicity?

Studies reveal that differences in health behaviors exist among racial and ethnic groups. Bolen and colleagues (1997) summarized findings from the 1997 Behavioral Risk Factor Surveillance System (BRFSS) of the distribution of access to health care, health-status indicators, health-risk behaviors, and use of clinical preventive services across five racial and ethnic groups (i.e., whites, blacks, Hispanics, American Indians or Alaska Natives, and Asian Americans or Pacific Islanders) and by state. BRFSS is an ongoing state-specific surveillance system about modifiable risk factors for chronic diseases and other leading causes of death among adults that are collected annually (Bolen, Rhodes, Powell-Griner, Bland, & Holtzman, 1997). The results of Bolen and colleagues' (1997) research showed that variations in risk for chronic disease and injury among racial and ethnic groups exist both within states and across states (see Table 1.2).

Social Circumstances

Social circumstances include factors such as socioeconomic status (SES), income, stress, discrimination, marriage and partnerships, and family roles. SES is made up of a combination of variables including occupation, education, income, wealth, place of residence, and poverty. These variables do not have a direct affect on health, but they do have an indirect effect. For example, low SES does not cause disease, but poor

TABLE 1.2   Medians and Ranges of Values for Health-Status Indicators, Health-Risk Behaviors, and Clinical Preventive Services, by Race or Ethnicity— Behavioral Risk Factor Surveillance System, 1997*

	Total %	White %	Black %	Hispanic %	American Indian or Alaska Native %	Asian American or Pacific Islander %
Cost as a barrier to obtaining health care	9.9	9.4	13.2	16.2	12.6	11.6
No routine physical examination	16.8	18.0	8.7	18.2	14.5	17.1
Obesity	16.6	15.6	26.4	18.2	30.1	4.8
No leisure-time physical activity	28.0	25.1	38.2	34.2	37.2	28.9
Alcohol Consumption						
Current drinking	53.5	55.4	40.4	50.8	50.5	38.2
Binge drinking	14.4	14.3	8.7	16.2	18.9	6.7
Cigarette smoking	23.3	23.6	22.8	23.1	41.3	10.7
Lack of safety belt use	30.7	30.0	37.6	30.3	40.9	18.6
Clinical Preventive Services						
Blood cholesterol checked	69.2	71.2	67.4	59.3	54.7	67.8
Papanicolaou test	84.8	84.7	91.1	80.9	†	†
Breast Cancer Screening						
Mammogram	73.7	73.7	76.1	63.5	†	†
Clinical breast examination	77.0	77.5	78.2	75.5	†	†
Mammogram plus clinical breast examination	66.4	67.6	67.8	57.8	†	†
Colorectal Cancer Screening						
Home-kit blood stool test	18.1	18.2	20.3	14.2	†	†
Sigmoidoscopy	30.1	30.4	28.2	22.4	†	†

* Lowest and highest state estimates.

† Median is not considered meaningful for the three or fewer states that had ≤50 respondents in this racial or ethnic category and is not shown.

Data source: Bolen, Rhodes, Powell-Griner, Bland, and Holtzman. (1997).

nutrition, limited access to health care, and substandard housing certainly do, and these are just a few of the many indirect effects. Discrimination does not cause poor health directly either, but it can lead to depression and high blood pressure.

One variable of social circumstances, poverty, can be measured in many ways. One approach is to measure the number of people who are recipients of federal aid programs, such as food stamps, public housing, and Head Start. Another method is through labor statistics, but the most common way is through the federal government's measure of poverty based on income. The federal government's definition of poverty is based on a threshold defined by income, and it is updated annually. In 2003, a person in the 48 contiguous states and the District of Columbia whose income was $8,980 or less was considered to be living in poverty, and a family of four with earnings of $18,400 or less was considered to be below the poverty level. For each additional person, the threshold increased by $3,140 (Federal Register, 2003). So how is poverty related to ethnicity?

The official poverty rate in 2003 was 12.5%, which equates to 35.9 million people (Denavas-Walt, Proctor, & Mills, 2004). The two-year average for 2002 and 2003 by race can be found in Table 1.3. Poverty is higher among certain racial and ethnic groups, and hence, it is a contributing factor to health disparities because poverty impacts many factors, such as where people live and their access to health care.

TABLE 1.3   Poverty Rates by Race and Hispanic Origin Using 2002 and 2003 Averages

Race and Hispanic Origin	Percentage in Poverty
Black alone	24.3%
American Indian and Alaska Native alone	23.9%
Hispanic origin	22.1%
Asian American alone	10.9%
White alone, not Hispanic	8.1%

When the race or origin is followed by the word "alone," it indicates that the person did not indicate any other race category.

Source: Denavas-Walt, Proctor, and Mills. (2004).

Education is an important indicator of health status. Higher education appears to lead to better health because it increases knowledge about health, helps to assert health-promoting behaviors to prevent disease and maintain health, and increases income, which helps determine where someone lives and other important factors related to health (McKenzie, et al., 2005). Education is related to higher social position, and there is a clear association between socioeconomic position and health. Further, the relationship between socioeconomic position and health holds not only at the individual level but also at the community level. That is, persons living in poor neighborhoods, even after accounting for their individual socioeconomic characteristics, tend to have worse health outcomes.

Racism is a factor of social circumstances, and there is an association between racism and health. One of the most prominent stressors may be racial discrimination. "Stress resulting from institutionalized racism and discrimination, be it real or perceived, blatant or muted, is an 'added pathogenic factor' that contributes to well-above average levels of hypertension, respiratory illness, anxiety, depression, and other ills in minority populations" (Williams, 2007). Because racial discrimination has profoundly shaped the experiences of racial groups, discrimination may be among the factors that shape health disparities. Evidence suggests that racial discrimination still occurs in the present day, especially in structurally important domains such as housing, education, and employment. Audit studies that send a white and a minority prospective tester with identical portfolios (e.g., similar income and job titles) to assess a given housing market have consistently found that whites are favored over minorities. Hispanics, for example, are more likely to be quoted a higher rent for a given unit than are their white counterparts. Other studies have shown that minorities are more likely to face discrimination in applying for a job or shopping.

Stress from discrimination may lead to illness. Kessler and colleagues (1999) suggested that discrimination is among the most important of all the stressful experiences that have been implicated as causes of mental health problems. Studies have reported that stress due to racial discrimination is associated with high blood pressure, mental health problems (Gee, 2002; Kessler, Mickelson, & Williams, 1999), and alcohol consumption (Yen & Syme, 1999).

Psychosocial conditions, including crowding, social disorganization, racial discrimination, fear, and economic deprivation, also may be sources of stress. One stressor that has received extensive attention is fear of crime, and minority neighborhoods tend to have higher crime rates. Perceptions of crime and disorder within an individual's community has been associated with numerous health outcomes, including anxiety, depression, posttraumatic stress disorder, and substance use.

Medical Care

The shortfalls for minorities in the health-care system in the United States can be categorized into three general areas: (1) lack of access to care, (2) lower quality of care, and (3) limited providers with the same ethnic background.

Lack of Access to Medical Care

Research has shown that without access to timely and effective preventive care, people may be at risk for potentially avoidable conditions, such as asthma, diabetes, and immunizable conditions (National Center for Health Statistics, 2006). It also is important for prompt treatment and follow-up to illness and injury. Access to health care is a problem for many Americans as the number of people who are uninsured continues to climb. According to the National Health Interview Survey, in the first half of 2007, 42.5 million Americans (14.3%) were uninsured (Cohen & Martinez, 2007). Access to health care is particularly problematic for minorities, because they have higher rates of being uninsured than whites. Indicators to access to care include having a regular place to go for medical care, whether a person receives his or her care in the right place (for example, whether care for a non-urgent condition is sought at a physician's office or in an emergency department), and the ability to pay for care (which includes having health insurance).

Access to care is unequal among ethnicities. Non-whites are more likely to lack insurance coverage. Approximately 31% of Hispanic or Latino persons were uninsured in the first part of 2007 compared to 10.2% of non-Hispanic whites, 14.4% of blacks, 13% of Asian Americans, and 23.6% of other and multiple races (Cohen & Martinez, 2007). According to the 2005 National Health Interview Survey, 77.1% of Hispanics have a usual place to go for health care compared to 85.7% of non-Hispanic blacks and 89.4% of non-Hispanic whites (National Center for Health Statistics, 2006 as cited in Cohen & Martinez, 2007). In 2004, the emergency department utilization rate for blacks was significantly higher than for whites (68.9 versus 35.2 per 100 persons) (National Center for Health Statistics, 2006 as cited in Cohen & Martinez, 2007).

Lower Quality of Care

When minorities do have access to care, research shows that unequal treatment exists, and minorities receive a lower quality of care even when social determinants and insurance status are controlled (Betancourt & Maina, 2004). A review by the

Institute of Medicine (2001) concluded that racial and ethnic minorities tend to receive lower quality health-care services than non-minorities, even when access-related factors, such as patients' insurance status and income, are controlled. The study committee found evidence that stereotyping, biases, and uncertainty on the part of health-care providers can contribute to unequal treatment. For example, minorities appear to have longer waiting times for kidney transplants and liver transplants and report less satisfaction with their medical visits. African-Americans and other minorities have been shown to be less likely to receive expensive and high-tech procedures and kidney dialysis and transplants (Williams, 2007). These same groups were more likely to receive lower-limb amputations for diabetes (Williams, 2007).

Limited Providers with the Same Ethnic Background

Ethnic minorities are poorly represented among physicians and other health care professionals. Although Hispanics, African Americans, and American Indians represent more than 25% of the United States population, they comprise fewer than 6% of doctors and 9% of nurses (Cooper & Powe, 2004). As a result, minority patients are frequently treated by professionals from a different racial or ethnic background. Many programs, funding agencies, and research studies suggest that more diversity is needed among health care professionals to improve quality of care and reduce health disparities, but is there evidence that racial concordance (patients being treated by people in the same ethnic group) accomplishes these goals?

Cooper and Powe (2004) conducted an extensive literature review about patient–provider concordance with regard to race and ethnicity, and they compared and contrasted these findings to the literature on patient–provider language concordance. They found that race-concordant visits were longer and had greater positive effects for patients than race-discordant visits. Patients in race-concordant visits reported higher levels of satisfaction, perceived their physicians as more participatory, regardless of the communication that occurred during the visit, and was associated with longer visits and measurably better communication. Few studies have focused on the utilization and health outcomes of race-concordant relationships. Regardless of whether race concordance is linked to health outcomes, there is support for the notion that increasing racial and ethnic diversity among physicians will provide ethnic minority patients with more choices and better experiences with care processes, including positive effects, longer visit durations, higher patient satisfaction, and better participation in care.

Cooper and Powe (2004) researched the under-representation of certain ethnic groups in health care professions and focused on four hypotheses:

1. *The service patterns hypothesis.* Health care professionals from racial and ethnic minority and socioeconomically disadvantaged backgrounds are more likely than others to serve racial and ethnic minority and socioeconomically disadvantaged populations, thereby improving access to care for vulnerable populations and, in turn, improving health outcomes.

2. *The concordance hypothesis.* Increasing the number of racial and ethnic minority health care professionals—by providing greater opportunity for minority patients to see a practitioner from their own racial or ethnic group or, for patients with limited English proficiency, to see a practitioner who speaks their primary language—will improve the quality of communication, comfort level, trust, partnership, and decision making in patient–practitioner relationships, thereby increasing use of appropriate health care services and adherence to effective programs, ultimately resulting in improved health outcomes.

3. *The trust in health care hypothesis.* Greater diversity in the health care workforce will increase trust in the health care delivery system among minority and socioeconomically disadvantaged populations and will thereby increase their propensity to use health services that lead to improved health outcomes.

4. *The professional advocacy hypothesis.* Health care professionals from racial and ethnic minority and socioeconomically disadvantaged backgrounds will be more likely than others to provide leadership and advocacy for policies and programs aimed at improving health care for vulnerable populations, thereby increasing health care access and quality, and ultimately health outcomes, for those populations.

The research generated the following findings (Cooper & Powe, 2004):

- Under-represented health professionals, particularly physicians, disproportionately serve minority and other medically underserved populations.
- Minority patients tend to receive better interpersonal care from practitioners of their own race or ethnicity, particularly in primary care and mental health settings.
- Non-English-speaking patients experience better interpersonal care, greater medical comprehension, and have a greater likelihood of keeping follow-up appointments when they see a language-concordant practitioner, particularly in mental health care.
- Insufficient evidence exists as to whether greater diversity in health care professionals leads to greater trust in health care or greater advocacy for disadvantaged populations.

CHAPTER SUMMARY

One of the great attributes of the United States is the diverse landscape. Known by some as a melting pot, immigrants (voluntary and forced) who have come to the United States and natives of this country have experienced different levels of cultural adaptation to blend into the dominant society. Some have retained their strong cultural ties to create a society of rich and diverse cultures filled with various beliefs, traditions, languages, and societal norms. Understanding and respecting this diverse landscape is a goal for the nation, specifically for the health care industry. Health care providers need to be knowledgeable about and sensitive to cultural differences to provide effective care and education.

The goal of this chapter is to provide an understanding of the foundations of multicultural health and the key terms and concepts associated with it, such as culture, race, assimilation, and cultural relativism. We want readers to have a general appreciation of how culture impacts health, the breadth and depth of health disparities, and their related causes. In the next chapter, we go further into the topic of culture and health by building upon these foundations.

REVIEW

1. What is the focus of multicultural health, and why is it important?
2. Is race a biological or social construct? Why is race important?
3. What is the difference between ethnicity and culture? What is the difference between race and ethnicity?
4. Explain cultural ethnocentricity and relativism.
5. Explain the difference between acculturation, assimilation, and bicultural.
6. Does the level of acculturation have a positive or negative affect on health? Explain.
7. What are health disparities and their causes?

CASE STUDY

The book titled *The Spirit Catches You and You Fall Down*, by Anne Fadiman, tells the story of Lia Lee, a Hmong child, with epilepsy, who lived in Merced, California. When 3-month-old Lia Lee arrived at the county hospital emergency room in Merced, a chain of events was set in motion from which Lia, her parents, and her doctors would never recover. Lia's parents, Foua and Nao Kao, were part of a large Hmong community in

Merced, refugees from the "Quiet War" in Laos. Her parents and doctors both wanted the best for Lia, but their ideas about the causes of her illness and its treatment were very different. The Hmong see illness and healing as spiritual matters that are linked to virtually everything in the universe, but the medical community marks a division between body and soul and concerns itself almost exclusively with the former. Lia's doctors attributed her seizures to the misfiring of her cerebral neurons; her parents called her illness "qaug dab peg"—the spirit catches you and you fall down— and ascribed it to the wandering of her soul. The doctors prescribed anticonvulsants; her parents preferred animal sacrifices. *The Spirit Catches You and You Fall Down* moves from hospital corridors to healing ceremonies, and from the hill country of Laos to the living rooms of Merced, uncovering in its path the complex sources and implications of two dramatically clashing worldviews.

Lia's doctors prescribed a complex regimen of medication designed to control her seizures. However, her parents believed that the epilepsy was a result of Lia "losing her soul" and did not give her the medication as indicated because of the complexity of the drug therapy and the adverse side effects. Instead, they did everything logical in terms of their Hmong beliefs to help her. They took her to a clan leader and shaman, sacrificed animals, and bought expensive amulets to guide her soul's return. Lia's doctors believed that her parents were endangering her life by not giving her the medication, so they called child protective services, and Lia was placed in foster care. Lia was a victim of a misunderstanding between these two cultures that were both intent on saving her. The results were disastrous: A close family was separated, and Hmong community faith in Western doctors was shaken.

Lia was surrounded by people who wanted the best for her and her health. Unfortunately, the involved parties disagreed on the best treatment because they understood her epilepsy differently. The separate cultures of Lia's caretakers had different concepts of health and illness.

This example illustrates how culture and health impact each other and at times clash. To help ensure good care for diverse patients, health-care providers must address cultural issues and respect the cultural values of each patient.

There are several issues to consider about this case:

- How can health care providers prepare for situations like Lia's?
- Should child protective services have been contacted?
- Were Lia's parents irresponsible?
- How did the parents' belief system impact Lia's health care?
- Were the parents' decisions morally and legally wrong?

GLOSSARY TERMS

multicultural health

culture

cultural competency

race

acculturation

ethnicity

ethnocentricity

cultural relativism

racism

discrimination

minority

cultural adaptation

dominant culture

assimilation

heritage consistency

health disparities

Healthy People 2010

REFERENCES

Babisch, W., Fromme, H., Beyer, A., & Ising, H. (2001). Increased catecholamine levels in urine in subjects exposed to road traffic noise: The role of stress hormones in noise research. *Environment International, 26*, 475–481.

Bashir, S. A. (2002). Home is where the harm is: Inadequate housing as a public health crisis. *American Journal of Public Health, 92*, 733–738.

Beck, B. D., & Weinstock, S. (1988). Age and nutrition. In: J. D. Brian (Ed.), *Variations in susceptibility to inhaled pollutants: Identification, mechanisms, and policy implications* (pp. 104–126). Baltimore: Johns Hopkins University Press.

Betancourt, J. R., & Maina, A. W. (2004, October). The Institute of Medicine Report: "Unequal Treatment": Implications for academic health centers. *The Mount Sinai Journal of Medicine, 71*(5).

Berry J., Trimble J., & Olmedo E. (1986). Assessment of acculturation. In: W. J. Lonner & J. W. Berry (Eds), *Field Methods in Cross-cultural Research* (pp. 291–324). Thousand Oaks, CA: Sage Publications.

Bolen, J. C., Rhodes, L., Powell-Griner, E. E., Bland, S. D., & Holtzman, D. (1997). National Center for Chronic Disease Prevention and Health Promotion. *State-specific prevalence of selected health behaviors, by race and ethnicity—Behavioral Risk Factor Surveillance System, 1997.* Retrieved March 24, 2008, from http://www.cdc.gov/mmwr/preview/mmwrhtml/ss4902a1.htm

Brenner, M. H. (1995). Political economy and health. In: B. C. Amick, S. Levine, A. R. Tarlov, & D. Chapman Walsh (Eds.), *Society and health* (pp. 211–246). New York: Oxford University Press.

Burt, C. W., McCaig, L. R., & Rechtsteiner, E. A. (2007). *Ambulatory medical care utilization estimates for 2005.* Retrieved December 26, 2007, from http://www.cdc.gov/nchs/data/ad/ad388.pdf

Campinha-Bacote, J. (1994). Cultural competence in psychiatric mental health nursing: A conceptual model. *Nursing Clinics in North America, 29*(1), 1–8.

Carter-Porras, O., & Baquest, C. (2002, September–October). Association of Schools of Public Health. What is a "health disparity"? *Public Health Reports, 117.*

Centers for Disease Control and Prevention. (1991). Behavioral risk factor survey of Vietnamese— California.

Centers for Disease Control and Prevention. (1997). Behavioral risk factor survey of Korean Americans—Alameda County, California, 1994. MMWR.

Centers for Disease Control and Prevention. (2004). *Fact sheet. Racial/ethnic health disparities.* Retrieved December 20, 2007, from http://www.cdc.gov./od/oc/media/pressrel/fs040402.htm

Centers for Disease Control and Prevention. (2007a). *Lesbian, gay, bisexual and transgender health.* Retrieved January 19, 2008, from http://www.cdc.gov/lgbthealth/index.htm

Centers for Disease Control and Prevention. Office of Minority Health and Health Disparities. (2007b). *Eliminating racial and ethnic health disparities.* Retrieved October 21, 2007, from http://www.cdc.gov/omhd/About/disparities.htm

Cohen, D. A., Mason, K., Bedimo, A., Scribner, R., Basolo, V., & Farley, T. A. (2003). Neighborhood physical conditions and health. *American Journal of Public Health, 93,* 467–471.

Cohen, R. A., & Martinez, M. E. (2007). Centers for Disease Control and Prevention. *Health insurance coverage: Early release of estimates from National Health Interview Survey, January–June 2007.* Retrieved December 26, 2007, from http://www.cdc.gov/nchs/data/nhis/earlyrelease/insur 200712.pdf

Cooper, L. A., & Powe, N. R. (2004). *Disparities in patient experiences, health care processes, and outcomes: The role of patient–provider racial, ethnic, and language concordance.* Retrieved January 19, 2008, from http://www.commonwealthfund.org/publications/publications_show.htm?doc_id=231670

Council of Economic Advisors For the President's Initiative on Race. (1998). Changing America: Indicators of Social and Economic Well-being by Race and Hispanic Origin. Retrieved January 19, 2008, from http://www.gpoaccess.gov/eop/ca/pdfs/toc.pdf.

Cubbin, C., Hadden, W. C., & Winkleby, M. A. (2001). Neighborhood context and cardiovascular disease risk factors: The contribution of material deprivation. *Ethnicity and Disease, 11,* 687–700.

Deaton, A., & Lubotsky, D. (2003). Mortality, inequality and race in American cities and states. *Social Science and Medicine, 56,* 1139–1153.

Denavas-Walt, C., Proctor, B. D., & Mills, R. J. (2004). US Census Bureau. Income, poverty, and health insurance: Coverage in the United States: 2003.

Evans, G. W., & Lepore, S. J. (1993). Household crowding and social support: A quasiexperimental analysis. *Journal of Personality and Social Psychology, 65,* 308–316.

Federal Register, No. 26, Vol. 68 pp. 6456–6458 (2003, February 7).

Fleming, I., Baum, A., & Weiss, L. (1987). Social density and perceived control as mediators of crowding stress in high-density residential neighborhoods. *Journal of Personality and Social Psychology, 52,* 899–906.

Gee, G. C., & Payne-Sturges, D. C. (2004, December). Environmental health disparities: A framework integrating psychosocial and environmental concepts. *Environmental Health Perspectives, 112*(17), 1645–1653. Retrieved November 11, 2007, from http://www.pubmedcentral.nih.gov/articlerender.fcgi?artid=1253653#b125-ehp0112-001645

Gee, G. C., & Takeuchi, D. T. (2004). Traffic stress, vehicular burden and well-being: A multilevel analysis. *Social Science and Medicine, 59,* 405–414.

Geronimus, A. T., Bound, J., & Waidmann, T. A. (1999). Poverty, time, and place: Variation in excess mortality across selected US populations, 1980–1990. *Journal of Epidemiology and Community Health, 53,* 325–334.

Geronimus, A. T., Bound J., Waidmann, T. A, Colen, C. G., & Steffick, D. (2001). Inequality in life expectancy, functional status, and active life expectancy across selected black and white population in the United States. *Demography, 38,* 227–251.

Goldberg, J., Hayes, W., & Huntley, J. (2004, November). Health Policy Institute of Ohio. Understanding health disparities.

Grieco, E. M., & Cassidy, R. C. (2001). *Overview of race and Hispanic origin* (US Census Bureau, Census 2000 Special Report Series C2KBR/01-1). Washington, DC: US Government Printing Office.

Hobbs, F., & Stoops, N. (2002). *Demographic trends in the 20th century* (US Census Bureau, Census 2000 Special Report Series CENSR-4). Washington, DC: US Government Printing Office.

Iceland, J., Weinberg, D. H., & Steinmetz, E. (2002). *Racial and ethnic residential segregation in the United States: 1980–2000* (US Census Bureau, Series CENSR-3). Washington, DC: US Government Printing Office.

Institute of Medicine. (2001). *Health and behavior: The interplay of biological, behavioral, and societal influences.* Washington, DC: National Academies Press.

Jacobs, D. E., Clickner, R. P., Zhou, J. Y., Viet, S. M., Marker, D. A., Rogers, J. W., et al. (2002). The prevalence of lead-based paint hazards in US housing. *Environmental Health Perspectives, 110,* 599–606.

Juckett, G. (2005, December 1). Cross-cultural medicine. *American Family Physician.* Retrieved January 6, 2008, from http://www.aafp.org/afp/20051201/2267.html

Kessler, R. C., Mickelson, K. D., & Williams, D. R. (1999). The prevalence, distribution, and mental health correlates of perceived discrimination in the United States. *Journal of Health and Social Behavior, 40*(3), 208–30.

LaVeist, T. A. (1993). Segregation, poverty, and empowerment: Health consequences for African Americans. *The Milbank Quarterly, 71,* 41–64.

Lee, C. (2002). Environmental justice: Building a unified vision of health and the environment. *Environmental Health Perspectives, 110*(Suppl. 2), 141–144.

Lee, S. K., Sobal, J., & Frongillo, E. A. (2000, July). Acculturation and health in Korean Americans. *Social Science and Medicine, 51*(2), 159–173.

Logan, J. R. (2003). Ethnic diversity grows, neighborhood integration lags. In: B. Katz & R. E. Lang (Eds.), *Redefining urban and suburban America* (pp. 235–256). Washington, DC: Brookings Institution.

Massey, D. (2001). Residential segregation and neighborhood conditions in US metropolitan areas. In: N. J. Smelser, W. J. Wilson, & F. Mitchell (Eds.), *America becoming: Racial trends and their consequences* (pp. 391–434). Washington, DC: National Academies Press.

Massey, D., & Denton, N. A. (1993). *American apartheid: Segregation and the making of the underclass.* Cambridge, MA: Harvard University Press.

Mazumdar, S., Mazumdar, S., Docuyanan, F., & McLaughlin, C. M. (2000). Creating a sense of place: The Vietnamese-Americans and Little Saigon. *Journal of Environmental Psychology, 20,* 319–333.

McGinnis, J. M., Williams-Russo, J. M., & Knickman, J. R. (2002). The case for more active policy attention to health promotion. *Health Affairs, 21*(2), 78–93.

McKenzie, J. F., Pinger, R. R., & Kotecki, J. E. (2005). *An introduction to community health.* Sudbury, MA: Jones and Bartlett.

Mohai, P., & Bryant, B. (1992). Environmental racism: Reviewing the evidence. In: B. Bryant & P. Mohai (Eds), *Race and the incidence of environmental hazards: A time for discourse* (pp. 163–176). Boulder, CO: Westview.

Morello-Frosch, R., Pastor, M., Porras, C., & Sadd, J. (2002). Environmental justice and regional inequality in southern California: Implications for future research. *Environmental Health Perspectives, 110*(Suppl. 2), 149–154.

Morland, K., Wing, S., Diez-Roux, A. V., & Poole, C. (2002). Neighborhood characteristics associated with the location of food stores and food service places. *American Journal of Preventive Medicine, 22*, 23–29.

Morrison, R. S., Wallenstein, S., Natale, D. K., Senzel, R. S., & Huang, L. L. (2000). "We don't carry that"—failure of pharmacies in predominantly nonwhite neighborhoods to stock opioid analgesics. *New England Journal of Medicine, 3426*, 1023–1026.

National Association of Chronic Disease Directors. (2006). Retrieved September 1, 2007, from www.chronicdisease.org

National Center for Health Statistics. (2006). *NCHS data on health insurance and access to care*. Retrieved December 26, 2007, from http://origin.cdc.gov/nchs/data/factsheets/healthinsurance.pdf

National Diabetes Education Program. (2005). *The diabetes epidemic among American Indians and Alaska Natives*. Retrieved October 21, 2007, from http://ndep.nih.gov/diabetes/pubs/FS_AmIndian.pdf

Northridge, M. E., Stover, G. N., Rosenthal, J. E., & Sherard, D. (2003). Environmental equity and health: Understanding complexity and moving forward. *American Journal of Public Health, 93*, 209–214.

Office of Minority Health. (n.d.). *Minority populations*. Retrieved January 11, 2008, from http://www.omhrc.gov/templates/browse.aspx?lvl=1&lvlID=5

Office of Minority Health. (2001). *National standards for culturally and linguistically appropriate services in health care*. Washington, DC: US Department of Health and Human Services.

Ouis, D. (2001). Annoyance from road traffic noise: A review. *Journal of Environmental Psychology, 21*, 101–120.

Perera, F. P., Illman, S. M., Kinney, P. L., Whyatt, R. M., Kelvin, E. A., Shepard, P., et al. (2002). The challenge of preventing environmentally related disease in young children: Community-based research in New York City. *Environmental Health Perspectives, 110*, 197–204.

Rios, R., Poje, G. V., & Detels, R. (1993). Susceptibility to environmental pollutants among minorities. *Toxicology and Industrial Health, 9*, 797–820.

Senior, P. A., & Bhopa, R. (1994). Ethnicity as a variable in epidemiological research. *British Medical Journal, 309*, 327–300.

Sexton, K., Olden, K., & Johnson, B. L. (1993). "Environmental justice": The central role of research in establishing a credible scientific foundation for informed decision making. *Toxicology and Industrial Health, 9*, 685–727.

Stephenson, M. (2000). Development and validation of the Stephenson Multigroup Acculturation Scale (SMAS). *Psychological Assessment, 12*, 77–88.

Tran, T. V., Fitzpatrick, T., Berg, W. R., & Wright, R., Jr. (1996). Acculturation, health, stress, and psychological distress among elderly Hispanics. *Journal of Cross Cultural Gerontology, 11*, 149–165.

Tylor, E. B. (1924). *Primitive culture: Researches into the development of mythology, philosophy, religion, language, art, and custom* (7th ed). New York: Brentano. (Original work published 1871)

US Census Bureau. (n.d.). *American fact finder*. Retrieved November 11, 2007, from http://factfinder.census.gov/servlet/QTTable?_bm=y&-geo_id=01000US&-qr_name=DEC_2000_SF1_U_DP1&-ds_name=DEC_2000_SF1_U

US Census Bureau. (2000). *The population profile of the United States: 2000 (Internet release)*. Retrieved October 21, 2004, from http://www.census.gov/population/www/pop-profile/profile2000.html

US Census Bureau. (2003). *Housing patterns*. Retrieved October 12, 2008, from http://www.census.gov/hhes/www/housing/resseg/tab7-1.html

US Department of Commerce. (1999). *Emerging minority marketplace*. Retrieved November 11, 2007, from http://faculty.washington.edu/mbarreto/courses/minoritypopulation2050.pdf

US Department of Health and Human Services. (2000). *Healthy People 2010: National health promotion and disease prevention objectives* (Conference ed. in 2 vols.) Washington, DC: Author.

Williams, D. R., Lavizzo-Mourey, R., & Warren, R. C. (1994). *The concept of race and health status in America*. Retrieved November 11, 2007, from http://www.pubmedcentral.nih.gov/picrender.fcgi?artid=1402239&blobtype=pdf

Williams, D. T. (2007). *Harvard public health review. Exposing the roots of health disparities*. Retrieved November 14, 2007, from www.hsph.harvard.edu/review/winter07/williams1.html

Winslow, C. E. A. (1920). The untilled field of public health. *Modern Medicine, 2*, 183–191.

Yen, I. H., & Syme, S. L. (1999). The social environment and health: A discussion of the epidemiologic literature. *Annual Review of Public Health, 20*, 287–308.

Zambrana, R. E., Scrimshaw, S. C. M., Collins, N., & Dunkel-Schetter, C. (1997). Prenatal health behavior and psychosocial risk factors in pregnant women of Mexican origin: The role of acculturation. *The American Journal of Public Health, 87*, 1022–1026.

CHAPTER 2

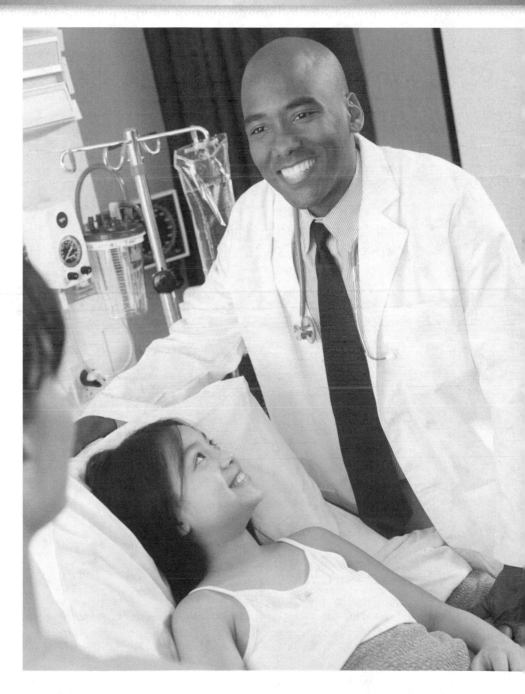

Cross-Cultural Concepts of Health and Illness

After all, when you come right down to it, how many people speak the same language even when they speak the same language?

—Russel Hoban

An understanding of the determinants of the different distribution of health problems among racial or ethnic groups is a prerequisite to the development and direction of effective programs and services to address them.

—Williams, Lavizzo-Mourey, & Warren (1994)

KEY CONCEPTS

- Worldviews
- Evil eye
- Shaman
- Susto
- Curandero
- Mal de ojo
- Sorcerers
- Vitalistic

- Ayurvedic medicine
- Humours
- Alternative medicine
- Reiki
- Homeopaths
- Naturopaths
- Advance directives
- Beneficence

CHAPTER OBJECTIVES

1. Explain the two overarching theories of the causes of illness and provide examples of each.
2. Explain the differences between the biomedical and holistic systems of care.
3. Provide at least three examples of cultural differences in verbal communication.
4. Provide at least three examples of cultural differences in nonverbal communication.
5. Explain two models of cultural competence.

Leaving the house with wet hair and drinking hot tea with honey are two commonly held beliefs by the dominant culture in the United States about how illness can occur and be cured, respectively. People from different cultures hold dissimilar beliefs about the causes and cures of illness, which impacts where one seeks care. But many others factors impact our health care experience, such as how we communicate about health, if we believe that we have control over our own health, and how health care decisions are made. These factors can be so deeply ingrained that they are almost invisible. Because of this invisibility, health care professionals can overlook these key differences and forget that not all people who reside within the United States have the same beliefs about health and illness. Therefore, it is essential to bring these issues to light, which is the purpose of this chapter.

In this chapter we begin with discussing theories about how illness occurs and different systems of care for when illness does occur. We then move into a discussion about **worldviews**. Worldviews incorporate how people perceive the world, which can have profound impacts on their health. Understanding the theories of causes of illness, pathways to care, and worldviews moves professionals to a higher level of cultural competence, which is discussed in the last section of this chapter.

THEORIES OF HEALTH AND ILLNESS

Theories about health and illness address the beliefs people hold about how to maintain health and the causes of illness. These ideologies are socially constructed and deeply ingrained in cultural beliefs and practices (Breslow, 2002). Ideas about health maintenance vary among cultures and include ideologies such as the consumption of a well-balanced diet, wearing of amulets, rewards for good behavior, and prayer. Illness causation ideologies include breach of taboo, soul loss, exposure to germs, **evil eye**, upset in the hot–cold balance of the body, or a weakening of the body's immune system.

Theories of illness causation derive from the underlying cognitive orientation of a cultural group, and therapeutic practice usually follows the same cultural logic (Breslow, 2002). These perspectives shape how people receive and respond to prevention programs, treatment, and health education messages. The theories of health and illness serve to create an understanding for the context of the illness so that the patient can frame the illness in a meaningful and logical manner. A meaningful context for illness usually develops from core cultural values and enables the patient to understand the illness in a logical manner and to regain some sense of control in a frightening situation that feels out of one's control (Breslow, 2002).

Anthropologists often divide theories of illness into two broad categories: personalistic and naturalistic (Breslow, 2002; Hopwood, 1997). In a personalistic system, illness is believed to be caused by the intentional intervention of an agent that may be a supernatural being (a deity or ancestral spirits) or a human being with special powers (a witch or sorcerer). The sick person's illness is considered to be a direct result of the harmful influence of these agents and is often linked to the ill person's behavior. In naturalistic causation, illness is explained in terms of a disturbed natural equilibrium. When the body is in balance with the natural environment, a state of health is achieved. When the balance no longer exists, then illness occurs. Often, people invoke both types of causation in explaining an episode of illness, and treatment may entail two corresponding types of therapy (Breslow, 2002).

Personalistic Theories

Personalistic theories of illness are linked to the person's misbehavior, which could be spiritual or moral in nature. The behavior could be related to not adhering to social norms, religious beliefs, or rituals, for example. If someone has violated a social or religious norm, he or she may have punishment invoked in the form of illness by the anger of a divine being or other agent, and the illness did not occur by accident (Breslow, 2002). Healers usually use supernatural means to understand what is wrong with their patients and to return them to health. Although there are many beliefs about how illness can occur under this ideology, a few of them are discussed here.

One method by which illness may be instilled is by spirit possession or damage, a supernatural being introducing a foreign object, or bewitching (O'Neil, 2005). The foreign objects could be rocks, bones, insects, arrowheads, small snakes, or even supernatural objects (O'Neil, 2005). It is believed that the foreign objects were intentionally put into an individual's body by witchcraft or some other supernatural means. The fact that there is no wound in the skin for the entry of the object supports the belief that supernatural actions were involved (O'Neil, 2005). This type of illness is cured by a **shaman**, a person who is not part of an organized religion and is in direct contact with the spirit world. The shaman will not make an incision into the skin; usually healing occurs by the shaman removing the object while in a trance state. Typically, shamans appeal to supernatural spirits for assistance, manipulate the patient's body, blow tobacco smoke over the site of the pain, and suck on the skin over the pain with a tube or by mouth to remove the object (O'Neil, 2005).

Susto is another type of personalistic illness. Susto literally means "fright" or "sudden fear" in Spanish. The fear leads to the person's soul being separated from the body. The presumed cause of the soul loss is due to incidents that have a destabilizing effect on an individual (e.g., being thrown from a horse, the unexpected barking of a dog, having a nighttime encounter with a ghost, or being in a social situation that causes fear or anger). The symptoms of susto can include nervousness, diarrhea, insomnia, loss of appetite, listlessness, and restlessness while sleeping. These symptoms are characteristic of what Western-trained medical professionals would likely attribute to excessive emotional stress or clinical depression (O'Neil, 2005). An example of this kind of illness is found among some Hispanics in the United States and Latin America. Treatments traditionally include rituals that are used to exhort the frightened soul back into the body. A **curandero** (folk curer) may jump over the victim's body or pass a chicken egg and special herbs over the patient's body to absorb some of the illness, and later the egg may be left where the soul loss occurred, along with gifts to appease the supernatural being who has the patient's soul. The patient may then be massaged and finally "sweated" on a bed placed over or near a hot stove (O'Neil, 2005). Another method used to induce sweating is covering the ill person with numerous blankets (O'Neil, 2005).

Another type of personalistic illness is caused by evil eye, or **mal de ojo** in Spanish. Evil eye is an old and widespread belief that someone can cause harm to another person by gazing or staring at the person or his or her property. There is an assortment of beliefs about evil eye and who it is cast by. Some people believe that evil eye can be cast by people they know, such as neighbors and kin, and others believe it is cast by strangers, witches, the devil, or by a jealous person on people of whom they are envious. Illness from evil eye results from the perception that some people are "stronger" than others and that their strength can harm "weak" people. In traditional Mexican and Central American culture, women, babies, and young children are thought of as being weak, and men as well as rich and politically powerful people of either gender are strong (O'Neil, 2005). When a strong person stares at a weak individual, the eyes of the strong person can intentionally or unintentionally drain the power and/or soul from the weak one. Proof that this may have occurred to someone is that he or she cries inconsolably without a cause and has diarrhea, disturbed sleep, vomiting, and/or a fever. The traditional cure in rural Mexico often involves a curandero sweeping a raw chicken egg over the body of a victim to absorb the power of the person with the evil eye. The egg may then be covered with a straw or palm cross and placed under the patient's head while he or she sleeps. The egg is later broken into a glass or bowl of water and examined. The shape of the yolk indicates if the person has been cured.

Illness also can be caused by people who have the power to make others ill, such as witches, practitioners of voodoo, and **sorcerers**. These malevolent human beings manipulate secret rituals and charms to cause illness in their enemies.

Preventing personalistic illness includes avoiding situations that can provoke jealousy or envy, wearing certain amulets, adhering to social norms and moral behaviors, adhering to food taboos and restrictions, and performing certain rituals. Recovery from an illness arising from personalistic causes usually involves the use of ritual and symbolism, most often by practitioners who are specially trained in these healing practices.

Naturalistic Theories

Naturalistic theories of disease causation tend to view health as a state of harmony between the person and his or her environment; when this balance is upset, illness will result (Breslow, 2002). The naturalistic explanation assumes that illness is due to impersonal, mechanistic causes in nature that can be potentially understood and cured by the application of the scientific method. Examples of causes of illness include an imbalance of hot and cold, an energy imbalance, or parasites.

The **vitalistic** system is built upon the ideology that illness is caused by an energy imbalance. The belief system has a long history and embraces the belief that disease is a result of an imbalance in vital energies, which distinguish living and nonliving matter. In **ayurvedic medicine** the vital force is called the *prana*, in the Chinese system it is called the *qi*, and in the Western tradition the vital forces were identified as **humours**. Later the ideology of germ theory took center stage. These four belief systems about the causes of illness are discussed here.

Ayurvedic Medicine

Ayurveda is an ancient naturalistic theory developed in the East. The term "ayurveda" is taken from the Sanskrit words *ayus*, meaning life or life span, and *veda*, meaning knowledge. Ayurveda is actively practiced in India today. The system links the body's *chakras*, or energy centers associated with organs of the body, with primal forces, *such as prana* (breath of life), *agni* (spirit of light or fire), and *soma* (manifestation of harmony). Ayurveda suggests that there are three primary principles that govern every human body. These principles are called *doshas*, which are derived from the five elements: earth, air, water, fire, and space. It is the doshas that regulate all actions of the body. When the doshas are balanced, we experience good health, vitality, ease, strength, flexibility, and emotional well-being. When the doshas fall out of balance, we experience energy loss, discomfort, pain, mental or emotional instability, and, ultimately, disease. Ayurvedic treatment focuses on rebalancing the doshas with methods such as breathing exercises, rubbing the skin with herbalized oil, meditation, yoga, mantras, and herbs.

Chinese Medicine

In China a similar system was developed with the underpinnings of the polar opposites *yin* (female, dark, cold) and *yang* (male, light, hot) in which one combines the interaction of body fluids and energy channels or meridians. This vitalist belief system is widespread in China, South Asia, and Southeast Asia. When vital forces within the body flow in a harmonious pattern, a positive state of health is maintained. Illness results when this smooth flow of energy is disrupted, and therapeutic measures are aimed at restoring a normal flow of energy in the body. In China this vital force is known as *chi* or *qi*; in India it is called *prana*. In China the ancient art of acupuncture is based on this understanding of the body. Acupuncture needles help to restore a proper flow of energy within the body.

Humoral Pathology

Humoral pathology, developed by Hippocrates (a Greek physician), was the basis of both ancient Greek and Roman medicine. It was part of the mainstream medical system in Europe and North America well into the nineteenth century (O'Neil, 2005).

The humoral system is an ancient belief system and is based on the idea that our bodies have four important fluids or humours, which are blood, phlegm, black bile, and yellow bile. These four fluids are related to seasons, internal organs, physical qualities (hot/cold; wet/dry) and human temperaments (see Table 2.1). Each humour is thought to have its own "complexion." For example, blood is hot and wet, and yellow bile is hot and dry. Different kinds of illnesses, medicines, foods, and most natural objects also have specific complexions.

Curing an illness involves discovering the complexion imbalance and rectifying it. A hot injury or illness must be treated with a cold remedy and vice versa (O'Neil, 2005). In the nineteenth century there was a radical transition from the humoural theory to the germ theory of disease as it involved new concepts, rules, and classifications, as well as the abandonment of old ones.

Germ Theory

Germ theory proposes that microorganisms are the cause of many diseases. Although highly controversial when first introduced, it is now a cornerstone of modern medicine

TABLE 2.1	Humour and Related Organ and Complexion				
Humour (Fluid)	**Associated Internal Organ**	**Associated Season**	**Associated Element**	**Normal Complexion**	**Temperament**
Blood	Liver	Spring	Air	Hot and wet	Sanguine (cheerfully confident; optimistic)
Phlegm	Brain and lungs	Winter	Water	Cold and wet	Phlegmatic (calm, sluggish; apathetic)
Black bile	Spleen	Fall	Earth	Cold and dry	Melancholic (in low spirits; gloomy)
Yellow bile	Gallbladder	Summer	Fire	Hot and dry	Choleric (easily angered)

and has led to innovations and concepts such as antibiotics and hygienic practices. Typical causes of illness according to this belief are (O'Neil, 2005):

- Organic breakdown or deterioration (e.g., tooth decay, heart failure, senility)
- Obstruction (e.g., kidney stones, arterial blockage due to plaque buildup)
- Injury (e.g., broken bones, bullet wounds)
- Imbalance (e.g., too much or too little of specific hormones and salts in the blood)
- Malnutrition (e.g., too much or too little food, not enough proteins, vitamins, or minerals)
- Parasites (e.g., bacteria, viruses, amoebas, worms)

Medical and nursing students in the United States are taught this kind of naturalistic explanation.

All theories of health and illness serve to create a context of meaning within which the patient can make sense of his or her bodily experience. A meaningful context for illness usually reflects core cultural values and allows the patient to bring order to the chaotic world of serious illness and to regain some sense of control in a frightening situation (Trollope-Kumar, 2002).

PATHWAYS TO CARE

The theory of illness with which a person identifies has an impact on where he or she seeks care. Within the United States there are two general systems of care to choose from: the biomedical (allopathic) approach and the holistic approach. The biomedical approach is often viewed as being scientific and focuses more on the physical components of illness than on the social aspects. Holistic medicine is viewed by some as being unscientific, and it is based on a psychosocial model of health care. A comparison of these two approaches can be found in Table 2.2. There are reasons why people select one health care delivery system over the other, and this decision-making process includes considerations such as culture, access to care, health beliefs, and affordability, but many people use both systems.

Biomedical Medicine

In the Western part of the world, the theoretical construct about the cause of illness is biomedicine (also known as conventional or allopathic medicine). The approach is built on the ideology that illness occurs when the human biological system goes out of balance and that microorganisms are the cause of many diseases. In biomedicine the body is viewed as a machine, and a core assumption of biomedicine is that scientific data should be the basis of diagnosis and treatment.

Care in the biomedical system is provided by a variety of types of professionals with diverse expertise and levels of training. Allopathic physicians, who are called doctors of medicine (MDs) and doctors of osteopathic medicine (DOs), are one type of clinician. MDs and DOs are licensed to provide the same services, have similar educational requirements, and are required to pass a licensing examination. There also are numerous allied health professionals, such as nurses, respiratory therapists, physical therapists, physician assistants, health educators, and radiologists.

Holistic Medicine

The holistic approach (also called **alternative medicine** or complementary medicine) has a long history and has been rapidly gaining in popularity worldwide. Holistic medicine is an approach to maintaining and resuming health that takes the body, mind, and spiritual being into consideration. Holistic medicine uses a variety of therapies, such as massage, prayer, herbal remedies, and **reiki**. More detail about these therapies is provided in Chapter 3.

It has been estimated that 62% of adults in the United States have used complementary medicine when prayer for health reasons was included (Barnes, Powell-Griner,

TABLE 2.2 Two Health Paradigms	
Allopathic	**Holistic**
Focuses on measurements: symptoms	Focuses on experience: causes and patterns
Disease as entity: pain avoiding	Disease as process: pain reading
General classified diagnosis	Specific individual needs
Health as commodity	Health as process
Technical tools	Integrated therapies
Remedial, combative, reactive	Preventive, corrective, proactive
Crisis oriented: occasional intervention	Lifestyle oriented: sustained maintenance
Radical, defensive	Natural, ecological
Medicine as counteragent	Medicine as coagent
Side effects: chemicals, surgery, radiation, replacement	Low risk: conservative, organic, purification, manipulation, correction
Emphasis on cure	Emphasis on healing
Speed, comfort, convenience	Restoration, regeneration, transformation
Practitioner as authority: pacifying	Practitioner as educator: activating
Patient as passive recipient	Patient as source of healing
Mechanical, analytical, biophysical	Systemic, multidimensional, body–mind–spirit
Best for infectious diseases, trauma, structural damage, organ failure, acute conditions	Best for degeneration, chronic stress and lifestyle disorders, toxemia, glandular weakness, systemic imbalances, immunity

Source: © Lonny J. Brown is the author of *Enlightenment in Our Time* (www.BookLocker.com/LonnyBrown), *Meditation—Beginners' Questions & Answers* (www.SelfHelpGuides.com), and *Self-Actuated Healing* (www.amazon.com). www.LonnyBrown.com

McFann, & Nahin, 2004). When prayer for health reasons was excluded, 36% of adults reported using complementary medicine during the past 12 months (Barnes, et al., 2004). In 1997, Americans paid $27 billion out of pocket for complementary medicine therapies (Fontanarosa & Lundberg, 1998).

Holistic providers have vast differences in their levels of training. These differences include length of training, certification and licensing requirements, and required experience. For example, people who study ayurvedic medicine in India often have four or more years of training, and in the United States it is often much less. Because of this broad spectrum of training and education requirements, it is essential to inquire about education and experience when seeking a provider. Providers include professionals such as **homeopaths**, **naturopaths**, acupuncturists, and hypnotherapists.

WORLDVIEW

Worldview refers to one's overall perspective from which one sees and interprets the world. It is a complex mixture of internalized motivations, perceptions, beliefs, and assumptions about human behavior that strongly affects how we interact with other people and objects in nature (O'Neil, 2005). Worldview includes feelings and attitudes that are mostly learned early in life and are not readily changed later (O'Neil, 2005). One's view of the world is made up of a collection of beliefs about life and the universe held by an individual or a group. Cultural groups have varied views of the world, and when they clash people may find the behavior of others to be offensive or confusing. Some of the prominent variances in worldviews include health beliefs, one's orientation toward time, use of space, social organization, and communication.

A person's worldview is closely linked with his or her cultural and religious background and has profound health care implications. For example, people with chronic diseases who believe in fatalism (predetermined fate) often do not adhere to treatment because they believe that medical intervention cannot affect their outcomes. Some of the major components of worldview that affect health care professionals are discussed in the following sections.

Time Orientation

Time is one of the most central differences that separates cultures. In the West, time tends to be seen as quantitative and is measured in units that reflect the march of progress. It is logical, sequential, and present focused, moving with incremental certainty toward a future. In the East, time feels like it has unlimited continuity, and it does not have a defined boundary. Birth and death are not such absolute ends because the universe continues, and humans, though changing form, continue as part of it.

Some cultures are present oriented, and others focus on the past or future. Overall, people in the United States are future oriented, but this emphasis appears to be shifting to a more present-focused society. Time perspective affects our health behaviors and expectations of health care behavior. In general, people understand that healthy behaviors in the present impact our health in the future, and future-oriented people are willing to make sacrifices now for future benefits. Present-focused people are not willing to make sacrifices for the future and engage in behaviors to satisfy their immediate desire regardless of the long-term consequences. Future-oriented individuals place value on getting screenings and preventive measures for future payoffs. Present-oriented cultures, including American Indians and African Americans, may see living in the moment as the priority and are not willing to forego immediate pleasures for future benefits. Cultures that are past oriented tend to value elders and honor traditions. For example, the Asian culture is generally past oriented, and they value and perform traditional healing practices, such as acupuncture and herbal remedies.

Space (Proxemics)

Another variable across cultures has to do with relating to space, which includes interpersonal distance and boundaries. North Americans tend to prefer a large amount of space, and Europeans tend to stand more closely together when talking and are accustomed to smaller personal spaces (LeBaron, 2003).

Violating these boundaries can lead to conflict, stress, anxiety, miscommunication, or discomfort. If someone is accustomed to standing or sitting very close when he or she is talking with another, that person may see the other's attempt to create more space as evidence of coldness, condescension, or a lack of interest. Those who are accustomed to more personal space may view attempts to get closer as pushy, disrespectful, or aggressive (LeBaron, 2003).

Also related to space is the degree of comfort we feel when furniture or other objects are moved. It is said that a German executive working in the United States became so upset with visitors to his office moving the guest chair to suit themselves that he had it bolted to the floor (LeBaron, 2003). Contrast this with United States and Canadian mediators and conflict-resolution trainers, whose first step in preparing for a meeting is not infrequently a complete rearrangement of the furniture (LeBaron, 2003).

Social Organization

Social organization refers to patterns of social interactions. Examples include how people interact and communicate, the kinship system, marriage residency patterns, division of labor, who has access to specific goods and knowledge, social hierarchy, religion, and economic systems. Three components of social organization that have an immense impact in health care are explored here: individualism versus collectivism, fate versus free will, and communication.

Individualism versus Collectivism

Individualism and collectivism are contrasting perspectives and values (see Table 2.3). Individualists see a person as a social unit, and each person has primary responsibility for him- or herself. In the United States the overarching culture values individualism, autonomy, and independence, and these qualities are rewarded and respected. If someone is successful, it is primarily because of these personal qualities.

Collectivism holds that a group (the nation, family, community, race, etc.) is a social unit (Stata, 1992), and dependence and connections with the group is valued. One's identity is determined by the groups with which he or she interacts and the relationships within those groups. People make decisions based on what is good for the group rather than what is good for the individual. Saving face is valued as well as showing respect for others. The needs and goals of the individual are subordinate to those of the larger group and should be sacrificed when the collective good so requires. Collectivists believe that achievement is a product of society (Stata, 1992). This view is often held by minority groups within the United States.

Why are these two opposing views important in health care? People from individualistic cultures make the decisions independently. In contrast, collectivist cultures

TABLE 2.3   Individualism versus Collectivism

Individualism	Collectivism
Focus on self rather than group	Focus on group rather than self
Guilt	Shame
Self-respect	Saving face
Behavior primarily regulated by likes and dislikes	Behavior primarily regulated by group norms
Conflict more acceptable	Conflict avoidance; emphasis on harmony and hierarchy
Person is basic unit of analysis and reality	Group is basic unit of analysis and reality
Focus on being unique	Focus on fitting in
Direct	Indirect
Achievement is a product of personal qualities	Achievement is a product of society
Priority given to promotion of own goals	Priority given to promotion of goals of others

will want to involve their families in the decision-making process, so health care professionals need to be aware of this aspect of worldview. Illness is considered to be a family event rather than an individual occurrence. In the United States, legal documents such as **advance directives** and durable powers of attorney are strategies to prolong autonomy in situations in which patients can no longer represent themselves (Searight & Gafford, 2005). Other cultures, however, deemphasize autonomy, perceiving it as isolating rather than empowering. These non-Western cultures believe that communities and families, not individuals alone, are affected by life-threatening illnesses and the accompanying medical decisions (Searight & Gafford, 2005).

Fate versus Free Will

Fate and free will refer to the degree to which people believe they are the masters of their own lives (free will) versus the degree to which they believe that they are subject to events outside our control (fate). Basically, fate and free will refer to the beliefs that people hold about their ability to change and maneuver the course of their lives and relationships. This concept also is called locus of control. People who believe that they have control over their health have an internal locus of control (free will belief), and people who believe that it is outside of their control (fate belief) have an external locus of control. In some ethnic groups, factors outside medical intervention, such as a divine plan and personal coping skills, may be more important for health and survival than medical intervention and health behaviors.

An example of why health care professionals need to consider this aspect of social organization is when health outreach workers in India attempted to provide children with free polio vaccinations, and they found that many of the parents refused the immunization because they believed that Allah would take care of the children's health. Providing preventive care and treatment can be challenging when people believe that fate will determine their health and that their health behaviors will not change what the master plan is for them.

COMMUNICATION

Communication is an interactive process that involves sending and receiving information, emotions, thoughts, and ideas through verbal and nonverbal means. It is the basis of human interaction. Effective communication enables health care professionals to accurately exchange information, establish relationships, and understand the person's needs and concerns. Effective communication is important in all facets of life, but in health care it can be the deciding factor between life and death.

Intercultural communication is sensitive to exchanging information across cultural boundaries in a way that preserves mutual respect and minimizes miscommunication and conflict. An example is that if communication is hindered, patients who utilize traditional remedies may be reluctant to inform their biomedical providers about them, leading to potentially dangerous interactions between medications prescribed by the two types of providers (Druss and Rosenheck, 1999 as cited in Taylor & Lurie, 2004).

In addition to better health outcomes, effective communication can lead to higher patient satisfaction, continued care, and better adherence to treatment recommendations while reducing conflict and errors, lost opportunities for encouraging health behavior changes, misinterpretations of treatment plans, damaged relationships (including a lost of trust) between the provider and patient or community member, and legal actions. All of these reasons illustrate why culturally competent communication is a vital component of health care.

Verbal Communication

As indicated in the quotation of Hoban at the beginning of this chapter, even people who speak the same language speak different languages. For example, in some age groups the word "fox" means attractive, but the term makes someone from a different generation think of the animal. People whose first language is English have a difficult time communicating, so imagine how difficult it must be to communicate with people in the United States when English is not someone's first language. According to the 2000 U.S. census, 18% of the total population aged 5 years and over, about 47 million people, reported that they speak a language other than English at home (Shin, 2003).

In addition to the risks of everyday language breeding possibilities for miscommunication, health care has a language of its own that can increase the chances of communication mishaps. Health care providers should avoid jargon and select words that people will understand without making them feel like you are talking down to them. Ask the receiver to summarize what you said to check for understanding and look for nonverbal cues that indicate when miscommunication has occurred. We describe a few cultural communication differences in the following paragraphs.

In some cultures, asking questions of health care providers is not an acceptable behavior. Patients from these cultures may be less likely to ask even clarifying questions and, subsequently, may not understand their condition or be able to follow their treatment plan, potentially resulting in a lower quality of care or even medical error.

Some cultures do not want to inform the patient about his or her health problem. This nondisclosure may be because of the belief that the discussion about illness may eliminate or reduce the patient's hope or induce depression or anxiety. Others believe that discussing the illness may make the person worse or that it is disrespectful. This issue also is a concern with regard to consent forms. The patient may believe that discussing the possible death or side effects of a medical procedure or medication may make it self-fulfilling and actually happen.

Some cultures protect patients from the emotional and physical harm caused by directly addressing death and end-of-life care. Many Asian and American Indian cultures value **beneficence** (physicians' obligation to promote patient welfare) by encouraging the patient's hope, even in the face of terminal illness (Searight & Gafford, 2005). Emotional reaction to news of serious illness also is considered to be directly harmful to health. It is thought that a patient who is already in pain should not also have to struggle with depression or stress. This negative emotional impact on health also appears to be one of the primary reasons that Chinese patients are less likely to sign their own do-not-resuscitate (DNR) orders (Searight & Gafford, 2005). This concern, together with Asian values of admiration for the elderly, may be especially pronounced in senior patients who, because of their frailty, are perceived as more vulnerable to being upset by bad news. In addition, the special status of the elderly in Asian cultures includes a value that they should not be burdened unnecessarily when they are ill.

As stated previously, there is a concern that direct disclosure of bad health news may eliminate patient hope. Bosnian respondents indicated that they expected physicians to maintain patients' optimism by not revealing terminal diagnoses (Searight & Gafford, 2005). Filipino patients may not want to discuss end-of-life care because these exchanges demonstrate a lack of respect for the belief that individual fate is determined by God (Searight & Gafford, 2005).

American Indian, Filipino, and Bosnian cultures emphasize that words should be carefully chosen because when they are spoken, they may become a reality (Searight & Gafford, 2005). Carrese and Rhodes (1995) noted that Navajo informants place a particularly prominent value on thinking and speaking in a "positive way." About one-half of their Navajo informants would not even discuss advance directives or anticipated therapeutic support status with patients because these discussions were considered to be potentially injurious.

Nonverbal Communication

Communication is more than just words, and much of the information that we convey is done nonverbally. Our system of nonverbal communication includes gestures, posture, silence, spatial relations, emotional expression, touch, and physical appearance (LeBaron, 2003). Our sense of what nonverbal behavior is appropriate is derived from our culture. Differences in nonverbal communication may lead to misunderstandings, misinterpretations about the person's character, damaged relationships, conflict, or escalating existing conflict.

Differences in nonverbal communication can be related to the following:

- Voice tone and volume
- Pace of speech
- Tolerance of silence
- Physical distance between speakers
- Posture
- Eye contact
- Gestures
- Direct versus indirect approaches
- Ways of greeting people
- Amount and location of touch

There are three general ways in which nonverbal communication can be received: (1) The nonverbal message may exist in both cultures but not have the same meaning, (2) the nonverbal message exists in the sender's culture but not in the receiver's culture, or (3) the nonverbal message exists in both cultures and has the same meaning. The following are examples of nonverbal gestures that have different meanings in various parts of the world (Gunawan, Bahasa, & BuahBatu Bandung, 2001).

- In Asian cultures smiling is used to show pleasure, and it also is used to cover emotional pain or embarrassment. When students are late to class or they can't answer questions from the teacher, they might smile to cover their embarrassment.
- When we are sad or angry, we can frown, scowl, or even cry. In Arab and Iranian cultures, people express grief openly and mourn out loud.
- The "ring" or "okay" gesture has different meaning in different countries. In the United States and other English-speaking countries, the ring or okay gesture means "everything is okay." In Japan it can mean money; in some Mediterranean countries it is used to infer that a man is homosexual; in Indonesia it means zero.
- The V sign has an "up yours" interpretation in Australia, New Zealand, and Great Britain. The palm faces toward the speaker for the insult version. In the United States, the V sign means victory, but the two fingers and the palm face out. Others may interpret the sign to mean the number two.
- In the United States, getting someone to come toward you by motioning with your index finger is common or acceptable; however, in the Philippines, Korea, and parts of Latin America, as well as other countries, the same gesture is considered to be rude. Indonesians extend one arm in front of them and, with the palm down, wave to the person to come.

- Eye contact is important because it shows intimacy, attention, and influence. People from some other cultures consider it to be rude and feel as though they are being disrespected or challenged.

CULTURAL COMPETENCE

Cultural competency occurs when an individual or organization has the ability to function effectively within the cultural context of beliefs, behaviors, and needs of the person or community that they serve. Campinha-Bacote (2009) defined cultural competence as, "the process in which the healthcare professional continually strives to achieve the ability and availability to effectively work within the cultural context of a client." Cultural competency requires a set of skills and knowledge that all health care professionals and organizations should strive to acquire. The ability to be culturally competent is on a continuum, with cultural destructiveness on one end of the continuum and cultural proficiency at the other end, as illustrated in Figure 2.1.

Being culturally competent does not mean that people need to know everything about every culture because that is not possible. What it does mean is that people are respectful and sensitive to cultural differences and can work with clients' cultural beliefs and practices. To be culturally competent, one needs to understand his or her own worldviews and those of the person or community while avoiding stereotyping, judgment, and misapplication of scientific knowledge. Becoming culturally competent is a process that health care professionals should continue to strive to achieve. Models have been developed to assist individuals and organizations with achieving this goal.

Cultural Competency Models

Models are tools that assist with understanding the causes of behaviors, predicting behaviors, and evaluating interventions. Older models focused more on individuals in isolation, but the more recent models take into consideration the social and physical environments. Cultural competency models help the learner understand the different components of cultural competency to help guide their interactions with people of different cultural groups and help them identify areas in which they may need to increase their education.

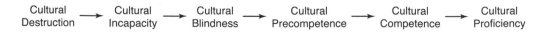

Cultural Destruction → Cultural Incapacity → Cultural Blindness → Cultural Precompetence → Cultural Competence → Cultural Proficiency

FIGURE 2.1 Cultural competency continuum.
Source: Adapted from University of Michigan Health System, Program for Multicultural Health.

The Process of Cultural Competence in the Delivery of Healthcare Services

Josepha Campinha-Bacote developed a model called The Process of Cultural Competence in the Delivery of Healthcare Services. This model of cultural competence is based on five constructs, which are cultural awareness, cultural knowledge, cultural skill, cultural encounters, and cultural desire.

1. *Cultural awareness* is defined as the process of conducting a self-examination of one's own biases towards other cultures and the in-depth exploration of one's cultural and professional background.
2. *Cultural knowledge* is defined as the process in which the healthcare professional seeks and obtains a sound information base regarding the worldviews of different cultural and ethnic groups as well as biological variations, diseases and health conditions, and variations in drug metabolism found among ethnic groups (biocultural ecology).
3. *Cultural skill* is the ability to conduct a cultural assessment to collect relevant cultural data regarding the client's presenting problem as well as accurately conducting a culturally-based physical assessment.
4. *Cultural encounter* is the process which encourages the healthcare professional to directly engage in face-to-face cultural interactions and other types of encounters with clients from culturally diverse backgrounds in order to modify existing beliefs about a cultural group and to prevent possible stereotyping.
5. *Cultural desire* is the motivation of the healthcare professional to "want to" engage in the process of becoming culturally aware, culturally knowledgeable, culturally skillful and seeking cultural encounters; not the "have to." (Campinha-Bacote, 2009)

The Purnell Model for Cultural Competence

The Purnell Model for Cultural Competence started as an organizing framework in 1991 when Dr. Larry Purnell discovered the need for both students and staff to have a framework for learning about their cultures and the cultures of their patients and families. This discovery was based on the ethnocentric behavior and lack of cultural awareness, cultural sensitivity, and cultural competence that existed. The purposes of the model are to provide a framework for health care providers to learn concepts and characteristics of culture and to define circumstances that affect a person's cultural worldview in the context of historic perspectives (Purnell, 2005).

The model (illustrated in Figure 2.2) is a circle in which an outlying rim represents global society, a second rim represents community, a third rim represents family, and an inner rim represents the person. Table 2.4 lists the four rings with their related definitions. The interior of the circle is divided into 12 pie-shaped wedges that depict cultural

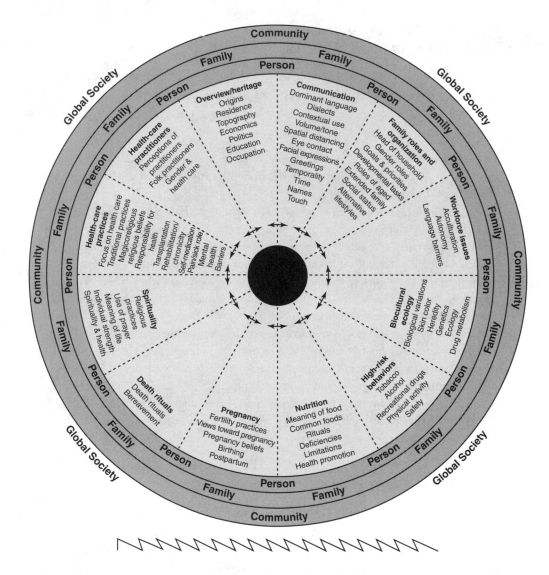

FIGURE 2.2 The Purnell Model for Cultural Competence.
Source: Reprinted with permission from Dr. Larry Purnell, University of Delaware.

domains and their concepts. The dark center of the circle represents unknown phenomena. Along the bottom of the model is a jagged line that represents the nonlinear concept of cultural consciousness. The 12 cultural domains (constructs) provide the organizing framework of the model. Health care providers can use this same process to understand their own cultural beliefs, attitudes, values, practices, and behaviors.

TABLE 2.4   The Rings of the Purnell Model for Cultural Competence

Ring	Definition
Global society	World communications and politics; conflicts and warfare; natural disasters and famines; international exchanges in business, commerce, and information technology; advances in the health sciences; space exploration; and the increased ability for people to travel around the world and to interact with diverse societies
Community	A group of people who have a common interest or identity and live in a specified locality
Family	Two or more people who are emotionally involved with each other and who may or may not be blood relatives
Person	A biopsychosociocultural human being who is constantly adapting

Source: Reprinted with permission from Dr. Larry Purnell, University of Delaware.

PROMOTING CULTURAL COMPETENCY

Promoting cultural competency within organizations is increasingly becoming a higher priority in the health care industry. The rationale for this includes the existence of health disparities, existing differences in access to care and quality of care among minorities, concerns about providing quality of care and legal actions, and credentialing. Standards for culturally competent care are provided in Chapter 5, but here we discuss ways to promote and assess your own level of cultural competence and that of your organization.

Implementing cultural competency programs is a nonlinear, multilevel, complex process. The paths to progression are varied. Areas for promoting cultural competency are related to policies, human resource development, and services. We have included two tools to assess the cultural competency at an individual level and at an organizational level. These types of assessments are a good place to start, and they will help identify areas in need of improvement.

Individual Assessment of Cultural Competence

As a member of the organization, the knowledge you have of yourself and others is important and reflected in the ways you communicate and interact. The individual assessment instrument in Table 2.5 was developed to assist you in reflecting upon and examining your journey toward cultural competence.

The following statements are about you and your cultural beliefs and values as they relate to the organization. Please check the ONE answer that BEST DESCRIBES your response to each of the statements.

TABLE 2.5 Individual Cultural Assessment

Individual Assessment	Almost Always	Often	Sometimes	Almost Never
1. I reflect on and examine my own cultural background, biases, and prejudices related to race, culture, and sexual orientation that may influence my behaviors.				
2. I continue to learn about the cultures of the consumers and families who are served in the program, in particular attitudes toward disability; cultural beliefs and values; and health, spiritual, and religious practices.				
3. I recognize and accept that the consumer and family members make the ultimate decisions even though they may be different compared to my personal and professional values and beliefs.				
4. I intervene, in an appropriate manner, when I observe other staff members engaging in behaviors that appear culturally insensitive or reflect prejudice.				
5. I attempt to learn and use key words and colloquialisms of the languages used by the consumers and families who are served.				
6. I utilize interpreters for the assessment of consumers and their families whose spoken language is one for which I am not fluent.				
7. I have developed skills to utilize an interpreter effectively.				
8. I utilize methods of communication, including written, verbal, pictures, and diagrams, that will be most helpful to the consumers, families, and other program participants.				

TABLE 2.5 (*Continued*)				
Individual Assessment	**Almost Always**	**Often**	**Sometimes**	**Almost Never**
9. I write reports, or any form of written communication, in a style and at a level that consumers, families, and other program participants will understand.				
10. I am flexible, adaptive, and will initiate changes that will better serve consumers, families, and other program participants from diverse cultures.				
11. I am mindful of cultural factors that may influence the behaviors of consumers, families, and other program participants.				

Source: Reprinted with permission from the Committee of the Association of University Centers on Disabilities (AUCD) Multicultural Council.

Organizational Assessment of Cultural Competence

Table 2.6 offers a means of assessing an organization's cultural competence. Some suggestions for achieving a culturally competent organization include the following:

- Maximize diversity among the workforce.
- Involve community representatives in the organization's planning and quality improvement meetings.
- Establish a cultural competency board to help guide the implementation of culturally sensitive prevention and treatment efforts.
- Provide ongoing training to staff members.
- Develop health materials for the target population that is written at the appropriate literacy level, in a variety of languages, and with culturally appropriate images—this includes materials such as educational brochures, consent forms, signage, postprocedural directions, and advance directives.
- Make on-site interpretation services available when possible, and be sure that all appropriate staff members are educated about how to use telephone interpretation services.
- Assess customer satisfaction and clinical outcomes regularly.
- Consider the health disparities that exist in your community when planning outreach efforts.

Please check the ONE answer that BEST DESCRIBES your response to each of the statements.

TABLE 2.6 Organizational Cultural Assessment

A. Organization	Yes	No	Don't Know
1. Cultural competence is included in the mission statement, policies, and procedures.			
2. A committee/task force/program area addresses issues of cultural competence.			
3. Partnerships with representatives of ethnic communities actively incorporate their knowledge and experience in organizational planning.			
4. The organization supports involvement with and/or utilization of the resources of regional and/or national forums that promote cultural competence.			

B. Administration	Almost Always	Often	Sometimes	Almost Never	Don't Know
1. Personnel recruitment, hiring, and retention practices reflect the goal to achieve ethnic diversity and cultural competence.					
2. Resources are in place to support initial and ongoing training for personnel to develop cultural competence.					
3. Position descriptions and personnel performance measures include skills related to cultural competence.					
4. Participants for all advisory committees and councils are recruited and supported to ensure the diverse cultural representation of the organization's geographic area.					
5. Personnel are respected and supported for their desire to honor and participate in cultural celebrations.					
6. Fiscal resources are available to support translation and interpretation services.					

TABLE 2.6 *(Continued)*

C. Clinical Services	Almost Always	Often	Sometimes	Almost Never	Don't Know
Important: If your organization does not provide these services, please check here and proceed to the next section. _____					
1. Clinical services are routinely and systematically reviewed for methods, strategies, and ways of serving consumers and their families in culturally competent ways.					
2. Cultural bias of assessment tools is considered when interpreting results and making recommendations.					
3. Translation and interpretation assistance is available and utilized when needed.					
4. Forms of communication (reports, appointment notices, telephone message greetings, etc.) are culturally and linguistically appropriate for the populations that are served.					
5. Pictures, posters, printed materials, and toys reflect the culture and ethnic backgrounds of the consumers and families who are served.					
6. When food is discussed or used in assessment or treatment, the cultural and ethnic background of the consumer and family is considered.					

(Continues)

TABLE 2.6 Organizational Cultural Assessment (*Continued*)					
D. Research and Program Evaluation	**Almost Always**	**Often**	**Sometimes**	**Almost Never**	**Don't Know**
Important: If your organization is not involved in these activities, please check here and proceed to the next section. _____					
1. Input on research priorities is sought from consumers and/or their families who represent diverse cultures.					
2. Research projects include subjects of diverse cultures that are representative of the targeted research population.					
3. The researchers include members of the racial/ethnic groups to be studied and/or individuals who have acquired knowledge and skills to work with subjects from those specific groups.					
4. Consumers and families who represent diverse cultures provide input regarding the design, methods, and outcome measures of research and program evaluation projects.					
E. Technical Assistance/Consultation					
Important: If your organization is not involved in these activities, please check here and proceed to the next section. _____					
1. Technical assistance/consultation activities are routinely and systematically reviewed for methods, strategies, and ways of serving communities in culturally competent ways.					

(Continues)

TABLE 2.6   *(Continued)*

	Almost Always	Often	Sometimes	Almost Never	Don't Know
2. When assessing the need for technical assistance/consultation in communities, input from members who reflect the diverse cultural makeup of these communities is sought and utilized.					
3. Efforts are made to involve consultants who have knowledge of and experience with the cultural group who requested the technical assistance/consultation.					
4. Evaluation from the recipients of technical assistance/consultation activities includes components of cultural competence.					

F. Education/Training	Almost Always	Often	Sometimes	Almost Never	Don't Know
Important: If your organization is not involved in these activities, please check here and proceed to the next section. _____					
1. Trainees/students are actively recruited from diverse cultures.					
2. Trainees/students from diverse cultures are mentored.					
3. Representatives of the diverse cultures are actively sought to participate in the planning and presentation of training activities.					
4. The training curriculum and activities incorporate content for the development of cultural competence.					
5. The training curriculum, materials, and activities are systemically evaluated to determine if they achieve cultural competence.					

(Continues)

TABLE 2.6 Organizational Cultural Assessment (*Continued*)					
G. Community/Continuing Education	Almost Always	Often	Sometimes	Almost Never	Don't Know
Important: If your organization is not involved in these activities, please check here. _____					
1. Participants are actively recruited from diverse cultures.					
2. Representatives of diverse cultures are actively sought to participate in the planning and presentation of these activities.					
3. The content and activities are culturally and linguistically appropriate.					
4. Participant evaluation of community/ continuing education activities includes components of cultural competence.					

Source: Reprinted with permission from the Committee of the Association of University Centers on Disabilities (AUCD) Multicultural Council.

When an individual, organization, or system has implemented change to progress toward cultural competency, the change process should be measured. This is important, because it can indicate the progress that has been made and identify areas that are in need of improvement. The measurement process itself can be a catalyst for change.

CHAPTER SUMMARY

We have all heard an abundance of stories about how illness can occur and how it can be cured. Some of these belief systems are ancient and are believed to be true, regardless of whether or not controversial evidence exists. These beliefs impact who we ask for medical advice and when. This is part of our worldview, which is our perception of how the world works. Health care professionals need to take these issues into consideration, and that is a step toward the progression of cultural competency.

In this chapter the authors identified several concepts that one needs to consider when working with people from different cultures. These concepts include different beliefs about how illness occurs, which impacts how, where, and when people seek medical care. Health care professionals should assess the person's worldview and tailor their approach and communication to successfully prevent and treat illness. Because of these differences, health care professionals need to become culturally competent. We have discussed what that means and provided tools to assess the level of cultural competency among individuals and organizations.

REVIEW

1. Explain the two overarching theories about the causes of illness.
2. Explain the two overarching systems of care in the United States and their differences.
3. What does worldview mean? Provide examples of why it is important to consider in health care.
4. Provide examples of differences in verbal and nonverbal communication methods among different cultures.
5. Explain the components of The Process of Cultural Competence in the Delivery of Healthcare Services model.
6. Explain the components of the Purnell Model for Cultural Competence.
7. List ways to improve cultural competency within an organization.

CASE STUDY

An interviewing medical student receives the pathology report from a recent endoscopy of his patient, a 78-year-old Japanese man. The report reveals adenocarcinoma of the stomach. The student is instructed to disclose the diagnosis to the patient. However, as the student approaches the patient's room, the patient's daughter stops him. The daughter demands to know the diagnosis and states that, if indeed it is cancer, her father should not be told. The daughter insists that she and her mother will decide what is best for her father. She argues that in her father's culture, family members make the decisions for the patient.

Consider the related questions:

- Is it the physician's duty to disclose the truth to her patient?
- How can the physician–patient relationship be preserved while taking into consideration the wishes of family members?
- What role should culture play in how a case is handled?

Source: Rosen, J., Spatz, E. S., Gaaserud, A. M. J., Abramovitch, H., Weinreb, B., Wenger, N. S., Margolis, C. Z. (2004). A new approach to developing cross cultural communication skills. *Medical Teacher, 26*(2), 126–132.

GLOSSARY TERMS

worldviews	ayurvedic medicine
evil eye	humours
shaman	alternative medicine
susto	reiki
curandero	homeopaths
mal de ojo	naturopaths
sorcerers	advance directives
vitalistic	beneficence

REFERENCES

Barnes, P. M., Powell-Griner, E., McFann, K., & Nahin, R. L. (2004). Complementary and alternative medicine use among adults: United States 2002. *Vital Statistics, 343*.

Betancourt, J. (2003). Cross-cultural medical education: Conceptual approaches and frameworks for evaluation. *Academic Medicine, 78*(6), 560–569.

Breslow, L. (Ed.). (2002). Theories of health and illness. *Encyclopedia of public health*. New York: Macmillan Reference. Retrieved September 9, 2007, from http://www.enotes.com/public-health-encyclopedia/theories-health-illness

Campinha-Bacote, J. (2008). *The process of cultural competence in the delivery of healthcare services.* Retrieved February 2, 2008, from http://www.transculturalcare.net/Cultural_Competence_Model.htm

Campinha-Bacote, J. (2009). The process of cultural competence in the delivery of healthcare services. Retrieved on March 10, 2009 from http://www.transculturalcare.net/Cultural_Competence_Model.htm

Candib, L. M. (2002). Truth telling and advance planning at the end of life: Problems with autonomy in a multicultural world. *Families, Systems & Health, 20*, 213–228. Retrieved December 30, 2007, from http://cms.nursingcenter.com/dev/prodev/ce_article.asp?tid=530681

Carrese, J. A., & Rhodes, L. A. (1995). Western bioethics on the Navajo reservation. Benefit or harm? *Journal of the American Medical Association, 274*, 826–829.

Council on Graduate Medical Education. (1999, March). *Physician education for a changing health care environment* (13th report). Washington, DC: Health Resources and Services Administration, US Department of Health and Human Services. Retrieved June 10, 2004, from http://www.cogme.gov/13.pdf

Drench, M. E., Noonan, A. C., Sharby, N., & Ventura, S. H. (2007). *Psychosocial aspects of health care.* Upper Saddle River, NJ: Pearson.

Druss, B. G., & Rosenheck, R. A. (1999). Association between use of unconventional therapies and conventional medical services. *Journal of the American Medical Association, 282*, 651–656.

Fontanarosa, P. B., & Lundberg, G. D. (1998). Alternative medicine meets science. *Journal of the American Medical Association, 280*(18), 1618–1619.

Gunawan, M. H., Bahasa, L., & BuahBatu Bandung, L. (2001). *Non-verbal communication: The "silent" cross-cultural contact with Indonesians.* Retrieved March 8, 2009 from http://www.ialf.edu/kipbipa/papers/MuhamadHandiGunawan.doc

Hopwood, A. (1997). The social construction of illness and its implications for complementary and alternative medicine. In: *Complementary therapies in medicine* (pp. 153–155). London: Pearson Professional.

Juckett, G. (2005, December 1). Cross-cultural medicine. *American Family Physician.* Retrieved January 6, 2008, from http://www.aafp.org/afp/20051201/2267.html

LeBaron, M. (2003). *Bridging cultural conflicts. A new approach for a changing world.* San Francisco: Jossey Bass.

Liu, J. M., Lin, W. C., Chen, Y. M., Wu, H. W., Yao, N. S., Chen, L. T., et al. (1999). The status of the do-not-resuscitate order in Chinese clinical trial patients in a cancer centre. *Journal of Medical Ethics, 25*, 309–314.

O'Neil, D. (2005). *Explanations of illness.* Retrieved December 30, 2007, from http://anthro.palomar.edu/medical/med_1.htm

Pew Health Professions Commission. (1995). *Critical challenges: Revitalizing the health professions for the twenty-first century.* San Francisco: UCSF Center for the Health Professions.

Purnell, L. (2002). The Purnell model for cultural competence. *Journal of Transcultural Nursing, 13*(3), 193–196. Retrieved December 26, 2008 from http://www.salisbury.edu/nursing/haitiancultcomp/purnellsmodel.htm

Purnell, L. (2005). The Purnell model for cultural competence. *Journal of Multicultural Nursing & Health.* Retrieved February 2, 2008, from http://findarticles.com/p/articles/mi_qa3919/is_200507/ai_n14825638/pg_1

Searight, H. R., & Gafford, J. (2005, February). Cultural diversity at the end of life: Issues and guidelines for family physicians. *American Family Physician.* Retrieved December 30, 2007, from http://www.aafp.org/afp/20050201/515.html

Shin, H. B. (2003). *Language use and English-speaking ability: 2000* (Census 2000 Brief). Retrieved September 1, 2007, from www.census.gov/prod/2003pubs/c2kbr-29.pdf

Smedley, B. D., Stith, A. Y., & Nelson, A. R. (Eds). (2002). Committee on Understanding and Eliminating Racial and Ethnic Disparities in Health Care, Board on Health Sciences Policy, Institute of Medicine. *Unequal treatment: Confronting racial and ethnic disparities in health care.* Washington, DC: National Academies Press.

Stata, R. (1992). *What is individualism.* Retrieved January 27, 2008, from http://rous.redbarn.org/objectivism/Writing/RaymieStata/WhatIsIndividualism.html

Stewart, M., Brown, J. B., Boon, H., Galadja, J., Meredith, L., & Sangser, M. (1999). Evidence on patient-doctor communication. *Cancer Prevention and Control, 3*(1), 25–30.

Taylor, S. L., & Lurie, N. (2004). The role of culturally competent communication in reducing ethnic and racial healthcare disparities. *The American Journal of Managed Care, 10,* SP1–SP4. Retrieved February 21, 2009 from http://www.ajmc.com/Article.cfm?Menu=1&ID=2686

Trollope-Kumar, K. (2002). Theories of health and illness. *Gale Encyclopedia of Public Health.* New York. Retrieved on March 10, 2009 from http://www.healthline.com/galecontent/theories-of-health-and-illness

Weech-Maldonado, R., Morales, L. S., Spritzer, K., Elliot, M., & Hays, R. D. (2001). Racial and ethnic differences in parents' assessments of pediatric care in Medicaid managed care. *Health Services Research, 36*(3), 575–595.

Williams, D. R., Lavizzo-Mourey, R., & Warren, R. C. (1994). The concept of race and health status in America. *Public Health Rep.* Jan–Feb, *109*(1): 26–41.

CHAPTER 3

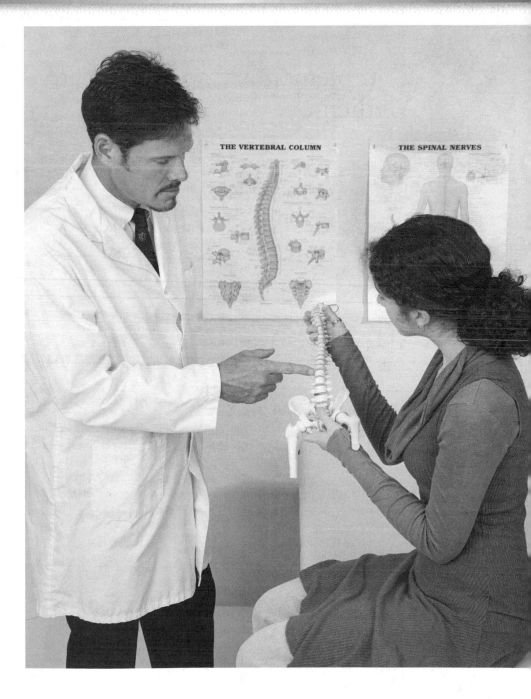

Complementary and Alternative Medicine

Everyone has a doctor in him or her; we just have to help it in its work.
The natural healing force within each one of us is the greatest force in getting well.
Our food should be our medicine.
Our medicine should be our food.

—Hippocrates

CHAPTER OBJECTIVES

1. Identify the difference between complementary and alternative medicine practices.
2. Understand the various types of CAM practices.
3. Discuss the potential benefits and risks of CAM practices.
4. Appreciate the cultural influences on CAM practices.

HISTORY OF COMPLEMENTARY AND ALTERNATIVE MEDICINE _____

It is not entirely clear when humans began to develop modalities to deal with pain, injury, and disease. However, we know that these practices have been in existence for ages. The various practices to treat disease and injury have been passed down through the centuries from person to person and family member to family member. The practices have been influenced by observation and experimentation, as well as religious, social, and cultural practices. Over time the various forms of these practices have taken on the unique characteristics of the people and cultures that utilize them.

Previously these practices have been termed "folk medicine" by the mainstream science-based medical professions. It was believed that with the advent of the scientific approach to medicine the various traditional folk medicine practices would die out. However, that has not been the case. As new cultures immigrated to the United States, so did their traditional healing practices. Increased interest in these traditional practices has spurred research into their efficacy and recharacterized them as complementary and alternative medical practices.

Complementary medicine is considered to be treatments that are utilized in conjunction with conventional Western medical therapies that are prescribed by a physician. Alternative medicine has been defined as practices used instead of conventional medical intervention. However, studies have found that people have been using both alternative medicine and mainstream medicine concurrently. Consequently, the concept of **integrative medicine**, where complementary and alternative medicine practices are incorporated into conventional care, came into being. Complementary and alternative medicine (CAM) is a broad range of modalities outside the traditional Western medicine approach to care. Folk medicine, or the use of traditional remedies, is considered to be a form of complementary and alternative medicine. Folk remedies thus include not only the remedies passed down in families but also long-existing practices, such as Chinese medicine, acupuncture, and naturopathy, to name a few.

The history of CAM in the United States is convoluted. Prior to the latter part of the nineteenth century, medical care was provided by lay healers, naturopaths, homeopaths, midwives, and botanical healers. The nineteenth century advances in science that included germ theory, antisepsis, and anesthesia spurred the trend to scientific medical education. After Abraham Flexner's 1910 report on the need for standardization in medical education, the demise of practices that were not in compliance with the accepted medical model began. As a result, nonconventional treatments were marginalized in the first half of the twentieth century. Then interest in whole foods and dietary supplements in the 1950s began a resurgence of interest in alternative medical practices. The traditional health practices of immigrant cultures exposed Americans to alternatives, and the counterculture movements of the 1960s began the interest in natural healing practices. In the 1970s, the holistic health approach began incorporating Eastern medical traditions with conventional medical practices (White House Commission, 2002).

This resurgent public interest in modalities, characterized as folk medicine, has encouraged medical practitioners to investigate their efficacy and impact on conventional medical practices. It has been noted that many folk medicine traditions have common features. Hufford (1988, 1997) noted that folk traditions tend to view the cause of disease as an imbalance or lack of harmony; they are based on personal responsibility and connections between health and the person's environment; they tend to be complex practices that involve a holistic approach to disease; and they often include an energy that provides harmony and balance.

Being aware of cultural differences in beliefs regarding disease and treatment is imperative to a medical practitioner because those who engage in CAM practices may also seek intervention from Western medicine. It has long been thought that those who are more likely to seek folk medicine remedies tend to be less acculturated to the American culture and have a number of shared characteristics (Pachter, 1994), including the following:

- Living in ethnic areas
- Preference for native language
- Educated in their country of origin
- Migration to and from country of origin
- Close contact with older persons with a high level of ethnic identity

Although that remains the majority view, recent studies have provided very different and interesting information about the utilization of CAM practices in the United States. In 1990 a study was conducted to determine the prevalence, cost, and pattern of use of CAM therapies in the United States. The study was limited to people with telephones who could speak English, so many ethnic groups were not well represented. Notwithstanding, the results were enlightening. One in three respondents reported using at least one CAM modality in the last year. The highest numbers were among nonblack people aged 25 to 49 years. Most were utilized for chronic conditions, and 83% also sought treatment for the same problem from their physician, although 72% did not inform their physician of the nontraditional treatment (Eisenberg, et al., 1993). The researchers concluded that the incidence of utilization of nontraditional therapies was much higher than anticipated, and further research on the issue was indicated.

A follow-up study was conducted in 1997 to determine any changes in the previous data. That study found an increase in the use of CAM from 36.3% to 46.3% of respondents. It also found that more visits were made to alternative practitioners in the previous year than to Primary care physicians ("Trends in Alternative Medicine Use in the United States, 1990–1997").

These studies provide insight into the prevalence of CAM usage in the United States. Although they were unable to evaluate utilization by many ethnic groups because of language barriers, the studies question the previous medical conceptions about utilization of CAM. Complementary and alternative medicine practices are being used not just by ethnic minorities but by those enculturated in the United States as well. The information about the broad use of CAM provides a backdrop for recent governmental action.

More recently, the National Institutes of Health National Center for Complementary and Alternative Medicine (NCCAM, 2002) conducted a study to determine the extent of CAM use in the United States. This study was conducted in 2002 and specifically investigated who was using CAM, what CAM practices were most prevalent, and why CAM was being used. The results were significantly different from the previous beliefs, which were previously discussed (see Table 3.1).

TABLE 3.1 Most Common CAM Practices	
Prayer/self	43%
Prayer/others	24.4%
Natural products	18.9%
Deep breathing	11.6%
Prayer group	9.6%
Meditation	7.6%
Chiropractic	7.5%
Yoga	5.1%
Massage	5.0%
Diets	3.5%

Source: NCCAM, 2002.

TABLE 3.2   Domains of CAM
Biologically-based practices. Uses substances found in nature, like herbs or vitamins in doses that are not used in mainstream medicine
Energy medicine. Uses energy fields that are believed to surround and penetrate the body
Manipulative and body-based practices. Uses manipulation and movement of body parts
Mind–body medicine. Uses techniques to enhance the mind's ability to impact the body
Source: NCCAM, 2002.

Initially, the study noted that 36% of Americans had used a CAM practice in the last year. The NCCAM study showed greater use in different populations than previously thought. People with higher education, and more women than men, were more likely to use CAM. Also, people who were hospitalized in the last year and who were former smokers were also more likely to seek CAM treatments (NCCAM, 2002). The mind–body domain (see Table 3.2) was the most common domain utilized when prayer was included in the CAM treatments. When prayer was not included, biologically-based practices were the most prevalent.

The reasons reported for using CAM treatments included improved health, although conventional medical treatment was the most prevalent response. Many respondents thought it would be interesting to try or that conventional medicine would not help their problem. Finally, some participants responded that they were advised to try a CAM modality by a conventional medical practitioner or that conventional treatment was too expensive (see Table 3.3).

TABLE 3.3 CAM Use by Race/Ethnicity		
	CAM with Megavitamins/Prayer	**CAM without Megavitamins/Prayer**
Asian	61.7%	43.1%
Black	71.3%	26.2%
Hispanic	61.4%	28.3%
White	60.4%	35.9%
Source: NCCAM, 2002.		

Prayer was the most commonly utilized CAM treatment for health problems, and race or ethnicity did not change that outcome (see Tables 3.1 and 3.3). Most respondents used CAM for their own health needs, and only 12% used it for the needs of others.

The NCCAM study did not examine the efficacy or safety of CAM treatments and acknowledged that few studies exist on those issues. Further, the current information is inconclusive. The NCCAM study recommended further research into the safety of the varied CAM practices and whether or not they work.

The White House Commission on Complementary and Alternative Medicine Policy was convened to evaluate CAM utilization in the United States and to make recommendations regarding future governmental action. It noted that the use of CAM is very prevalent in the United States patient population, which indicates a patient interest in exploring therapeutic options for chronic conditions that are not offered by conventional medicine. The Commission produced 25 recommendations for further action by the government and private enterprises, which deal with coordination of research, education and training of health practitioners, CAM information and development and dissemination, access and delivery, coverage and reimbursement, and coordinating federal efforts (see Table 3.4). The Commission and its recommendations are clear indicators of the interest and concern regarding CAM practices in the United States today.

With the White House Commission's recommendations, the National Institutes of Health's National Center for Complementary and Alternative Medicine has created a strategic plan to specifically address racial and ethnic health disparities in the utilization of CAM practices. The report notes that little is known about the use of CAM in minority populations, and research is needed to determine the extent of use by specific groups of CAM, conventional medicine, or a combination of the two. To accomplish these objectives, NCCAM will conduct research in areas that include the following:

- Review epidemiologic studies of CAM use in racial and ethnic populations.
- Develop research methods to study CAM in minority populations.
- Study the use of traditional, indigenous medicine systems.
- Conduct outcome research on CAM in minority populations.

Understanding that many CAM therapies arise from cultures from which American minorities come, it is necessary to better understand those practices and how they are utilized by minority populations. With that in mind, we will now turn our attention to specific CAM therapies in practice in the United States today.

TABLE 3.4   White House Commission on Complementary and Alternative Medicine Policy Recommendations and Actions

Coordination of Research

Recommendation 1: Federal agencies should receive increased funding for clinical, basic, and health services research on CAM.

Recommendation 2: Congress and the Administration should consider enacting legislative and administrative incentives to stimulate private sector investment in CAM research on products that may not be patentable.

Recommendation 3: Federal, private, and nonprofit sectors should support research on CAM modalities and approaches that are designed to improve self-care and behaviors that promote health.

Recommendation 4: Federal, private, and nonprofit sectors should support new and innovative CAM research on core questions posed by frontier areas of scientific study associated with CAM that might expand our understanding of health and disease.

Recommendation 5: Investigators engaged in research of CAM should ensure that human subjects participating in clinical studies receive the same protections as are required in conventional medical research and to which they are entitled.

Recommendation 6: The Commission recommends that state professional regulatory bodies include language in their guidelines stating that licensed, certified, or otherwise authorized practitioners who are engaged in research on CAM will not be sanctioned solely because they are engaged in such research if they:

1. Are engaged in well-designed research that is approved by appropriately constituted Institutional Review Boards.

2. Are following the requirements for the protection of human subjects.

3. Are meeting their professional and ethical responsibilities. All CAM and conventional practitioners, whether or not they are engaged in research, must meet whatever State practice requirements or standards govern their authorization to practice.

Recommendation 7: Increased efforts should be made to strengthen the emerging dialogue among CAM and conventional medical practitioners, researchers, and accredited research institutions; federal and state research, health care, and regulatory agencies; the private and nonprofit sectors; and the general public.

Recommendation 8: Public and private resources should be increased to strengthen the infrastructure for CAM research and research training at conventional medical and CAM institutions and to expand the cadre of basic, clinical, and health services researchers who are knowledgeable about CAM and have received rigorous research training.

TABLE 3.4   (*Continued*)

Recommendation 9: Public and private resources should be used to support, conduct, and update systematic reviews of the peer-reviewed research literature on the safety, efficacy, and cost–benefit of CAM practices and products.

Education and Training of Health Care Practitioners

Recommendation 10: The education and training of CAM and conventional practitioners should be designed to ensure public safety, improve health, and increase availability of qualified and knowledgeable CAM and conventional practitioners and enhance the collaboration among them.

Recommendation 11: The federal government should make available accurate, useful, and easily accessible information on CAM practices and products, including information on safety and effectiveness.

Recommendation 12: The quality and accuracy of CAM information on the Internet should be improved by establishing a voluntary standards board, a public education campaign, and actions to protect consumers' privacy.

Recommendation 13: Information on the training and education of providers of CAM services should be made easily available to the public.

Recommendation 14: CAM products that are available to U.S. consumers should be safe and meet appropriate standards of quality and consistency.

Recommendation 15: Provision of the Federal Food, Drug and Cosmetic Act, as modified by the Dietary Supplement Health and Education Act of 1994, should be fully implemented, funded, enforced, and evaluated.

Recommendation 16: Activities to ensure that advertising of dietary supplements and other CAM practices and products is truthful and not misleading should be increased.

Recommendation 17: The collection and dissemination of information about adverse events stemming from the use of dietary supplements should be improved.

Access and Delivery

Recommendation 18: The Department of Health and Human Services should evaluate current barriers to consumer access to safe and effective CAM practices and to qualified practitioners and should develop strategies for removing those barriers to increase access and to ensure accountability.

Recommendation 19: The federal government should offer assistance to states and professional organizations in (1) developing and evaluating guidelines for practitioner accountability and competence in CAM delivery, including regulation of practice, and (2) periodically reviewing and assessing the effects of regulations on consumer protection.

(*Continues*)

TABLE 3.4   White House Commission on Complementary and Alternative Medicine Policy Recommendations and Actions (*Continued*)

Recommendation 20: States should evaluate and review their regulation of CAM practitioners and ensure their accountability to the public. States should, as appropriate, implement provisions for licensure, registration, and exemption that are consistent with the practitioners' education, training, and scope of practice.

Recommendation 21: Nationally recognized accrediting bodies should evaluate how health care organizations under their oversight are using CAM practices and should develop strategies for the safe and appropriate use of qualified CAM practitioners and safe and effective products in these organizations.

Recommendation 22: The federal government should facilitate and support the evaluation and implementation of safe and effective CAM practices to help meet the health care needs of special and vulnerable populations.

Recommendation 23: Evidence should be developed and disseminated regarding safety, benefits, and cost-effectiveness of CAM interventions, as well as the optimum models for complementary and integrated care.

Recommendation 24: Insurers and managed care organizations should offer purchasers the option of health benefit plans that incorporate coverage of safe and effective CAM interventions provided by qualified practitioners.

Recommendation 25: Purchasers, including federal agencies and employers, should evaluate the possibility of covering benefits or adding health benefit plans that incorporate sage and effective CAM interventions.

Source: White House Commission on Complementary and Alternative Medicine Policy, 2002.

COMPLEMENTARY AND ALTERNATIVE HEALTH CARE MODALITIES

The White House Commission on Complementary and Alternative Medicine Policy noted that the major CAM systems have common characteristics that include focusing on individual treatment, a holistic approach to care, promotion of self-care and self-healing, and addressing spiritual influences on health. The Commission then created a classification model for CAM systems, which listed the various practices by their major domains (see Table 3.5). We will discuss the major modalities of complementary and alternative medicine and those that address specific cultural practices.

TABLE 3.5 CAM Systems of Health Care

I. Alternative health care systems
Ayurvedic medicine
Chiropractic
Homeopathic medicine
American Indian medicine (e.g., sweat lodge, medicine wheel)
Naturopathic medicine
Traditional Chinese medicine (e.g., acupuncture, Chinese herbal medicine)

II. Mind–body interventions
Meditation
Hypnosis
Guided imagery
Dance therapy
Music therapy
Art therapy
Prayer and mental healing

III. Biological-based therapies
Herbal therapies
Special diets (e.g., macrobiotics, extremely low fat or high carbohydrate diets)
Orthomolecular medicine (e.g., megavitamin therapy)
Individual biological therapies (e.g., shark cartilage, bee pollen)

IV. Therapeutic massage, body work, and somatic movement therapies
Massage
Feldenkrais
Alexander method

V. Energy therapies
Qigong
Reiki
Therapeutic touch

VI. Bioelectromagnetics
Magnet therapy

Source: White House Commission on Complementary and Alternative Medicine Policy, 2002.

Ayurvedic Medicine

Ayurveda, a Sanskrit word meaning science of life, was originally described in the ancient Hindu texts called Vedas. It was the major health care practice of India for thousands of years until the British raj emphasized its replacement with Western medical practices.

TABLE 3.6   The Doshas
Vata. Composed of air and ether
Pita. Composed of fire and water
Kapha. Composed of water and earth

It has experienced a resurgence of interest since Indian independence from Great Britain in the 1940s and, more recently, through the popular writer Dr. Deepak Chopra.

This ancient practice is based on the theory that the five great elements, ether, air, fire, water, and earth, are the basis for all living systems. The five elements are in constant interaction and are constantly changing. The elements combine in pairs to form **doshas**, the three vital energies that regulate everything in nature (see Table 3.6).

The doshas are combined at the time of conception in combinations unique to each individual. This combination is known as **prakriti**. A person's physiology, personality, intellect, and weaknesses are governed by two dominant doshas. If the doshas become imbalanced, the flow of prana, life energy, and agni, digestion, becomes upset. It is these imbalances that result in illness.

Ayurvedic practitioners seek to balance the doshas through herbal remedies, yoga, meditation, and massage. For example, Panchakarma is a remedy that consists of a purification process to remove impurities and restore balance to the doshas. Medicinal remedies are derived from minerals, herbs, and vegetables (Peters & Woodham, 2000).

Yoga

Yoga is an ancient system of exercises and breathing techniques designed to encourage physical and spiritual well-being. It incorporates a number of guidelines for well-being, including good nutrition and hygiene. The physical practice of yoga consists of going through asanas, or physical postures to improve the physical body and calm the nerves. Pranayamas are breathing techniques and meditations designed to improve spiritual well-being.

Some yoga practitioners teach that centers of energy, known as chakras, are connected to the nerves and spinal cord. It is believed that certain asanas and meditations can positively influence the chakras, improving physical and mental health. The exercise and relaxation techniques utilized in yoga are practiced by many people every day.

Homeopathy

Homeopathy is based on the **Law of Similars**, first postulated by the Greek healer Hippocrates. This concept that "like cures like" is premised on the belief in the body's ability to heal itself. This is accomplished by giving a person a substance that creates the symptoms of a disease in a healthy person. It is believed that this stimulates the body's natural healing properties to cure the disease.

Modern homeopathic practice was begun by German Samuel Hahnemann in the late eighteenth century from his experiments to cure malaria. His treatment concepts quickly spread throughout Europe and the United States. By 1900, 15% of U.S. physicians were homeopathic practitioners (Freeman, 2004). Not unlike other CAM practices, homeopathy suffered from the efforts of mainstream American medicine in the early twentieth century to squash its practice. However, homeopathy continued in other parts of the world and today is actively practiced in India, Germany, France, and Great Britain, and its practice has reemerged in the United States. Homeopathy is premised on three fundamental principles: the Principle of Similars, the Principle of Infinitesimal Dose, and the Principle of the Specificity of the Individual.

The **Principle of Similars** is based on the like cures like concept. If a substance is given to a healthy person and causes symptoms of a disease, then administering a smaller dose will cure the disease. This occurs through stimulation of the body's natural healing powers. Interestingly, this concept underlies Louis Pasteur's and Jonas Salk's work on immunity and vaccinations, the idea that exposure to a small amount of a disease will cause the body to create immunity to the disease. Also, allergies are often treated in mainstream Western medicine by exposing the patient to small amounts of an allergen to create resistance.

The **Principle of Infinitesimal Dose**, or the law of potentization, is the idea that the more a substance is diluted, the more potent it becomes for treatment. This reduces side effects from more potent doses, and practitioners believe that the more dilute a remedy, the longer its effect will last with fewer doses and the more effective the overall treatment will be. To achieve proper dilution, plant substances are dissolved in mixtures of alcohol and water and stored over a period of time so that the materials dissolve. The resultant solution is then repeatedly diluted in a process termed "potentization." This is a concept that raises questions regarding the effectiveness of homeopathy because through this process, little, if any, of the original substances are left in the ultimate remedy.

Finally, the **Principle of Specificity of the Individual** states that any condition must be matched to the distinctive symptoms of the person. This is termed "profiling" and involves evaluating the patient's physical, emotional, and mental characteristics to

TABLE 3.7   Hering's Laws of Cure
Constantine Hering was the father of American homeopathic practice. He developed the theory that healing progresses in a distinct pattern:
First, from the deepest part of the body to the extremities
Second, from the emotional and mental to the physical
Third, from the upper body to the lower body
Healing progresses in reverse order from the most recent problem to the oldest.

match his or her current condition to the correct remedy. Homeopathic practitioners have large resource materials to assist them in matching the person's symptoms to the proper remedy (see Table 3.7).

Homeopathic treatments have undergone study with varying results. Although there is disagreement on the mechanics of homeopathic treatment, studies have shown that homeopathic treatment can positively impact allergies, fibromyalgia, migraine, rheumatoid arthritis, and other conditions (Freeman, 2004).

Case Review and Analysis

Kistin and Newman (2007) reported a case wherein a healthy 28-year-old who had three previous pregnancies and one live birth began labor. She had no complications during her pregnancy, and she and her husband had created a birth plan with their doula, a birth coach. They desired a natural birth if at all possible.

The woman's labor proceeded well, and natural methods were used to stimulate labor. The well-being of the baby and mother were frequently monitored by the staff. A tablet of Caulophyllum 30C, a homeopathic remedy made from the herb blue cohosh, was given to help establish active labor. After nine hours of labor, the woman gave birth to a healthy baby boy. Kistin and Newman (2007) addressed the significance of this case as follows:

> The most recent Centers for Disease Control and Prevention (CDC) birth statistics from 2003 report that 20.6% of pregnant women undergo medical induction for labor, and an additional 17.0% are medically augmented. The methods for labor induction in hospital settings generally include intravenous oxytocin, oral or vaginal prostaglandins, and/or intracervical Foley bulb placement. Of these methods, intravenous oxytocin is the most widely-used agent.

Induction of labor for women with PROM at term reduces the risk of infectious morbidity without increasing the risk for cesarean or operative vaginal delivery. Induction of labor with oxytocin, however, is not without risk and may be associated with more complications in certain subpopulations, such as nulliparous women and women with an unripe cervix. Also, the use of oxytocin for induction of labor involves necessary additional interventions, including intravenous needle placement, continuous external or internal fetal monitoring, internal uterine pressure catheter, epidural anesthesia, and Foley catheter insertion, each of which carries added risks for the mother and fetus, as well as an additional monetary cost.

When induction of labor is indicated, women may be more accepting of a natural or nonpharmacologic method, and as with any intervention, it makes sense to use the least invasive, most effective method available. Homeopathic labor stimulants are potentially viable alternatives to oxytocin and prostaglandins for inducing and augmenting labor. Blue cohosh (*Caulophyllum thalictroides*) and black cohosh (*Actaea racemosa* [formerly *Cimicifuga racemosa*]) have been used as homeopathic labor stimulants around the world, especially in Europe and India. In the United States, there has been an upsurge in the use of homeopathic remedies, and a recent survey describing the use of complementary therapies among nurse–midwives in North Carolina reported that 30% recommend homeopathic substances for use during pregnancy. There is a rich history of positive experience with these remedies, but the evidence for the efficacy and safety is largely narrative and anecdotal. The purpose of this case study is to explore the role of homeopathic substances as potential alternatives to commonly used induction agents and to encourage further, rigorous clinical research into the safety and efficacy of use.

Reprinted from Kistin, S. J. & Newman, A. D. (2007). Introduction of labor with homeopathy: A case report. *Journal of Midwifery and Women's Health*, 52(3), 5, with permission from Elsevier.

Traditional Chinese Medicine

"Traditional Chinese medicine" is the term used for a group of ancient healing practices that date back some 2,000 years to 200 BC. The concepts utilized have been adapted by the Koreans, Japanese, and Vietnamese into their own versions of treatment. The system includes, among other treatments, herbalism, acupuncture, *qigong*, and t'ai chi ch'uan.

Traditional Chinese medicine, or TCM, is based on diagnosis from the pattern of symptoms rather than on endeavoring to identify a specific illness. It is believed that the cause of disease must be cured, not just its symptoms. TCM considers a person's body, mind, spirit, and emotions as part of one complete whole rather than individual parts that are to be treated separately.

The Theories of Traditional Chinese Medicine

TCM is based on a number of interrelated theories: the theory of Qi, the theory of the Five Elements, the theory of Yin and Yang, and the Meridian theory. These theories inform the treatment modalities that include acupuncture, herbal medicine, t'ai chi ch'uan, and *qigong*.

The Theory of Qi   **Qi**, pronounced "chee," is the vital life force that animates all things. Qi flows through the 12 meridians that run through the body. Physical, emotional, and mental harmony rely on the flow of qi. Qi has two parts, energy or power, and conscious intelligence. These parts are found in organ systems and allow them to perform their physical and energetic functions. Qi can also be described by how it functions. Qi creates all movement, protects the body, provides for harmonious transformation, such as water being turned into urine, keeps the organs and body parts in proper position, and warms the body. This theory holds that qi:

- Is spiritual in origin
- Makes up and moves through all living things
- Is available in infinite quantities, is positive in nature, and is important to all aspects of health
- Is present both inside the body and on its surface
- Flows throughout the body in specific channels
- Has its flow disturbed by negative thoughts or feelings

Qi deficiency can result in problems, such as what Western medicine calls chronic fatigue syndrome or a fever. Qi stagnation, where the energy cannot flow correctly, can result in what Western medicine calls pain.

The Five Elements Theory   The **five elements** are based on the perception of the relationships between all things. These patterns are grouped and named for the five elements: wood, fire, earth, metal, and water. This theory states that the five organ systems are each tied to a particular element and to a broader group of phenomena that are associated with their elements, including the seasons, colors, emotions, and foods (see Table 3.8). This theory illustrates the interrelatedness between all things.

Each of the elements gives energy to one element and controls another element. When control and energy are properly balanced, a state of wellness exists. If the relationships become unbalanced, health problems will emerge.

TABLE 3.8	The Characteristics of the Five Elements				
	Fire	**Earth**	**Metal**	**Water**	**Wood**
Season	Summer	Indian summer	Autumn	Winter	Spring
Taste	Bitter	Sweet	Pungent	Salty	Sour
Emotion	Joy	Worry	Grief	Fear	Anger
Body	Heart	Spleen	Lungs	Kidneys	Liver
	Small intestine	Stomach	Large intestine	Bladder	Gallbladder
	Tongue	Mouth	Nose	Hair	Tendons
	Blood vessels	Muscles	Skin	Bones	Eye
Energy/control	Melts metal	Dries water	Cuts wood	Douses fire	Breaks earth
	Water douses it	Wood breaks it	Fire melts it	Earth dries it	Metal cuts it

The Yin and Yang Theory   The **yin and yang** theory holds that everything is made up of two polar energies. Neither can exist without the other, and they never separate. It is the principle of interconnectedness and interdependence. Yin and yang describe how things function in relation to one another and the important principle of harmony where things blend together into a whole.

Yin is female and associated with the moon and night, late afternoon, cold, rest, responsiveness, passivity, darkness, interiority, downwardness, inwardness, and decrease. Yang is male and associated with the sun and daytime, early morning, heat, stimulation, movement, activity, excitement, vigor, light, exteriority, upwardness, outwardness, and increase (see Figure 3.1).

The Meridian Theory   **Meridians** are channels through which qi, blood, and information flow to all parts of the body. There are 12 meridians in the body; 6 are yin and 6 are yang. Although each meridian is attributed to, and named for, an organ or body function, the network of meridians connects the meridians to one another and all parts of the body, and they connect the body to the universe. When qi flows easily, the body is balanced and healthy. The meridians work to regulate the energy functions of the body and keep it balanced and in harmony.

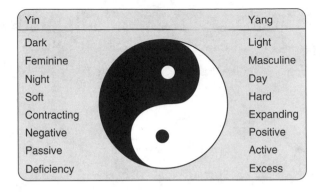

Yin	Yang
Dark	Light
Feminine	Masculine
Night	Day
Soft	Hard
Contracting	Expanding
Negative	Positive
Passive	Active
Deficiency	Excess

FIGURE 3.1   The symbol of yin and yang is a circle with two equal and opposite halves.

The Treatment Modalities of Traditional Chinese Medicine

Traditional Chinese Medicine encompasses many different treatment modalities. Here we will explore some of the treatment options utilized.

Acupuncture   **Acupuncture** is *one* of the most researched and accepted complementary practices in the United States today. It is experiencing greater acceptance by traditional medical practitioners, and research of its efficacy in treating various conditions has been undertaken, although it has proven to be a difficult subject to study. Even though the research was challenging, the National Institutes of Health Consensus Conference on Acupuncture (1998) concluded that acupuncture is effective for various conditions, such as postoperative and chemotherapy-induced nausea and vomiting, and noted that it could be useful for treating a number of conditions, such as head or back pain and alcohol dependence.

Acupuncture involves stimulating specific points along the meridians to achieve a therapeutic purpose. The usual practice involves inserting a needle into one of the acupoints along a meridian associated with that organ or function. Besides puncturing the skin, practitioners also use other methods, including pressure, heat, friction, or electrical stimulation of the needle.

The TCM theory is that acupuncture works by bringing healing energy, qi, to the affected part of the body through the meridians. The stimulation of the appropriate meridian can assist in bringing the affected organ into balance.

Chinese Herbal Therapies Another significant aspect of traditional Chinese medicine is the use of herbal remedies. Although it is not as prevalent in the United States as acupuncture, the use of herbal remedies is widespread in China and other Asian countries as well as among immigrants from Asian countries. Like acupuncture, herbal remedies are used to bring balance back to the body. Herbs are classified according to the five elements and their yin and yang properties to determine how they will be used. Herbs are combined according to their properties to treat a particular disharmony. They are usually administered as teas, pills, powders, or creams. Safety and efficacy issues related to herbal remedies are discussed in the "Herbal Remedies" section.

Qigong The term *qigong* translates to "energy work." It is a part of traditional Chinese medicine that involves movement, breathing, and meditation, and it is intended to improve the flow of qi throughout the body. *Qigong* is an ancient technique that is practiced by millions of people every day. It involves a number of basic postures that are involved in daily practice, and a master can tailor the techniques to address specific problems.

The ancient noncombative martial art, **t'ai chi ch'uan**, is a form of *qigong*. The purpose of t'ai chi ch'uan is to improve the flow of qi through the body to encourage balance and harmony.

Case Review and Analysis

The following cases were reported on Acupuncture.com by two practitioners of acupuncture and traditional Chinese medicine in a discussion of the treatment of Alzheimer disease, stroke, and Parkinson disease (Chen & Zhang, 1997).

- *Case #1.* An 83-year-old female had a stroke two years ago. When she was first seen, she hobbled into the clinic, did not answer questions, and fell asleep. Clinical observation showed an extremely deficient and deep pulse. Her tongue was pink and slightly dusky with a greasy, yellow-green coat, which was much thicker on the left side. The patient was started on a regimen of Neuro Plus (Nao Wei Kang Wan) daily and received acupuncture treatment twice weekly. With treatment she improved rapidly. She can now lift her feet, smile, respond somewhat, and stay awake throughout the entire treatment. After four months of treatments she is able to speak, and her friends are happy because she can now talk with them on the phone.

- *Case #2.* The patient is a 64-year-old retired male who had complaints of poor attention span, hand tremor, stiff tongue, inability to hold a rice bowl or chopsticks, poor balance, difficulty walking, and partial urinary and fecal incontinence with frequent urination. A CT scan showed cerebral atrophy. The patient's condition dramatically improved after taking Neuro Plus (Nao Wei Kang Wan). His hand tremors stopped within a few days, and he felt more energetic. His walking improved and frequency of urination decreased. The patient stated that the treatment was like a "magic bullet."

Musculoskeletal Manipulation and Chiropractic

The modern practice of **chiropractic** has its origins in ancient practices. Many cultures have incorporated musculoskeletal manipulation in their healing practices, including the Chinese, Japanese, Indians, Egyptians, Mayans, Arabs, and American Indian tribes. The Greek healer and father of medicine, Hippocrates, included chapters on manipulation in his works on medicine. In Europe during the Middle Ages and Renaissance, bonesetters practiced musculoskeletal manipulation (Freeman, 2004).

The most prevalent contemporary practice of musculoskeletal manipulation is chiropractic, although musculoskeletal manipulation continues in other practices, such as osteopathic medicine. The term "chiropractic" is derived from Greek and translates to "done by hand." In its simplest terms, chiropractic diagnoses and treats disorders of the muscular, nervous, and skeletal systems with special emphasis on the spine. Spinal adjustment is the predominate treatment tool.

Begun in the late nineteenth century by Daniel David Palmer, an immigrant from Canada, chiropractic is founded on the belief that the spine is the key to health and that spinal misalignments affect the function of the entire body. Through manipulation, normal nerve function throughout the spine and nerves is restored and health is improved.

Chiropractic practice has three basic tenets (Chisolm, 2007):

1. The body has a powerful self-healing ability.
2. The body's structure (primarily that of the spine) and its function are closely related, and this relationship affects health.
3. Chiropractic therapy is concerned with the goals of normalizing this relationship between structure and function and assisting the body as it heals.

Early chiropractic theory held that misaligned vertebrae, called subluxation, disrupted nerve function, which could lead to disease and pain. Currently, the belief that the spine has a primary function in health remains, but theories have changed to accommodate advances in knowledge of physiology. Also, chiropractors emphasize that they do not treat disease but, rather, promote the body's ability to heal itself.

The hallmark treatment modality of chiropractic care is spinal manipulation, known as "adjustment." This term refers to any number of techniques utilized to correct misalignment of the spine and nerves, improving the patient's condition. Adjustment is utilized to correct subluxations and return the spine, and body, to better function. Additional therapies, such as heat and ice, massage, ultrasound or electrical stimulation, and traction, may be added depending on the person's need. It is not uncommon for chiropractic care to be combined with other CAM practices, such as homeopathy, naturopathy, or traditional Chinese medicine.

Chiropractic care is sought for any number of problems. The most common complaints are back pain, neck pain, and headache. Although chiropractic care is sought at greater and greater frequency for these chronic conditions, the scientific research has not definitively determined its efficacy.

Some chiropractic practitioners have utilized chiropractic techniques to treat a number of nonmusculoskeletal problems. The research on the efficacy of these interventions is scarce. It indicates that chiropractic may be helpful for menstrual pain, colic, and carpal tunnel syndrome, but it is contraindicated in the treatment of vascular problems, arteriosclerosis, tumors, arthritis, and metabolic disorders, among others.

Chiropractic is attractive to many people for the treatment of acute musculoskeletal injuries as well as chronic pain conditions. In the United States today, chiropractors are the second largest group of primary care providers, and chiropractic is the most widely utilized CAM modality in the country (Eisenberg, et al., 1993).

Naturopathy

Naturopathy, or natural medicine, has its origins in the late nineteenth century in Germany based on the ancient belief in the healing power of nature and that natural organisms have the ability to heal themselves and maintain health. Naturopaths believe that the body strives to maintain a state of equilibrium, known as homeostasis, and unhealthy environments, diets, physical or emotional stress, and lack of sleep or fresh air can disrupt that balance (see Table 3.9).

Naturopathic Treatments

Naturopaths believe that the body attempts to maintain optimum health. When homeostasis is upset, they utilize any number of treatments to return the body to balance.

TABLE 3.9   The Six Key Principles of Naturopathy
1. Promote the healing power of nature.
2. Do no harm.
3. Treat the whole person.
4. Treat the cause.
5. Prevention is the best cure.
6. The physician is a teacher.

Source: National Center for Complementary and Alternative Medicine. (2007a).

All treatments are designed to enhance the body's ability to heal itself. Modalities include diet, yoga, manipulation, massage, hydrotherapy, and natural herbs. Naturopathic practitioners take a holistic approach to treatment and focus on the cause of a disruption of homeostasis rather than treating only symptoms.

Herbal Remedies   Plants used for medicinal purposes are classified as medicinal herbs. Herbs have been used to treat diseases for centuries. Many conventional medications were originally developed from herbs. Naturopaths use herbs to restore homeostasis through treating the cause of diseases. Today the use of herbal remedies is the fastest growing CAM therapy.

Herbal preparations use either whole plants or parts of plants. Many herbalists believe in synergy, the idea that whole plants are more effective than their individual parts. Herbal remedies are prepared in pill or liquid form for ingestion or as tinctures, creams, or ointments for external use.

The World Health Organization estimates that 80% of the world's population uses some form of herbal remedies for their care (Freeman, 2004). The 10 most popular natural products in the United States are listed in Table 3.10. Consequently, the safety of herbal remedies is a concern because herbs can be dangerous in the wrong dose or when mixed with other herbs or medications.

In the United States, herbal products are sold as dietary supplements. They are regulated by the U.S. Food and Drug Administration (FDA) as foods. This means that they do not have to meet the same standards as drugs and over-the-counter medications for proof of safety, effectiveness, and what the FDA calls Good Manufacturing Practices (see Table 3.11).

TABLE 3.10   Ten Most Popular Natural Products

Echinacea, 40.3%. Used to stimulate the immune system for colds and chronic infections

Ginseng, 24.1%. Used to lower blood pressure and blood sugar and to increase energy

Gingko biloba, 21.1%. Used to aid memory and diminish dementia symptoms

Garlic supplements, 19.9%. Used to lower cholesterol and blood pressure

Glucosamine, 14.9%. Used for joint pain and degeneration

St. John's wort, 12.0%. Used for depression

Peppermint, 11.8%. Used for gastrointestinal complaints

Fish oils/omega fatty acids, 11.7%. Used to prevent cardiovascular disease

Ginger supplements, 10.5%. Used for nausea, especially in pregnancy and motion sickness

Soy supplements, 9.4%. Used for menopause, osteoporosis, and memory problems

The percentage reflects the number of Americans who use natural products.
Source: National Center for Complementary and Alternative Medicine. (2007b).

TABLE 3.11   About Dietary Supplements

Dietary supplements were defined in a law passed by Congress in 1994. A dietary supplement is a product that contains vitamins, minerals, herbs or other botanicals, amino acids, enzymes, and/or other ingredients intended to supplement the diet. The U.S. Food and Drug Administration has special labeling requirements for dietary supplements and treats them as foods, not drugs. Dietary supplements must meet all of the following conditions:

- It is a product (other than tobacco) intended to supplement the diet, which contains one or more of the following: vitamins, minerals, herbs or other botanicals, amino acids, or any combination of these ingredients.

- It is intended to be taken in tablet, capsule, powder, softgel, gelcap, or liquid form.

- It is not represented for use as a conventional food or as a sole item of a meal or diet.

- It is labeled as being a dietary supplement.

Source: National Center for Complementary and Alternative Medicine. (2009).

When considering using herbal remedies, it is important to consult a professional who is informed about the use of these remedies. Because a product is labeled "natural" does not mean it is safe or does not have harmful effects, or the product may not be recommended for a person's specific situation, such as pregnancy. It should be remembered that these remedies can act in the same way as many prescription or over-the-counter drugs and can cause side effects or interfere with the actions of other medications. As with any medication, herbal remedies are not without hazards, and their use must be properly monitored.

Case Review and Analysis

The patient was a 48-year-old woman who had rheumatic fever in the past that caused her to have an irregular heartbeat and damage to her mitral valve. She had a procedure done to repair the mitral valve and was placed on a blood thinning medication (known as an anticoagulant) to slow blood clotting after the procedure.

The patient was discharged home and began taking herbal preparations she had previously received from an herbalist. After a few weeks she became very ill with fevers, shortness of breath, and malaise. She was readmitted to the hospital, and it was determined that she was overanticoagulated and her blood was clotting much too slowly. She reported the herbs she had been taking, and it was suspected that she was suffering from an interaction between the herbs and the anticoagulant medication.

The physician researched the herbal preparations she had been taking and determined that one of the ingredients was danshen, which is an herbal remedy often used for heart-related complaints and is a component of many herbal preparations. It is known for its potency and its ability to potentiate the effect of the anticoagulant medication the patient was taking.

The herbal preparations were discontinued, and the patient was treated for the problems related to being overanticoagulated. She had a full recovery, although it took a number of weeks for her blood clotting to stabilize (Yee, Chan, & Sanderson, 1997).

Hydrotherapy   **Hydrotherapy** is another treatment used by naturopathic practitioners based on the therapeutic effects of water. It was initially used in Germany and was thought to assist in ridding the body of waste and toxins. Hot and cold baths, compresses, wraps, and showers were used. Modern treatment uses the same modalities.

Water is known for its impact on the body. Cold water makes surface blood vessels restrict and inhibits inflammation, thus it reduces swelling and sends more blood to the internal organs. Hot water dilates blood vessels and is associated with relaxation and increased blood flow that relaxes muscles and stiffness. Some therapies use both hot and cold water either alternately or at the same time on different areas of the body.

Mind–Body Interventions

Mind–body interventions encompass an array of practices aimed at the relationship between the person's mind and physical function. These practices vary from emphasis on spiritual relations to psychological and emotional well-being.

Spirituality

In the NCCAM study (2007b) when prayer was included as a CAM therapy, it was the most often identified CAM practice used by respondents. Walker (2005) noted that the study provided further information regarding the importance of prayer to the respondents as follows:

- Respondents who used prayer for health reasons: 45%
- Respondents who prayed for their own health: 43%
- Respondents who had others pray for them: 25%
- Respondents who participated in a prayer group for health reasons: approximately 10%

Spiritual practices regarding health are not just limited to prayer. Beliefs in the ability of the supernatural to heal surfaced in shamanism thousands of years ago. Recorded history regarding spiritual healing includes Egyptian belief in the healing power of a particular holy site and Greek and Roman temples built to the healing gods. These types of practices are not unknown today. Shamanic traditions continue today in Africa, Central and South America, and among some American Indian tribes. Christians continue to make pilgrimages to holy sites that are believed to heal, like Lourdes. Scientific research has determined that spiritual practices positively impact health and increases longevity (Freeman, 2004). However, there is disagreement as to the mechanism of these benefits.

Spirituality is often described as a belief in a higher power, something beyond the human experience. Closely related but distinctive is religion, which is the acceptance of the specific beliefs and practices of an organized religion. A person may be spiritual without being religious, or they may be both. Research has shown that both spirituality and religious beliefs have positive effects on health (Freeman, 2004).

The scientific explanation for the positive influence of spirituality on health stems from a number of theories. One is the placebo effect, a beneficial response to a treatment that can't be explained on the basis of the treatment provided. Often the placebo effect is a response to suggestion of positive impact and the patient's belief in the treatment. Another scientific explanation for the positive impact of spirituality involves neurochemical or other physiologic changes.

Conversely, the religious explanation for the positive influence of prayer is due to connection to God and divine intervention in healing. Prayer, a petition to or contemplation of God, is the vehicle by which that divine connection is made. Prayer can be further subdivided into petitionary or intercessional prayer. Petitionary prayer is on one's personal behalf, and intercessional prayer is on behalf of another. Some form of prayer for connection with the Almighty is utilized in almost all cultures and religious tenets. Although there is disagreement between the scientific and religious worlds regarding the exact action of spirituality's and prayer's impacts on health, there is accord that they are beneficial.

Meditation   **Meditation** refers to a group of mental techniques intended to provide relaxation and mental harmony, quiet one's mind, and increase awareness. It has been a practice in many cultures for thousands of years. Meditative practices are found in Christian, Jewish, Buddhist, Hindu, and Islamic religious traditions. Although meditation found its origins in religious practices, it is currently utilized for nonreligious purposes, such as improved emotional and physical health. Meditation is utilized to decrease stress and anxiety, decrease pain, improve mood, and positively impact heart disease and the symptoms of physical illness. Scientific research indicates that meditation decreases oxygen consumption, decreases heart and respiratory rates, and influences brain wave and hormone activity (Freeman, 2004).

Various techniques are used by different groups and religions. All techniques have some common factors, namely, use of a quiet location, assuming a comfortable position, focusing one's attention by concentrating on one's breath or a mantra (word or sound), and having an open attitude by not allowing distractions to disrupt focus. There are two common types of meditation practices: mindfulness meditation and transcendental meditation.

Mindfulness meditation originated in the Buddhist traditions. It is the concept of increasing awareness and acceptance of the present. During meditation one observes

TABLE 3.12   Relaxation Technique
1. Find a quiet place to sit.
2. Sit in a comfortable position with your feet on the floor, hands relaxed, and eyes closed.
3. Take three slow, deep breaths.
4. Begin to relax your muscles starting with your toes and progressing upward to your feet and ankles, then lower legs, then upper legs, etc., until you reach your face and head. Sometimes it is helpful to actually contract the muscles and then allow them to relax.
5. Breathe through your nose, concentrating on the breath going in and out. As you exhale, say a word in your mind like "calm" or "one."
6. Continue to concentrate on your breathing for 10 to 20 minutes. At the end of the time, sit quietly for a few minutes and gradually begin to arouse.
There is no failure in meditation. The benefit comes from maintaining a positive attitude and allowing relaxation to happen and ignoring distracting thoughts by gently pushing them from your mind when they appear.

thoughts and images in a nonjudgmental manner with the goal of learning to experience thoughts and feelings with greater balance and acceptance. This technique has been used to treat posttraumatic stress disorder, drug abuse, and chronic pain. It has also been found to increase cognitive function in the elderly.

Transcendental meditation found its origins in the Indian Vedic tradition. This practice is designed to allow the practitioner to experience ever finer levels of thought until the source of thought is experienced. A mantra is used to focus the mind, and the choice of mantra is vital to success. Transcendental meditation allows the mind to reach a quiet state and strives to create a state of relaxed alertness.

Transcendental meditation has been found to stimulate what is termed the "relaxation response," which is responsible for decreased blood pressure, muscular relaxation, decreased heart and respiratory rate, and a decrease in lactate levels, which are associated with anxiety. Research shows that a number of relaxation meditation techniques include four parts: a mental focus, passive attitude, decreased muscle tone, and a quiet environment (Freeman, 2004). One relaxation technique is described in Table 3.12.

Studies have shown that transcendental meditation has a positive affect on blood pressure, cardiovascular disease, and overall health. Mindfulness meditation is useful in the treatment of chronic pain and certain psychological disorders. The only situation where meditation is considered to be unsafe is in serious mental disorders like psychosis and schizophrenia. Otherwise, meditation has been determined to be a safe practice for almost everyone.

Hypnosis

Another mind–body intervention is hypnosis. As a technique, hypnosis has been present in many cultures for centuries. Its modern practice began with Franz Anton Mesmer in the eighteenth century, who studied and described "animal magnetism." It was from his efforts that the term "mesmerize" arose.

Hypnotism is a state of attentive, focused concentration associated with the suspension of some peripheral awareness. A person under hypnosis is induced to a state of deep relaxation and is susceptible to suggestions. Referencing a number of studies, Freeman (2004) described the major elements of a hypnotic state as:

- *Absorption*. The capacity to focus intently on a focal point or a theme
- *Relaxation*. Controlled alteration of the person's attention
- *Dissociation*. Capacity to compartmentalize different aspects of experience
- *Suggestibility*. Capacity for heightened responsiveness to instructions

Modern hypnosis is conducted by practitioners who are trained to induce a hypnotic state. It is believed that up to 90% of the population is capable of being hypnotized. Some people are more susceptible to hypnosis than others, as reflected in a classification system from low to high susceptibility. Although the great majority of the population is capable of being hypnotized, practitioners agree that people cannot be hypnotized against their will or without their consent. Although many theories exist regarding exactly how hypnosis works, no definitive determination has been made about its mechanism.

One of the earliest modern uses of hypnosis was for pain control during surgery prior to the advent of anesthesia. Hypnosis has been used very successfully for all types of pain control, and numerous studies have documented that effect. It is believed that hypnosis reduces anxiety, which contributes to the experience of pain, but, again, no definitive information exists on exactly how it works. Besides pain, hypnosis has been shown to be useful in the treatment of a number of conditions, especially those that are mediated or exacerbated by emotional overtones, such as irritable bowel syndrome, fibromyalgia, asthma, anticipatory or pregnancy-induced nausea, phobias, addictive behaviors, and anxiety.

Energy Therapies

Energy therapies focus on energy fields that are believed to have healing properties. We have discussed some of these already, such as qi in traditional Chinese medicine and the doshas in ayurvedic medicine. In these varied practices it is believed that vital energy exists and flows both outside and within the human body. Therapists in these modalities work with this energy, commonly called biofield, to either restore its flow or utilize it to restore health.

There are two classifications of energy therapy. The first, **veritable energy**, refers to the use of energy fields that can be physically experienced and/or measured. These include modalities such as magnet, sound, or light. **Putative energy** employs biofields for therapeutic effect and has not been measurable to current methods. These therapies include healing touch, therapeutic touch, and reiki. Kirlian photography, often called aura imaging, has been theorized to capture this energy; however, it is not apparent just what Kirlian photography actually represents. In the following sections, we will discuss a few of these modalities that have not been addressed elsewhere in this chapter.

Magnet Therapy

Magnet therapy involves the use of electromagnetic energy that is always present. The therapy often involves the application of static magnets over areas of pain. This is often accomplished by bracelets for arthritis or magnetic pads. Practitioners believe that this application impacts the body's natural magnetic field, thereby decreasing pain. No research on the efficacy of these treatments is available.

Pulsating electromagnetic therapy has been used by medical practitioners for many years. It is prescribed to treat nonunion fractures, and it is thought to improve arthritis and multiple sclerosis.

Healing (Laying on of Hands)

Healing, often called laying on of hands, has been characterized as both an energy and spiritual healing practice. In either event, it is an ancient practice that has modern application in many cultures and beliefs. In this therapy, a healer, known as a "worker," channels healing energy to the patient to stimulate natural healing. This can occur either in person or at a distance. Healing and laying on of hands is common to many cultures. Edgar Cayce was a well-known American practitioner of healing. He was reported to place himself into a trance and heal others who requested his

TABLE 3.13   Types of Healing Practices
Aura healing. A healer sees energy fields around a person, which indicate his or her state of health, then the healer touches the person and visualizes healing auras.
Spiritual healing. A healer connects with his or her internal energy, which connects the healer to a greater energy, and channels the energy to the patient.
Faith healing. A healer channels energy, and the patient must believe in the healer's ability or the power of the deity to heal.
Spiritualist healing. A healer establishes a connection to an entity in the spirit world that heals through the healer.

intercession either in person or at a distance. Today many people are proponents of what is termed "new age" philosophies, which have theories involving the existence of energy fields that have beneficial properties (see Table 3.13).

CHAPTER SUMMARY

This chapter has discussed complementary and alternative health care modalities that are associated with a number of cultures. Many are ancient practices that continue to exist despite the efforts of modern Western medicine to marginalize them. Although research on the efficacy of many of these practices is scarce, the prevalence of use indicates a need for further investigation of the risks and benefits of these practices.

REVIEW

1. Describe the advantages and disadvantages of three of the CAM modalities discussed in this chapter.
2. Discuss how meditation could be used in Western health care practice.
3. Describe the relationship between ethnic cultures and CAM in the United States.
4. Discuss how to inquire about CAM modalities used by patients during an initial interview.

GLOSSARY TERMS

complementary medicine
integrative medicine
doshas
prakriti
yoga
homeopathy
Law of Similars (Principle of Similars)
Principle of Infinitesimal Dose
Principle of Specificity of the Individual
qi
five elements
yin and yang
meridians
acupuncture

Qigong
t'ai chi ch'uan
chiropractic
naturopathy
hydrotherapy
spirituality
meditation
mindfulness meditation
transcendental meditation
veritable energy
putative energy
magnet therapy
healing

REFERENCES

American Medical Association. (1997). Report 13 of Council on Scientific Affairs. Retrieved March 26, 2008, from http://www.ama-assn.org/ama/pub/category/13611.html

Chen, J., & Zhang, H. (1997). *Treatment of neurodegenerative disorders. Alzheimers, stroke and Parkinson's disease.* Retrieved April 25, 2008, from http://acupuncture.com/conditions/alzandparkinson.htm

Chisolm, S. (2007). *The health professions: Trends and opportunities in US health care.* Sudbury, MA: Jones and Bartlett.

Eisenberg, D. M., Kessler, R.C., Foster, C., Norloci, F.E., Calkins, D.R and Delbanco, T.L. (1993, January 28). Unconventional medicine in the United States: Prevalence, costs and patterns of use. *The New England Journal of Medicine, 328,* 246–252.

Freeman, L. (2004). *Complementary and alternative medicine: A research-based approach* (2nd ed). St. Louis, MO: Mosby.

Hufford, D. J. (1988). Contemporary folk medicine. In N. Gevitz (Ed.), *Other healers: Unorthodox medicine in the United States.* Baltimore: Johns Hopkins University Press.

Hufford, D. J. (1997). Folk medicine and health culture in contemporary society. *Primary Care, 24,* 723–741.

Kistin, S., & Newman, A. (2007, May–June). Induction of labor with homeopathy: A case report. *Journal of Midwifery & Women's Health, 52*(3), 303–307. Retrieved April 25, 2008, from http://www.sciencedirect.com/science?_ob=ArticleListURL&_method=list&_ArticleListID =880293199&_sort=d&view=c&_acct=C000050221&_version=1&_urlVersion=0&_userid= 10&md5=357920d842ed02d9d59f2af944e52d36

National Center for Complementary and Alternative Medicine. (2002). *Office of Special Populations strategic plan to address racial and ethnic health disparities.* Retrieved April 28, 2008, from http://nccam.nih.gov/about/plans/healthdisparities

National Center for Complementary and Alternative Medicine. (2007a). *Backgrounder: An introduction to naturopathy.* Retrieved April 24, 2008, from http://www.nccam.nih.gov/health/naturopathy

National Center for Complementary and Alternative Medicine. (2007b). *The use of CAM in the United States.* Retrieved April 24, 2008, from http://www.nccam.nih.gov

National Center for Complementary and Alternative Medicine. (2009). *Using dietary supplements wisely.* Retrieved January 25, 2009, from http://nccam.nih.gov/health/supplements/wiseuse.htm

National Institutes of Health. (1998). National Institutes of Health consensus conference: Acupuncture. *Journal of the American Medical Association, 280,* 1518.

Pachter, L. M. (1994, March 2). Culture and clinical care. *Journal of the American Medical Association, 271*(9), 127–131.

Peters, D., & Woodham, A. (2000). *Encyclopedia of natural healing.* New York: Dorling Kindersley.

Trends in alternative medicine use in the United States, 1990–1997. Results of a follow-up national survey. (1998). *Journal of the American Medical Association, 280,* 1569–1575.

Walker, D. (2005). *Prayer and spirituality in health: Ancient practices, modern science.* Retrieved April 26, 2008, from http://nccam.nih.gov/news/newsletter/2005_winter/prayer.htm

What is traditional Chinese medicine? (2008). Retrieved April 12, 2008, from http://www.tcmworld.org/what_is_tcm/

White House Commission on Complementary and Alternative Medicine Policy. (2002). *Chapter 10: Recommendations and actions.* Retrieved March 27, 2008, from http://www.whccamp.hhs.gov/fr10.html

Yee, C., Chan, J., & Sanderson, J. (1997). Chinese herbs and warfarin potentiation by "Danshen." *Journal of Internal Medicine, 241,* 337–338.

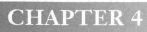

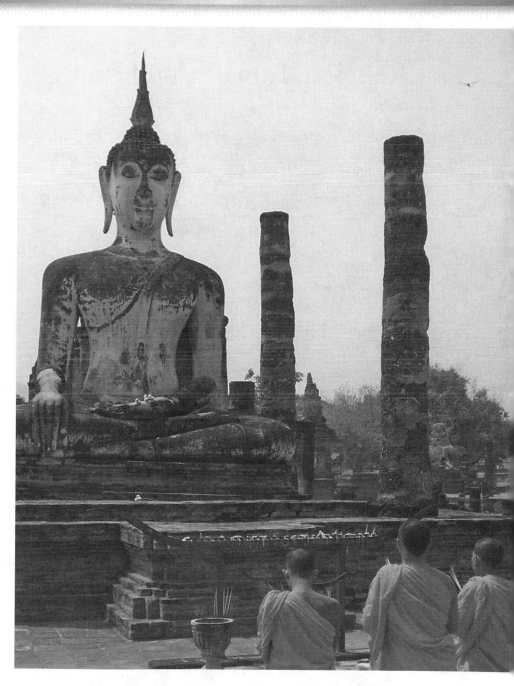

CHAPTER 4

Religion, Rituals, and Health

Nothing is so conducive to good health as the regularity of life without haste and without worry which the rational practice of religion brings in its train.

—James J. Walsh

To prevent disease or to cure it, the power of truth, of divine Spirit, must break down the dream of the material senses.

—Mary Baker Eddy

KEY CONCEPTS

- Rituals
- Euthanasia
- Karma
- Ahimsa
- Living will

- Religion and health behaviors
- Religion and health outcomes
- Religion and medical decisions
- Shrines
- Animal sacrifice

CHAPTER OBJECTIVES

1. Describe the role that religion plays in the lives of Americans.
2. Explain how religion impacts health behaviors and the rationale behind these choices.
3. Describe ways that religion can have positive and negative effects on physical and mental health.
4. Explain how religion impacts medical decisions and the rationale behind these choices.
5. Describe religious differences in birthing and death rituals.

Have you ever prayed for a loved one or yourself when ill? If so, you fall within the majority of Americans. A national survey conducted by the federal government and published in 2004 found that 43% of Americans prayed for their own health, and 24% reported that other people were praying for their health (Dember, 2005). Seventy-nine percent of adults in the United States believe that spiritual faith can help people recover from illness, injury, or disease (McNicol, 1996).

Religion has a significant role in the United States and in the health of Americans. It has an impact on their social lives and health behaviors and, hence, their physical and mental well-being. Religion is a belief in and respect for a supernatural power or powers, which is regarded as creator and governor of the universe, and a personal or institutionalized system grounded in such belief and worship. Religion is divergent from spirituality, although there is overlap, because many people find spirituality in the form of religion. For many people spirituality means the life force within each one of us, and it refers to an individual's attempt to find meaning and purpose in life. Most of the research has focused on health and religion, as opposed to health and spirituality, primarily because religion is associated with behaviors that can be quantified (e.g., how often one prays or attends a place of worship), it can be categorized by type of religion, and there is more agreement about its meaning.

Religion and **rituals** overlap, but not all rituals are related to religion. Therefore, we discuss the two items separately in this chapter, but the reader should be aware that some rituals are related to religious practices, such as baptism, and other rituals are not tied to religion, such as the burning of ghost money when a person dies (a tradition in China). In the first part of the chapter we discuss religion and move into rituals, but the separation is not definitive. The opening topic is religion in America, and then we move into the subject of how religion impacts health. The second section of the chapter focuses on rituals related to health. Because these topics have such a vast scope, only the more common religious practices within the United States are covered.

RELIGION IN THE UNITED STATES

In 1999, about 95% of the population in the United States reported a belief in God or a higher power (Miller & Thoresen, 2003). In 2005, 57% of Americans said religion is very important in their lives, and another 28% said it is fairly important (Winseman, 2005). Church and synagogue attendance also reflects the importance of religion. Researchers have asked Americans how often they attend their place of worship, and since it was instituted in 1992, the question has produced consistent results (Saad, 2003). The survey results for 2003 are presented in Table 4.1. The most common self-identified religions in the United States can be found in Table 4.2.

Religion and ethnicity are linked, but it is important to not assume a person's religion based on his or her ethnicity. For example, in a 2002 study, 57% of people who identified themselves as Hispanic stated that they identified with the Catholic religion,

TABLE 4.1	Frequency of Church and Synagogue Attendance

How often do you attend church or synagogue: at least once a week, almost every week, about once a month, seldom, or never?

Once a Week	Almost Every Week	About Once a Month	Seldom	Never	No Opinion
31%	14%	14%	30%	10%	1%

Source: Saad, L. (2003).

which leaves 43% identifying with other religions or no religion (Kosmin, Mayer, & Keysar, 2001). It also is not safe to assume that a person strictly adheres to the practices of a religion. Adherence to religious practices exists on a continuum, with some strictly adhering to all of the guidelines and some having looser ties.

TABLE 4.2	Top 10 Religions in the United States, 2001

Religion	Percentage of United States Population in 2000	2001 Estimated Adult Population
1. Christianity	76.5%	159,030,000
2. Nonreligious/secular	13.2%	27,539,000
3. Judaism	1.3%	2,831,000
4. Islam	0.5%	1,104,000
5. Buddhism	0.5%	1,082,000
6. Agnostic	0.5%	991,000
7. Atheist	0.4%	902,000
8. Hinduism	0.4%	766,000
9. Unitarian Universalist	0.3%	629,000
10. Wiccan/pagan/druid	0.1%	307,000

Source: Adapted from Adherents.com.

RELIGION AND HEALTH BEHAVIORS

Lifestyle represents the single most prominent influence over our health today. It has been estimated that about 40% of the causes of early death are related to health behavioral patterns (Cottrell, Girvan, & McKenzie, 2006). As a result, the United States is seeing the need for more emphasis on prevention and behavior modification. People with religious ties have been shown to engage in healthier behavioral patterns, and these positive lifestyle choices lead to improved health and longer lives. The question is, Why do people with stronger religious ties have better health? The answer includes several possible factors, such as proscribed behaviors, social relationships, and improved coping mechanisms.

Health behaviors encouraged or proscribed by particular religions are one possible explanation for how religion can positively affect health. Some religions prohibit tobacco, alcohol, caffeine, and premarital sex, and some encourage vegetarianism, for example.

Social relationships are another potential explanatory factor for the connection between religion and improved health indicators. Social ties can provide both support and a sense of connectedness. Many churches and temples offer activities such as workshops, health fairs, and crafts fairs, which provide social interactions. Social relationships also are tied to coping mechanisms, because they provide support in multiple forms during times of stress. For example, they may provide financial support to people who have incurred a tragedy, such as a disability, loss of job, and house fire. Religious organizations also conduct fundraisers for families who have had a death or personal tragedy in the family. Churches and temples assist elders by providing transportation or taking communion or food to the homebound. Friendships and a sense of purpose also are methods of support.

Now that we have explained some possible reasons for religion impacting health, we are going to focus on specific behaviors.

Dietary Practices

Dietary practices have a long history of being incorporated into religions around the world. Some religions prohibit followers from consuming certain foods and drinks all of the time or on certain holy days; require or encourage specific dietary and food preparation practices and/or fasting (going without food and/or drink for a specified time); or prohibit eating certain foods at the same meal, such as dairy and meat products. Other religions require certain methods of food preparation and have special rules about the use of pans, plates, utensils, and how the food is to be cooked. Foods and drinks also may be a part of religious celebrations or rituals.

The restriction of certain foods and beverages may have a positive impact on the health of those engaged in such practices. For example, restricting consumption of animal products, such as beef and pork or all animal products, may reduce the risk of health problems. Many religions, such as Hinduism and Buddhism, practice or promote vegetarianism, and these diets have been shown to have several health effects, such as the reduction of heart disease, cancer, obesity, and stroke. Some religions help prevent obesity through beliefs that gluttony is a sin, only take what you need, and the need for self-discipline. Table 4.3 presents a list of religions, their related dietary practices and restrictions, and the rationale behind them.

Religions may incorporate some element of fasting into their practices. In many religions, the general purpose for fasting is to become closer to God, show respect for the body (temple) that is a gift from God, understand and appreciate the suffering that the poor experience, acquire the discipline required to resist temptation, atone for sinful acts, and/or cleanse evil from within the body (Advameg Inc., 2008). Fasting may be recommended for specific times of the day; for a specified number of hours; on designated days of the week, month, or year; or on holy days.

During times of fasting, most but not all religions permit the consumption of water. Water restriction can lead to a risk of dehydration. Some fasters may not take their medication during the fast, which may put their health at risk. Prolonged fasting and/or restrictions from water and/or medications may pose health risks for some followers. Because of these health risks, certain groups are often excused from fasting. These groups include people with chronic diseases, frail elderly, pregnant and lactating women, people who engage in strenuous labor, young children, and malnutritioned individuals.

Use of Stimulants and Depressants

In addition to foods, some religions prohibit or restrict the use of stimulants. A stimulant is a product (including medications), food, or drink that stimulates the nervous system and alters the recipient's physiology. Stimulants include substances that contain alcohol or caffeine, including tea, coffee, chocolate, and energy drinks. Caffeine is prohibited or restricted by many religions because of its addictive properties. Many religions also restrict spices and certain condiments, such as pepper, pickles, or foods with preservatives, because they are believed to be harmful by nature and flavor the natural taste and effect of foods (Advameg Inc., 2008).

Some religions prohibit the use of stimulants and depressants, but others use them during ceremonies. For example, Roman Catholics, Eastern Orthodox Christians, and certain Protestant denominations use wine as a sacramental product to represent

TABLE 4.3   Religions and Their Related Food and Substance Practices and Restrictions and Related Rationales

Type of Religion	Practice or Restriction	Rationale
Buddhism	• Vegetarian diet is desirable. • All foods in moderation.	• Natural foods of the earth are considered to be the most pure. • Encourage nonviolence (some Buddhists believe that the cause of human aggression is violence against animals).
Eastern Orthodox Christianity	• Restrictions on meat and fish. • Fasting selectively. • The ritual of the transubstantiation (changing) of bread and wine into the body and blood of Jesus Christ is believed to occur at communion.	• Observance of Holy Days includes fasting and restrictions to increase spiritual progress.
Hinduism	• Beef is forbidden. • Vegetarian diet is advocated. • Alcohol is avoided. • Numerous fasting days—may depend on the person's caste (or social standing) and the occasion.	• Cows are sacred and cannot be eaten, but the products of the "sacred" cow are pure and desirable. • Fasting promotes spiritual growth.
Islam	• Pork and certain birds are forbidden. • Alcohol is prohibited. • Coffee, tea, and stimulants are avoided. • Fasting from all food and drink during specific periods.	• Eating is for good health. • Failure to eat correctly minimizes spiritual awareness. • Fasting has a cleansing effect of evil elements.
Judaism	• Consumption of certain foods, including dairy products and fish, is subject to restrictions; for example, pork and shellfish are prohibited, and so is consuming meat and dairy at the same meal. • Leavened food is restricted. • Foods must be prepared in the right way to be kosher; for example, animals that provide meat must be slaughtered correctly. • Fasting is practiced.	• Land animals that do not have cloven hooves and that do not chew their cud are forbidden as unclean (e.g., hare, pig, camel). • The kosher process is based upon the Torah. • The Passover commemorates the birth of the Jewish nation, and the food eaten helps to tell the story of the exodus; for example, bitter herbs recall the suffering of the Israelites under Egyptian rule.

(Continues)

TABLE 4.3	**Religions and Their Related Food and Substance Practices and Restrictions and Related Rationales** (*Continued*)	
Mormonism	• Caffeinated and alcoholic beverages are forbidden. • All foods should be consumed in moderation. • Fasting is practiced.	• Caffeine is addictive and leads to poor physical and emotional health. • Fasting is the discipline of self-control and honoring God.
Protestantism	• Few restrictions of food or fasting observations. • Moderation in eating, drinking, and exercise is promoted.	• God made all animal and natural products for humans' enjoyment. • Gluttony and drunkenness are sins to be controlled.
Rastafarianism	• Meat and fish are restricted. • Vegetarian diets only, with salts, preservatives, and condiments prohibited. • Herbal drinks are permitted; alcohol, coffee, and soft drinks are prohibited. • Marijuana used extensively for religious and medicinal purposes.	• Pigs and shellfish are unclean, they are viewed as scavengers. • Foods grown with chemicals are unnatural and prohibited. • Biblical texts support the use of herbs (marijuana and other herbs).
Roman Catholicism	• Meat is restricted on certain days. • Fasting is practiced. • The ritual of the transubstantiation (changing) of bread and wine into the body and blood of Jesus Christ is believed to occur at communion. • Fast for at least one hour prior to communion.	• Restrictions are consistent with specified days of the church year.
Seventh-day Adventist	• Expects adherence to kosher laws. • Pork is prohibited, and meat and fish is avoided. • Recommends vegetarian diet. • Alcohol and illegal drugs are discouraged. • Avoid caffeinated beverages.	• Diet is related to honoring and glorifying God.

Source: Adapted from Advameg Inc. (2008).

the blood of Christ in communion services (Advameg Inc., 2008). Rastafarians introduced marijuana into their religious rites because they consider it to be the "weed
of wisdom", and they believe it contains healing ingredients (Advameg Inc., 2008).
American Indians use tobacco and the hallucinogenic peyote as part of their spiritual
ceremonies.

Other Health Behaviors

Research in adults and adolescents also has suggested a strong association between
religious involvement and behaviors for which there is no specific religious teaching.
For example, a national study of high school seniors in the United States found that
religious students were more likely than their nonreligious peers to wear seatbelts, eat
breakfast, eat fruit and green vegetables, get regular exercise, and sleep at least
seven hours a night (Wallace & Forman, 1998 as cited in Williams & Sternthal, 2007).
This research indicates that religious participation could have a general effect on
lifestyle and not only a direct effect from the rules of the religion. Strawbridge and
colleagues (2001) reviewed 28 years of data about people who lived in Alameda County,
California, and they found that those who attended weekly services were more likely
to quit poor health behaviors or adopt healthier behaviors (Hamilton, n.d.). In the
same study, they found that weekly attendance also was associated with less depression and higher marital stability (Hamilton, n.d.).

RELIGION AND HEALTH OUTCOMES

As a result of religion's effects on health behaviors, it is not surprising that religion
has been shown to have positive effects on both physical and mental health. Over the
last several decades, a notable body of empirical evidence has emerged that examines
the relationship between religion or religious practices and a host of outcomes. Most
of the outcomes have been positive, but it is important to note that religion does not
always have favorable effects on health. Next we briefly describe the potential negative effects and then move into a detailed description of the positive effects.

Religion can negatively impact health, because it has sometimes been used to justify hatred, aggression, and prejudice (Lee & Newberg, 2005). Religion can be judg-
mental, alienating, and exclusive. It also may cause the development of stressful social
relations, and failure to conform to community norms may evoke open criticism by
other congregation members or clergy. Feelings of religious guilt and the failure
to meet religious expectations or cope with religious fears can contribute to illness

(Trenholm, Trent, & Compton, 1998). Parents' reliance on faith healing instead of appropriate medical care has led to negative outcomes and death for many children (Asser & Swan, 1998). Also, people may not participate in healthy behaviors because they believe that their health is in God's hands, so their behaviors will not change God's plan. This is referred to as a fatalistic attitude.

In terms of positive effects, there is an abundant amount of research that supports religion's constructive effect on health outcomes. A meta-analysis of 49 studies regarding religious coping found that positive forms of religious coping were related to lower levels of depression, anxiety, and distress, and negative forms of religious coping were associated with poorer psychological adjustment (Ano & Vasconcelles, 2005 as cited in Williams & Sternthal, 2007). Studies of adolescent behavior have found that higher levels of religious involvement are inversely related to alcohol and drug use, smoking, sexual activity, depressive symptoms, and suicide risk (Williams & Sternthal, 2007). These studies also found that spirituality and religion are positively related to immune system function. A review of 35 studies of the relationship between religion and health-related physiological processes found that both Judeo–Christian and Eastern religious practices were associated with reduced blood pressure and improved immune function; moreover, Zen, yoga, and meditation practices correlated with lower levels of stress hormones and cholesterol and better overall health outcomes in clinical patient populations (Seeman, Dubin, & Seeman, 2003 as cited in Williams & Sternthal, 2007).

Literature Review

In an important publication, Duke University researchers Harold Koenig and colleagues Michael McCullough and David Larson (2000) have systematically reviewed much of the research on religion and health. This lengthy and detailed review of hundreds of studies focuses on scholarship from refereed journals. In sum, the review demonstrates that the majority of published research is consistent with the notion that religious practices or religious involvement are associated with beneficial outcomes in mental and physical health (Johnson, Tompkins, & Webb, 2008). These outcome categories include hypertension, mortality, depression, alcohol use or abuse, drug use or abuse, and suicide. Reviews of additional social science research also confirm that religious commitment and involvement in religious practices are significantly linked to reductions not only in delinquency among youth and adolescent populations but also in criminality among adult populations. The following is a summary of the findings from an extensive literature review conducted by Johnson, Tompkins, and Webb (2008). This information is reprinted with permission from the Baylor Institute for Studies of Religion.

Hypertension

Hypertension, which afflicts 50 million Americans, is defined as a sustained or chronic elevation in blood pressure. It is the most common of cardiovascular disorders and affects about 20% of the adult population. Though there is strong evidence that pharmacologic treatment can lower blood pressure, there remains concern about the adverse side effects of such treatments. For this reason, social epidemiologists are interested in the effects of socioenvironmental determinants of blood pressure. Among the factors shown to correlate with hypertension is religion. In recent years, epidemiological studies have found that individuals who report higher levels of religious activities tend to have lower blood pressure. Johnson, Tompkins, and Webb's (2008) review of the research indicates that 76% of the studies found that religious activities or involvement tend to be linked with reduced levels of hypertension (see Table 4.4).

Mortality

A substantial body of research reveals an association between intensity of participation in religious activities and greater longevity. Studies reviewed for the report done by Johnson, Tompkins, and Webb (2008) examined the association between degree of religious involvement and survival (see Table 4.4). Involvement in a religious community is consistently related to lower mortality and longer life spans. Johnson, Tompkins, and Webb's (2008) review of this literature revealed that 75% of these published studies conclude that higher levels of religious involvement have a sizable

TABLE 4.4   Results of Religion and Health Outcomes Studies

	Hypertension	Mortality	Depression	Suicide	Sexual Behavior	Alcohol Use	Drug Use	Delinquency
Beneficial outcomes	76%	76%	67%	87%	97%	88%	91%	76%
NA/mixed outcomes	20%	21%	27%	14%	3%	10%	8%	17%
Harmful outcomes	4%	3%	7%	0%	0%	3%	2%	2%

The data represents the percentage of published studies that were reviewed.
Source: Johnson, B. R., Tompkins, R. B., and Webb, D. (2008). Reprinted with permission from The Baylor Institutes for Studies of Religion.

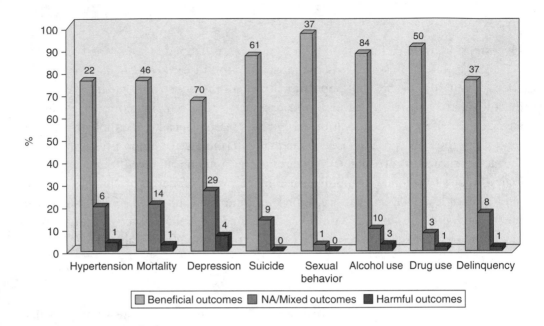

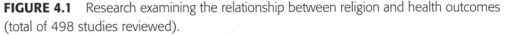

FIGURE 4.1   Research examining the relationship between religion and health outcomes (total of 498 studies reviewed).
Source: Johnson, B. R., Tompkins, R. B., and Webb, D. (2008). Reprinted with permission from The Baylor Institutes for Studies of Religion.

and consistent relationship with greater longevity (see Figure 4.1). This association was found to be independent of the effect of variables such as age, sex, race, education, and health. In a separate analysis, McCullough and colleagues conducted a meta-analytic review that incorporated data from more than 125,000 persons and similarly concluded that religious involvement had a significant and substantial association with increased length of life (McCullough, Hoyt, Larson, Koenig, & Thoresen, 2000 as cited in Johnson, Tompkins, and Webb, 2008). In fact, longitudinal research in a variety of different cohorts also has documented that frequent religious attendance is associated with a significant reduction in the risk of dying during study follow-up periods ranging from 5 to 28 years.

Depression

Depression is the most common of all mental disorders, and approximately 330 million people around the world suffer from it. People with depression also are at increased risk for use of hospital and medical services and for early death from physical causes. Over 100 studies that examined the religion–depression relationship were reviewed by Johnson, Tompkins, and Webb (2008), and they found that religious involvement tends to be associated with less depression in 68% of these articles (see Figure 4.1). People who are frequently involved in religious activities and who highly value their religious faith are at reduced risk for depression. Religious involvement seems to play an important role in helping people cope with the effects of stressful life circumstances. Prospective cohort studies and quasi-experimental and experimental research all suggest that religious or spiritual activities may lead to a reduction in depressive symptoms. These findings have been replicated across a number of large, well-designed studies and are consistent with much of the cross-sectional and prospective cohort research that has found less depression among more religious people (see Table 4.4).

Suicide

Suicide now ranks as the ninth leading cause of death in the United States. This is particularly alarming when one considers that suicides tend to be underestimated due to the fact that many of these deaths are coded as accidental. A substantial body of literature documents that religious involvement (e.g., measured by frequency of religious attendance, frequency of prayer, and degree of religious salience) is associated with less suicide, suicidal behavior, and suicidal ideation, as well as less tolerant attitudes toward suicide across a variety of samples from many nations. This consistent inverse association is found in studies using both group and individual-level data. In total, 87% of the studies reviewed on suicide found these beneficial outcomes (see Figure 4.1).

Promiscuous Sexual Behaviors

Out-of-wedlock pregnancy, often a result of sexual activity among adolescents, is largely responsible for the nearly 25% of children aged 6 years or younger who are below the federal poverty line. According to the Centers for Disease Control, unmarried motherhood is also associated with significantly higher infant mortality rates. Further, sexual promiscuity significantly increases the risk of contracting sexually transmitted diseases. Studies in the Johnson, Tompkins, and Webb (2008) review generally show that those who are religious are less likely to engage in premarital sex or extramarital affairs or to have multiple sexual partners (see Table 4.4). In fact, approximately 97% of the studies that were reviewed reported significant correlations between increased religious involvement and lower likelihood of promiscuous sexual behaviors (see Figure 4.1). None of the studies found that increased religious participation or commitment was linked to increases in promiscuous behavior.

Drug and Alcohol Use

The abuse of alcohol and illicit drugs ranks among the leading health and social concerns in the United States today. According to the National Institute on Drug Abuse, approximately 111 million persons in the United States are current alcohol users. About 32 million of these people engage in binge drinking, and 11 million Americans are heavy drinkers. Additionally, some 14 million Americans are current users of illicit drugs. Both chronic alcohol consumption and abuse of drugs are associated with increased risks of morbidity and mortality. Johnson, Tompkins, and Webb (2008) reviewed over 150 studies that examined the relationship between religiosity and drug use ($n = 54$) or alcohol use ($n = 97$) and abuse. The vast majority of these studies demonstrate that participation in religious activities is associated with less of a tendency to use or abuse drugs (87%) or alcohol (94%). These findings are consistent regardless of the population under study (i.e., children, adolescents, and adult populations) or whether the research was conducted prospectively or retrospectively (see Table 4.4). The greater a person's religious involvement, the less likely he or she will be to initiate alcohol or drug use or have problems with these substances if they are used (see Table 4.4). Only four of the studies that were reviewed reported a positive correlation between religious involvement and increased alcohol or drug use. Interestingly, these four tended to be some of the weaker studies with regard to methodological design and statistical analyses.

Delinquency

There is growing evidence that religious commitment and involvement helps protect youth from delinquent behavior and deviant activities. Recent evidence suggests that such effects persist even if there is not a strong prevailing social control against delinquent behavior in the surrounding community. There is mounting evidence that religious involvement may lower the risks of a broad range of delinquent behaviors, including both minor and serious forms of criminal behavior. There is also evidence that religious involvement has a cumulative effect throughout adolescence and thus may significantly lessen the risk of later adult criminality. Additionally, there is growing evidence that religion can be used as a tool to help prevent high-risk urban youths from engaging in delinquent behavior. Religious involvement may help adolescents learn prosocial behavior that emphasizes concern for other people's welfare. Such prosocial skills may give adolescents a greater sense of empathy toward others, which makes them less likely to commit acts that harm others. Similarly, when individuals become involved in deviant behavior, it is possible that participation in specific kinds of religious activities can help steer them back to a course of less deviant behavior and, more important, away from potential career criminal paths.

Research on adult samples is less common but tends to represent the same general pattern—that religion reduces criminal activity by adults. An important study by T. David Evans and colleagues found that religion, indicated by religious activities, reduced the likelihood of adult criminality as measured by a broad range of criminal acts (Johnson, Tompkins, and Webb, 2008). The relationship persisted even after secular controls were added to the model. Further, the finding did not depend on social or religious contexts. A small but growing body of literature focuses on the links between religion and family violence. Several recent studies found that regular religious attendance is inversely related to abuse among both men and women. As can be seen in Figure 4.1, 78% of these studies report reductions in delinquency and criminal acts to be associated with higher levels of religious activity and involvements.

Summary

In sum, Johnson, Tompkins, and Webb's (2008) review of the research on religious practices and health outcomes indicates that, in general, higher levels of religious involvement are associated with reduced hypertension, longer survival, less depression, lower level of drug and alcohol use and abuse, less promiscuous sexual behaviors, reduced likelihood of suicide, lower rates of delinquency among youth, and reduced criminal activity among adults. As can be seen in Figure 4.1, this substantial body of empirical evidence demonstrates a very clear picture: People who are most involved in religious activities tend to fare better with respect to important and yet diverse outcome factors. Thus, aided by appropriate documentation, religiosity is now beginning to be acknowledged as a key protective factor, reducing the deleterious effects of a number of harmful outcomes.

Well-Being

Well-being has been referred to as the positive side of mental health. Symptoms for well-being include happiness, joy, satisfaction, fulfillment, pleasure, contentment, and other indicators of a life that is full and complete (Koenig, H. G., McCullough, M. & Larson, D. B., 2001, as cited in Johnson, Tompkins, and Webb, 2008). Many studies have examined the relationship between religion and the promotion of beneficial outcomes (see Table 4.5). Many of these studies tend to be cross-sectional in design, but a significant number are important prospective cohort studies. As reported in Figure 4.2, Johnson, Tompkins, and Webb (2008) found that the vast majority of these

TABLE 4.5	Results of Religion and Well-Being Outcomes Studies			
	Well-Being	**Hope**	**Self Esteem**	**Educational Attainment**
Beneficial outcomes	81%	81%	68%	87%
NA/mixed outcomes	16%	16%	30%	10%
Harmful outcomes	4%	0%	5%	5%

The data represents the percentage of published studies that were reviewed.
Source: Johnson, B. R., Tompkins, R. B., and Webb, D. (2008). Reprinted with permission from The Baylor Institutes for Studies of Religion.

studies, some 81% of the 99 studies reviewed, reported some positive association between religious involvement and greater happiness, life satisfaction, morale, positive affect, or some other measure of well-being. The vast number of studies on religion and well-being have included younger and older populations as well as African Americans and Caucasians from various denominational affiliations. Only one study

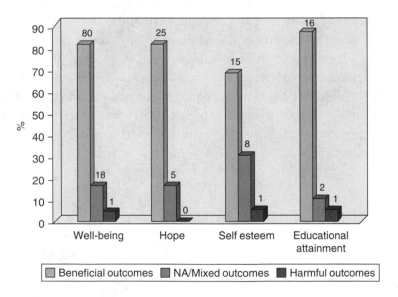

FIGURE 4.2   Research examining the relationship between religion and well-being outcomes (total of 171 studies reviewed). *Source:* Johnson, B. R., Tompkins, R. B., and Webb, D. (2008). Reprinted with permission from The Baylor Institutes for Studies of Religion.

found a negative correlation between religiosity and well-being, and this study was conducted in a small, nonrandom sample of college students.

Hope, Purpose, and Meaning in Life

Many religious traditions and beliefs have long promoted positive thinking and an optimistic outlook on life. Not surprisingly, researchers have examined the role religion may or may not play in instilling hope and meaning or a sense of purpose in life for adherents. Researchers have found, on the whole, a positive relationship between measures of religiosity and hope in varied clinical and nonclinical settings. In total, 25 of the 30 studies reviewed (83%) document that increases in religious involvement or commitment are associated with having hope or a sense of purpose or meaning in life (see Figure 4.2). Similarly, studies show that increasing religiousness also is associated with optimism as well as larger support networks, more social contacts, and greater satisfaction with support. In fact, 19 out of the 23 studies reviewed by Johnson, Tompkins, and Webb (2008) conclude that increases in religious involvement and commitment are associated with increased social support (see Table 4.5).

Self-Esteem

Most people would agree that contemporary American culture places too much significance on physical appearance and the idea that one's esteem is bolstered by their looks. Conversely, a common theme of various religious teachings is that physical appearance, for example, should not be the basis of self-esteem. Religion provides a basis for self-esteem that is not dependent upon individual accomplishments, relationships with others (e.g., who you know), or talent. In other words, a person's self-esteem is rooted in the individual's religious faith as well as the faith community as a whole. Of the studies Johnson, Tompkins, and Webb (2008) reviewed, 65% conclude that religious commitment and activities are related to increases in self-esteem (see Figure 4.2).

Educational Attainment

The literature on the role of religious practices or religiosity on educational attainment represents a relatively recent development in the research literature. In the last decade or so, a number of researchers have sought to determine if religion hampers or enhances educational attainment. Even though the development of a body of evidence is just beginning to emerge, some 84% of the studies reviewed concluded that religiosity or religious activities are positively correlated with improved educational attainment (see Figure 4.2).

Summary

To summarize, a review of the research on religious practices and various measures of well-being reveals that, in general, higher levels of religious involvement are associated with increased levels of well-being, hope, purpose, meaning in life, and educational attainment. As can be seen in Figure 4.2, this substantial body of evidence shows quite clearly that those who are most involved in religious activities tend to be better off on critical indicators of well-being. Just as the studies reviewed earlier (see Table 4.4 and Figure 4.1) document that religious commitment is a protective factor that buffers individuals from various harmful outcomes (e.g., hypertension, depression, suicide, delinquency, etc.), there is mounting empirical evidence to suggest that religious commitment is also a source for promoting or enhancing beneficial outcomes (e.g., well-being, purpose or meaning in life). This review of a large number of diverse studies leaves one with the observation that, in general, the effect of religion on physical and mental health outcomes is remarkably positive. These findings have led some religious health care practitioners to conclude that further collaboration between religious organizations and health services may be desirable. In an extensive literature review conducted by Johnson, Tompkins, and Webb (2008), Peterson (1983) noted that "we are convinced that a church with a vigorous life of worship, education, and personal support together with the promotion of wellness has more of an impact on the health of a community than an addition to the hospital or another doctor in town. Right now this is a hunch; in five years, we'll have the data to prove it" (p. 15). This enthusiasm notwithstanding, more research utilizing longitudinal and experimental designs is needed to further address important causal linkages between organic religion and myriad social and behavioral outcomes.

RELIGION AND MEDICAL DECISIONS

Medical decisions such as abortion, the use of birth control, allowance of blood transfusion, utilization of chemotherapy, advance directives, and euthanasia are difficult and life altering. Many people turn to religion to guide them with this process. Koenig (2004) stated that in a study of patients who visited the pulmonary disease clinic at the University of Pennsylvania, 66% of patients indicated that religious beliefs would influence their medical decisions should they become seriously ill, and 80% indicated that they would be receptive to inquiries about their religious beliefs. Religions provide guiding principles or direct rules about medical decisions. In this section we focus on two areas of medical decisions, beginning- and end-of-life decisions, but it is important to note that religion also affects many decisions between these two polar opposite life stages.

Beginning-of-Life Decisions

The beginning-of-life decisions, specifically abortion and birth control usage, have been a source of contradiction not only in religion, but in the United States legal system as well. Debates about whether abortion should be legal or not, when abortion can be performed, adolescents' access to birth control, and sex education in the schools are just a few of the legal and moral debates that continue today. Although laws regulate decisions about abortion and contraception use to some degree, so does religion.

Abortion

A central issue surrounding the morality of abortion is related to the core question about when life begins. Does it begin when the egg is fertilized, when the soul enters the fetus, when consciousness occurs, when the embryo becomes embedded in the uterine wall, when the fetus moves, or when the birth occurs? The answer to this question depends on whom you ask, and the answer one gives will shape his or her views on the morality of abortion. Some religions prohibit abortion on the basis of it being viewed as murder, bringing about bad karma, and it being an act of violence regardless of when or why the abortion takes place.

Many religions will approve of abortion under certain circumstances. These circumstances may include:

- The health of the mother being at risk if the pregnancy is continued
- The child may be born with a disability that will cause suffering
- In the case of rape or incest

Birth Control

With the exception of the emergency contraceptive, decisions surrounding the use of birth control center around the debate about the purpose of sexual intercourse. Is it for procreation or other reasons? The usage of birth control is prohibited for reasons such as men are not permitted to waste "their seed" and/or that it is a violation of the design built into the human race by God. Some religions permit the use of hormonal birth control methods such as pills, patches, injections, and implants, but they do not allow the use of birth control methods that block or destroy sperm, such as condoms and vasectomies. Condom use may be permitted to protect one from sexually transmitted infections, and birth control may be allowed when a woman needs a rest between pregnancies, when pregnancy poses a risk to the mother or baby, or when the man cannot financially support another child.

End-of-Life Decisions

In "The Parable of the Mustard Seed," the Buddha teaches a lesson that is valid for all cultures; human beings receive no exemption from mortality. Deep in the throes of grief after the death of her son, a woman seeks wisdom from the Buddha, who says that he does indeed have an answer to her queries. Before giving it, however, he insists that she must first collect a mustard seed from every house that has not been touched by death. She canvasses her entire community but fails to collect a single seed. Returning to the Buddha, she understands that, like all other living beings, we are destined to die.

Death is inevitable, but modern technology has changed the process through life-extending technologies. Organ transplantation, respirators, antibiotics, surgical procedures, and feeding tubes enable life to be prolonged. Other technologies, such as lethal injections, may hasten death. The decision to use these technologies is an individual choice. In some situations, the utilization of technology to prolong life may be contradictory to another fundamental human value, such as going against God's will. Human beings struggle with not overstepping these boundaries or playing God with life and death.

Decisions surrounding continuing treatment, discontinuing treatment, or hastening death are difficult and agonizing. As individuals and their families face these controversial questions and as many states consider revising their laws about end-of-life choices, religious traditions and values can offer guidance and insight, if not solutions, for some.

In the remainder of this section we cover the more controversial and general decisions, but there are many other end-of-life decisions to consider, such as burial versus cremation, timing of the burial, length of the mourning process, appropriate dress and behavior before and during the service and after the burial, and permission to conduct an autopsy.

Organ Donation

Organ donation is the removal of tissues of the human body from a person who has recently died or from a living donor for the purpose of transplanting or grafting them into other persons. Religion and organ donation is changing. Some religions that previously prohibited organ donation are now altering their views and seeing it as an act of compassion, but some continue to prohibit organ donation. Many of these latter religions prohibit organ donation because of their beliefs of life after death and resurrection. Some religions will consent to an organ donation if they are certain that it is for the health and welfare of the transplant recipient, but if the outcome is questionable, then the donation is not encouraged.

Euthanasia

Euthanasia is a Greek term that means "good death." Also called mercy killing, it is the act or practice of ending the life of an individual who is suffering from a terminal illness or an incurable condition by lethal injection or the suspension of extraordinary medical treatment. The person who is suffering from the painful and incurable disease or incapacitating physical disorder is painlessly put to death. Because there is no specific provision for it in most legal systems, it is usually regarded as either suicide (if performed by the patient) or murder (if performed by another person, which includes physician-assisted suicide).

Murder and suicide are against the belief systems of most religions, so in those systems it would be considered morally wrong (in some religions, such as Hinduism, suicide is acceptable if it is done by fasting because it is nonviolent). Other reasons for religious opposition is the concern for patients who may be in vulnerable positions because of their illness or their lack of social and economic resources. There is fear that patients who cannot afford expensive treatment, for example, will be pressured to accept euthanasia. There also is great concern about the moral nature of the doctor's professional self.

Karma and rebirth are other considerations for not supporting euthanasia. Karma is the total effect of a person's actions and conduct during the successive phases of the person's existence, regarded as determining the person's destiny. Karma extends through one's present life and all past and future lives as well. In Hinduism and Buddhism, human beings are believed to be captured in endless cycles of rebirth and reincarnation. In both traditions, all living creatures (humans, animals, plants, etc.) represent manifestations of the laws of karmic rebirth. To honor these laws, one must show great respect for the preservation of life and noninjury of conscious beings. Acts that are destructive of life are morally condemned by the principle of **ahimsa**, which is the conceptual equivalent of the Western principle of the sanctity of life. Religions may permit physicians to hasten death through legal injection but not by withholding care.

On the other side of the issue, most religions also consider acts of compassion and concern about the dignity of the dying person to be part of humanity. Concern for the welfare of others as one is dying is a consideration, because it can be seen as a sign of spiritual enlightenment. A person can decide to forego treatment to avoid imposing a heavy burden of caregiving on family or friends. He or she may also stop treatment to relieve loved ones of the emotional or economic distress of prolonged dying.

These two different perspectives lead to the dilemma of whether euthanasia is an act of compassion or murder. Religions answer the question differently, and debate exists within religions. This personal and difficult decision obviously needs to be made on an individual basis, but health care professionals should be aware of the conflicting perspectives and the rationale behind them.

Advance Directives and End-of-Life Care

Advance directives are legal documents that enable a person to convey his or her decisions about end-of-life care ahead of time. Advance directives include the **living will** and durable power of attorney, and they provide a way for patients to communicate their wishes to their family, friends, and health care professionals and to avoid confusion later in the event that the person becomes unable to do so.

A living will is a set of instructions that documents a person's wishes about medical care intended to sustain life. People can accept or refuse medical care. There are many types of life-sustaining care that should be taken into consideration when drafting a living will, such as:

- The use of life-sustaining equipment, such as dialysis and breathing machines
- Resuscitation if breathing or heartbeat stops
- Artificial hydration and nutrition (tube feeding)
- Withholding food and fluids
- Organ or tissue donation
- Comfort care

A durable power of attorney for health care is a document that names your health care proxy. The proxy is someone you trust to make health care decisions if you are unable to do so. Survey data suggest that about 20% of the United States population has advance directives, with significantly lower rates among Asian Americans, Hispanics, and blacks (Searight & Gafford, 2005). For example, about 40% of elderly white patients indicated that they have an advance directive, compared with only 16% of elderly blacks (Searight & Gafford, 2005). The low rates of advance directive completion among nonwhites may be because of distrust of the health care system, health care disparities, cultural perspectives on death and suffering, and family dynamics, such as parent–child relationships (Searight & Gafford, 2005). For example, whites may be concerned about dying patients undergoing needless suffering, and black physicians and patients are more likely to think of suffering as spiritually meaningful and being a display of religious faith (Searight & Gafford, 2005). Collectivist groups, such as Hispanics, may be reluctant to formally appoint a specific family member to be in charge because of concerns about isolating these persons or offending other relatives. Instead, a consensually-oriented decision-making approach appears to be more acceptable in this population. Among Asian Americans, aggressive treatment for elderly family members is likely to be frowned upon because family members should have love and respect for their parents and ancestors and because of their high respect for the elderly.

RITUALS

A ritual is a set of actions that usually are very structured and have a symbolic value or meaning. The performance of rituals are usually tied to religion or traditions, and their forms, purposes, and functions vary. These include compliance with religious obligations or ideals, satisfaction of spiritual or emotional needs of the practitioners, to ward off evil, to ensure the favor of a divine being, to maintain or restore health, demonstration of respect or submission, stating one's affiliation, obtaining social acceptance, or for the pleasure of the ritual itself. A ritual may be performed on certain occasions, at regular intervals, or at the discretion of individuals or communities. It may be performed by an individual, a small group, or the community, and it may occur in arbitrary places or specified locations. The rituals may be performed in private or public, or in front of specific people. The participants may be restricted to certain community members, with limitations related to age, gender, or type of activity (hunting and birthing rituals).

Rituals are related to numerous activities and events, such as birth, death, puberty, marriages, sporting events, club meetings, holidays, graduations, and presidential inaugurations, but rituals are not only related to major events. Handshaking, saying hello and good-bye, and taking your shoes off before entering a home are rituals. These actions and their symbolism are neither arbitrarily chosen by the performers nor dictated by logic or necessity, but they either are prescribed and imposed upon the performers by some external source or are inherited unconsciously from social traditions.

The biomedical system contains numerous rituals, including its own language filled with scientific terminology, jargon, and abbreviations (i.e., MRI, CAT scan). There are formal rules of behavior and communication, such as how physicians should be addressed and where the patient should sit. There are rituals such as hand washing, how to perform a physical examination, how to make a hospital bed, and how to document information in patient charts. The values and expectations include being on time for your appointment and adhering to the treatment regimen. People who are unaccustomed to this culture and these rituals can experience difficulty with them, and this includes maneuvering through the complex health insurance system, which is laden with unfamiliar rituals and rules. This can be particularly challenging if English is the patient's second language and if the patient did not come from a place with a similar system, such as socialized medicine.

In addition to rituals within health care systems, there are numerous rituals that are related to health. These rituals are discussed here to help prompt people who are working in health care to ask about, be sensitive to, and not be surprised about these key differences.

Objects as Rituals

There are numerous items that people wear to maintain their health. These may include amulets that may be worn on a necklace or strung around the neck, wrist, or waist. For example, people from Puerto Rico may place a bracelet on the wrist of a baby to ward off evil eye. In addition to being worn, amulets may be placed in the home. For example, items such as written documents, statues, crosses, or horseshoes may be hung on the home to protect the family's health as well as other factors. It is important to ask about removing these objects first because removal may cause great stress and concern for the person.

Shrines

For centuries people have described certain places as being holy or magic, as having a concentrated power, or having the presence of spirit. Ancient legends, historic records, and contemporary reports tell of extraordinary, even miraculous, happenings at these places. Different sacred sites have the power to heal the body, enlighten the mind, increase creativity, develop psychic abilities, and awaken the soul to a knowing of its true purpose in life. **Shrines** are located at some of these sacred sites. A shrine was originally a container, usually made of precious materials, but it has come to mean a holy or sacred place. Shrines may be enclosures within temples, home altars, and sacred burial places. Secular meanings have developed by association, and some of the associations are related to health and healing. People visit numerous shrines that represent health to maintain or restore health. Some examples of these shrines are Our Lady of La Leche, Our Lady of San Juan, and St. Peregrine. These shrines can be associated with healing for a specific disease or condition or with healing in general.

Animal Sacrifice

Animal sacrifice is not only practiced for food consumption but is believed to be needed for one to build and maintain a personal relationship with the spirit. It is also believed that it brings worshippers closer to their Creator or spirit and makes them aware of the spirit in them. Sacrifices are performed for events such as birth, marriage, and death. They are also used for healing. Animals are killed similarly to that of a kosher slaughter. Animals are cooked and eaten following all rituals, except in some healing and death rituals the animal is not eaten because it is believed that the sickness is passed into the dead animal.

Birthing Rituals

The birth of an infant is a life-altering event that is surrounded by many traditional and ancient rituals. These rituals are often related to protecting the health of the child, which includes protecting him or her from evil spirits. The rituals are related to events prior to, during, and after the birth. Because the rituals are so numerous, we have listed the general variations, but the list is not exhaustive.

Prior to birth:
- Food restrictions
- Wearing of amulets
- The fulfilling of food cravings
- Exposure to cold air
- Avoidance of loud noises or viewing certain types of people (i.e., deformed people)

During labor:
- How the placenta is discarded
- Silent birth (some cultures require that no words or sounds are spoken by the woman and/or family members)
- People present during labor
- Utilization of a midwife
- Place of delivery
- Medications used

After birth:
- Breastfeeding
- Amulets (placed on the baby, crib, or in the newborn's room)
- Female and male circumcision

- Baptism
- Animal sacrifice
- Cutting of child's lock of hair
- Bathing of baby
- Food restrictions
- When the naming of the baby occurs
- Rubbing the baby with oils or herbs
- Acceptance of postpartum depression
- Woman's and child's confinement period

Death Rituals

Responses to death vary widely across different cultures. Although some cultures may perform the same or similar rituals, they may have different meaning among the cultures. The rituals, in part, are related to beliefs about the meaning of life and life after death. Is death the end of existence or a transition to another life? Rituals play a role in behaviors, such as how people discuss death, respond to death, handle the deceased's body, the behaviors that occur at the funeral, and the mourning process.

Some general variations include:

- The method of disposing of the body
- Open versus closed casket
- The length of the mourning process and appropriate behavior
- Dress, including colors, at the funeral ceremony and afterwards
- Food restrictions or traditions
- Appropriate emotional responses
- The role of the family
- Use of prayer
- What is buried with the body
- Rituals engaged in before, during, and after the ceremony (i.e., burning of ghost money or candles, use of flowers)
- Animal sacrifice

CHAPTER SUMMARY

Religion plays a major role in the lives of Americans. It shapes our health behaviors and has been shown to have an overall positive effect on health behaviors. Religion also guides people when making difficult and sometimes life-altering decisions.

With technological advances, medical decisions can be complicated. Some people find the answers within their religion, but many people within religious sectors have differences in opinions. It is important for health care professionals not to assume someone's religion based upon their ethnicity and not to assume that everyone strictly adheres to the religious practices.

In this chapter we discussed how important religion is in the lives of Americans as well as the reasons why religion can impact health behaviors and decisions. We have discussed some reasons why people who are religious may have positive health habits and outcomes as well as the potential negative effects of religion. We ended the chapter with a discussion about rituals that are related to health. Many of those rituals are tied to religious beliefs, and health care professionals should make an effort to make provisions to adhere to these rituals.

REVIEW

1. Provide examples of how religion shapes health behaviors and the rationale behind them.
2. Explain some of the positive and negatives effects religion can have on health outcomes.
3. Provide examples of medical decisions that are made based on religion and the rationale behind them.
4. Explain issues that health care professionals should take into consideration related to beginning- and end-of-life transitions.

CASE STUDY

This case focuses on a Hasidic Judaism patient with cystic fibrosis and her family. Hasidic Judaism, sometimes referred to as Hasidic, refers to members of a Jewish religious movement founded in the eighteenth century in eastern Europe, which maintains that God's presence is in all of one's surroundings and that one should serve God in one's every deed and word. As you read through this story, pay particular attention to the multiple cultural and religious factors that influence this child's medical management.

Judy Cohen is 6 years old. Much of her life in the Hasidic Jewish community revolves around the neighborhood synagogue, her extended family, and their Hasidic Jewish community. She lives with her parents and four siblings in a house packed closely against her grandparents' house next door. The Cohen house is awash in the smells of Mrs. Cohen's cooking, the sounds of Yiddish prayer and conversation, and the laughter of children. The Cohens speak English fluently, but they prefer to speak their native language. They speak English only when necessary.

Judy's mother stays home to care for Judy and her four siblings, ages 3, 7, 9, and 10 years. Judy's father, Mr. Cohen, works for a family business. His job does not provide medical coverage, so the family is covered by Medicaid insurance. When the father is not working, he is usually praying, socializing, and consulting with the rabbi at the synagogue.

When she was 12 months old, Judy was diagnosed with cystic fibrosis (CF), which is an inherited chronic disease that affects the lungs and digestive system. At the time, the medical team that specialized in CF recommended that her siblings have sweat tests, which is the test used for diagnosing cystic fibrosis. Judy's parents declined because they believed that their children's health was in God's hands. Judy's condition was stable then, and she and her mother attended regularly scheduled appointments with the CF team. Judy's father, although he was concerned, did not usually come to Judy's appointments.

When Judy was 18 months old, she went to the clinic with an increased cough and weight loss. The team recommended that she be hospitalized. Judy's parents initially declined but agreed a week later after her cough had worsened.

At age 4 years, Judy again went into the hospital for pneumonia. Mr. and Mrs. Cohen reluctantly agreed to the hospital admission. When Judy appeared to be responding to the intravenous antibiotics, her parents convinced the medical team to allow Judy to complete her regimen of antibiotics at home. When she was home, the family did have their daughter complete the course of antibiotics that was recommended, but they refused visiting nurse services because they did not want the neighbors to know about Judy's illness.

When Mrs. Cohen became pregnant with her fifth child, the medical team strongly suggested that she go for genetic counseling and possibly testing. After discussing the issue with their rabbi, Mr. and Mrs. Cohen decided not to have genetic testing. Again, they believed that "whatever will be, will be" and that the unborn child's health was in God's hands.

Today, Judy went to the clinic for a routine follow-up appointment. This is her first visit since beginning school. Her respiratory status is good, but she's having more frequent stools. After being questioned, Mr. and Mrs. Cohen admit that they don't want the school to give Judy the required enzymes, which are recommended so that she can digest her food. They haven't told anyone at school that Judy has CF.

There are several issues to consider about this case:

- What are the various ways in which religious beliefs can affect the understanding of illness?
- How did the Cohen's Hasidic belief system impact Judy's treatment?
- What are some of the main tenets of Hasidic Judaism?
- Do you believe that the Cohens should have been required to have genetic testing done?
- Do you think the Cohens mishandled Judy's illness?

Source: Cross Cultural Health Care. (2003).

GLOSSARY TERMS

rituals	living will
euthanasia	shrines
karma	animal sacrifice
ahimsa	

REFERENCES

Adherents.com. (2005). *Largest religious groups in the United States of America*. Retrieved February 22, 2008, from www.adherents.com/rel_USA.html#religions

Advameg Inc. (2008). *Religion and Dietary Practices*. Retrieved on March 15, 2009 from http://www.faqs.org/nutrition/Pre-Sma/Religion-and-Dietary-Practices.html

Ano, G. G., & Vasconcelles, E. B. (2005). Religious coping and psychological adjustment to stress: A meta-analysis. *Journal of Clinical Psychology, 61,* 461–480.

Asser, S. M., & Swan, R. (1998). Child fatalities from religion-motivated medical neglect. *Pediatrics, 101,* 625–629.

Cottrell, R. R., Girvan, J. T., & McKenzie, J. F. (2006). *Principles and foundations of health promotion and education*. San Francisco: Pearson Benjamin Cummins.

Cross Cultural Health Care. (2003). *The case of Rivka Cohen*. Retrieved June 16, 2008, from http://support.mchtraining.net/national_ccce/case4/case.html

Dember, A. (2005, July 25). A prayer for health. *Boston Globe*. Retrieved February 3, 2008, from http://www.boston.com/news/globe/health_science/articles/2005/07/25/a_prayer_for_health/

Hamilton, S. R. (n.d.). American Society on Aging. *Studies show religious attendance brings added longevity*. Retrieved February 21, 2008, from www.asaging.org/at/at-226/religious.html

Johnson, B. R., Tompkins, R. B., & Webb, D. (2008). *Assessing the effectiveness of faith-based organizations: A review of the literature*. Waco, TX: Baylor University.

Koenig, H. G. (2004, December). Religion, spirituality, and medicine: Research findings and implications for clinical practice. *Southern Medical Journal, 97*(12), 1194–1200.

Koenig, H. G., McCullough, M. E., & Larson, D. B. (2000). *Handbook of religion and health*. New York: Oxford University Press.

Kosmin, B. A., Mayer, E., & Keysar, A. (2001). *American religious identification survey 2001*. Retrieved December 10, 2007, from www.gc.cuny.edu/faculty/research_studies/aris.pdf

Lee, B. Y., & Newberg, A. B. (2005). Religion and health: A review and critical analysis. *Zygon, 40*, 443–468.

McCullough, M. E., Hoyt, W. T., Larson, D. B., Koenig, H. G., & Thoresen, C. E. (2000). Religious involvement and mortality: A meta analytic review. *Health Psychology, 19*, 211–222.

McNicol, T. (1996, April 7). Where religion and medicine meet: The new faith in medicine. *USA Weekend*.

Miller, W. R., & Thoresen, C. E. (2003). Spirituality, religion, and health: An emerging research field. *American Psychologist, 58*, 24–35.

Peterson, B. (1983). Renewing the church's health ministries: Reflections on ten years' experience. *Journal of Religion and the Applied Behavioral Sciences, 17*.

Saad, L. (2003). *Religion is very important to majority of Americans*. Retrieved December 20, 2007, from http://www.gallup.com/poll/9853/Religion-Very-Important-Majority-Americans.aspx

Searight, H. R., & Gafford, J. (2005, February). Cultural diversity at the end of life: Issues and guidelines for family physicians. *American Family Physician*. Retrieved December 30, 2007, from http://www.aafp.org/afp/20050201/515.html

Seeman, T. E., Dubin L. F., & Seeman, M. (2003). Religiosity/spirituality and health. A critical review of the evidence for biological pathways. *American Psychologist, 58*, 53–63.

Strawbridge, W. J., Shema, S. J., Cohen, R. D. (2001). Religious attendance increases survival by improving and maintaining good health behaviors, mental health, and social relationships. *Annals of Behavioral Medicine, 23*, 68–74.

Trenholm, P., Trent, J., & Compton, W. C. (1998). Negative religious conflict as a predictor of panic disorder. *Journal of Clinical Psychology, 54*, 59–65.

Wallace, J. M., Jr., & Forman, T. A. (1998). Religion's role in promoting health and reducing risk among American youth. *Health Education and Behavior, 25*, 721–741.

Williams, D. R., & Sternthal, M. J. (2007). Spirituality, religion and health: Evidence and research directions. *The Medical Journal of Australia*. Retrieved February 22, 2008, from http://www.mja.com.au/public/issues/186_10_210507/wil11060_fm.html

Winseman, A. L. (2005). *Religion "very important" to most Americans*. Retrieved December 20, 2007, from http://www.gallup.com/poll/20539/Religion-Very-Important-Most-Americans.aspx

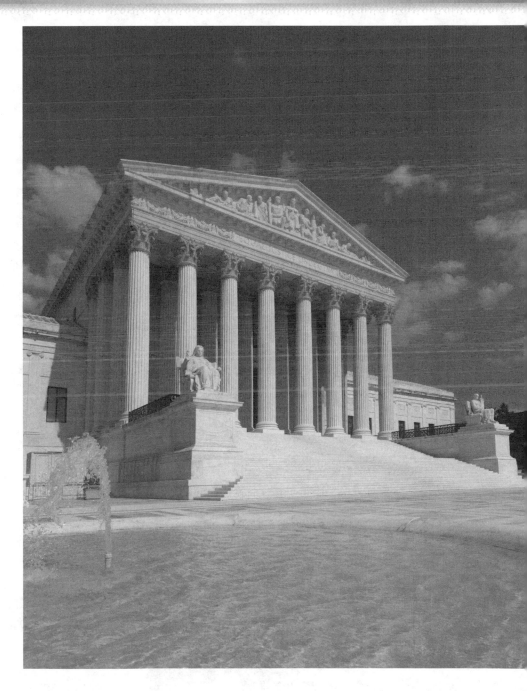

CHAPTER 5

Multicultural Health: Legal and Ethical Impacts

Give me your tired, your poor,
Your huddled masses yearning to breathe free,
The wretched refuse of your teeming shore.
Send these, the homeless, tempest-tossed to me.
I lift my lamp beside the golden door.

—Inscription on the base of the Statue of Liberty

KEY CONCEPTS

- Hill-Burton Act
- Ethics
- Morality
- Values
- Respect

- Autonomy
- Veracity
- Fidelity
- Nonmaleficence
- Justice

CHAPTER OBJECTIVES

1. Explain the interaction between cultural considerations and legal requirements.
2. Describe the fundamental rights embodied in the Constitution that relate to culture.
3. Describe laws impacting cultural practices.
4. Explain legal protections for cultural practices.
5. Explain the ethical principles impacting culture and health care practices.

The numerous ethnic groups that comprise the population of the United States are subject to both the protections and obligations of the laws of the federal government and the state within which they reside. Those laws can protect the members of a cultural or ethnic group from discrimination or can place cultural or ethnic practices at odds with legal requirements.

The United States Constitution is the source of all law for the country. It describes the structure and function of government and ensures that government does not intrude upon the fundamental rights of individual citizens. Those fundamental rights are found in the first 10 amendments to the Constitution and are known collectively as the Bill of Rights. Included among those fundamental rights are the rights to free speech and assembly, the right to the free exercise of religion, and the right to privacy. Individual rights are further expressed in the subsequent amendments to the Constitution. Notably absent from the list is the right to privacy. However, the U.S. Supreme Court has found that fundamental right to exist in the penumbra of rights embodied in the Bill of Rights (*Griswold v. Connecticut*, 1965).

Specifically, a fundamental right to engage in the practices or rituals that arise from cultural or ethnic origins does not exist. However, many of those practices are of a religious or private nature and are, arguably, protected.

For the government to impose upon a fundamental right, it must have a compelling reason. The most frequent basis for governmental action is its Constitutional responsibility to protect the general welfare of the citizens, commonly called the police powers. Therefore, when addressing governmental interjection into cultural issues, compelling interests of the two sides are often at stake: the fundamental rights of the members of the cultural group versus the responsibility of governments to protect the population at large.

The government also provides protection for cultural groups from discrimination in health care, employment, and public accommodations. Legislatures, either federal or state, create laws to protect those who might not otherwise be able to protect themselves from harm or discriminatory practices. Regulations are created by administrative agencies to ensure that members of cultural groups are able to access health care services and receive appropriate health care. In the remainder of this chapter we will explore both of these governmental functions.

Finally, there are private and quasi-governmental organizations that impact the relationship between culture, ethnicity, and health care. In this chapter we will explore these various areas of interplay as well as discuss the application of ethical principles to cultural health issues.

LAWS IMPACTING CULTURAL PRACTICES AND HEALTH

Many cultures have traditions and practices that involve health and healing. The members of the cultural group are familiar with the healing practices and find them normative. However, those practices can often conflict with the state and federal laws intended to protect the welfare of the community.

Unlicensed Practices

Every state licenses those who engage in the provision of health care services. Physicians, nurses, pharmacists, dentists, and so on must meet certain state-mandated requirements for education and testing before receiving a license to practice their profession. Again, the state's concern is protecting its citizens from unsafe practitioners. Those who attempt to practice the healing arts without obtaining the requisite license and complying with the licensing laws are prosecuted for the unlicensed practice of the particular profession. Penalties for unlawful practice can be stiff and include both prison time and monetary penalties.

Practitioners of culturally-related healing traditions must be aware and cautious of these types of laws. An example of a common area where these laws come in conflict with cultural practices is midwifery. Many cultures have customs regarding childbirth. Those who assist the mother in the delivery must be aware of the state's laws regarding that practice. For many years the practice of midwifery was banned by the great majority of states on the premise propounded by the medical associations that medical care during childbirth was safer for the mother and infant. Although those ideas have changed, and many states now sanction the practice of midwifery, the midwife must comply with licensing laws or risk sanctions for the unlawful practice of medicine or nursing. Therefore, traditional practitioners must be informed about both the legal requirements and liabilities that exist in their practice.

Another area of cultural practice that attracts scrutiny is the use of herbs and other natural products in the treatment of illness or disease. We are all familiar with the availability of herbal dietary supplements that are available in practically every store in the country. In ethnic areas of many cities in the United States, shops offer various products common to ethnic or cultural tradition. On the surface it appears that no difference exists between those herb shops and the over-the-counter dietary supplements at the local drug store. However, herbal treatments are often treated differently than dietary supplements.

Ethnic healers and herbalists risk running afoul of licensing laws in the manner in which they apply their healing practices. If the healer is merely making available various herbs or natural products to the public, then they are no different than over-the-counter preparations at the local drug store. However, it is when the healer begins to evaluate and diagnose symptoms and prescribe treatment that they are considered to be invading the domain of medical practitioners and become subject to sanctions for unlicensed practice.

Take, for example, Lee Wah. Mr. Lee was a healer in the ancient Chinese traditions. Mr. Lee had a patient that presented to his herb shop, described her ailment to him, and he prescribed certain herbs for the problem. He then chose the herbs and prepared them for her use. Mr. Lee was convicted of the unlicensed practice of medicine and was imprisoned (*People v. Lee Wah*, 1886).

Mexican Americans are very familiar with curanderas, traditional Mexican healers. Curanderas have dealt with illness in rural areas of Mexico for hundreds of years. It is not unexpected, then, that they should continue those practices within Mexican communities in the United States. However, the licensing laws apply to their practices as well. When a curandera visited an ill person in his home and prescribed a mixture of rhubarb, soda, glycerin, and spirits of peppermint for the patient's ailment, he was found to be in violation of the licensing laws (*People v. Machado*, 1929).

Many states now have licensing or registration requirements for herbal practitioners, and anyone engaging in those activities should consult local and state regulations to determine what rules they must comply with.

Ethnic Remedies

The remedies utilized by traditional healers are often prepared by the healer or herbalist or are brought to the United States from the native country. These remedies are subject to government oversight and regulation to ensure safety. The U.S. Food and Drug Administration (FDA) is responsible for ensuring the safety of all foods, drugs, and medical devices marketed and distributed in the United States. How the FDA views a particular remedy, and therefore the amount of regulation applicable to it, depends on how that remedy is classified.

Pharmaceutical products are subject to stringent regulation and testing both before and after approval by the FDA for placement on the market. These drugs are researched for mass production and distribution. No traditional ethnic remedy has ever been taken through the rigorous process for FDA approval.

Because traditional folk remedies contain ingredients such as vitamins, minerals, herbs, or other botanicals and substances such as enzymes and glandular and organ tissues, they are more likely to be viewed as dietary supplements and subject to less stringent regulation. The Dietary Supplement Health and Education Act of 1994 (DSHEA) established the FDAs current authority to regulate dietary supplements. A dietary supplement is a product taken by mouth that contains a "dietary ingredient" intended to supplement the diet. Those ingredients often are the very things that were previously noted as the components of ethnic remedies.

According to the DSHEA, a producer is responsible for determining that the dietary supplements it manufactures or distributes are safe and that any representations or claims made about them are substantiated by adequate evidence to show that they are not false or misleading. The dietary supplements do not need approval from the FDA before they are marketed (Center for Food Safety and Applied Nutrition, 2001). After a dietary supplement is on the market, the FDA has the responsibility to monitor its safety and, if it is found to be unsafe, to take action to remove it from the market. Further, a product may not be sold as a dietary supplement and promoted as a treatment, prevention, or cure for a specific disease or condition. Such an action would be considered the distribution of an illegal drug (Center for Food Safety and Applied Nutrition, 2001).

Although most ethnic healers would not consider their practices to include marketing a dietary supplement, nonetheless a traditional healer who provides any type of remedy is technically subject to these regulations and could be held responsible for their violation.

On a more local level, the state and county health departments are responsible for ensuring the health of the local community. It is not unusual for local health departments to investigate traditional healing practitioners for the unauthorized practice of medicine or the provision of remedies as treatments rather than as dietary supplements. Recently, health investigators in Houston, Texas, investigated the lead poisoning of siblings where the children had been given a traditional Mexican remedy for stomach ailments that was found to be 90% lead (Rhor, 2008). Serious consequences for the health and welfare of an unwary population such as this demand governmental involvement to protect the general welfare.

LEGAL PROTECTIONS FOR ETHNIC MINORITIES

As the law requires certain behavior, it also provides protection to those who are not able to protect themselves. It is a basic tenet of the U.S. Constitution that the minority be protected from discrimination by the majority. This principle has experienced uneven application in the past.

Historical Perspectives

It is an unfortunate necessity that any discussion of health care, ethnicity, and minorities must address the significant history of discrimination in the United States.

After the abolition of slavery in the late nineteenth century, hospitals, and medical practices were segregated, and minority physicians were often denied hospital privileges to treat patients. When ethnic patients were admitted to hospitals, it was to racially segregated sections of the hospital (Watson, 1997, 2001). That pattern of segregation in health care became institutionalized and was sanctioned by the U.S. Supreme Court in its infamous 1896 decision wherein the Court determined that separate but equal accommodations for minorities was constitutional (*Plessy v. Ferguson*, 1896).

Legal redress for discriminatory practices through the courts was often frustrating, and reparation was slow in coming. However, following on the heels of the Supreme Court's decision in *Brown v. Board of Education*, wherein it was held that racially separate but equal schools were unconstitutional, change in the health care arena began in 1963 when the Fourth Circuit of the U.S. Court of Appeals held unconstitutional the "separate but equal" provision of the Hill-Burton Act of 1946 (*Simkins v. Moses H. Cone Memorial Hospital*, 1963).

The Hospital Survey and Construction Act of 1946, known as the **Hill-Burton Act**, provided federal assistance to state governments for the construction and modernization of hospitals and other health care facilities. The original statute required recipient hospitals to make services available "to all persons residing in the territorial area of the application, without discrimination on account of race, creed, or color," but it made an exception "in cases where separate hospital facilities [were] provided for separate population groups," so long as equitable provisions were made to ensure that services were of like quality for each such group (Engelman Lado, 2001). The Simkins decision essentially made separate but equal hospitals illegal, much as *Brown v. Board of Education* determined that separate but equal schools were unconstitutional (Watson, 1997). Subsequently, the Hill-Burton Act has been revised and now provides specific protections for ethnic minorities in the reception of services. The Hill-Burton Act and the Simkins case will be discussed in greater detail later.

The Civil Rights Act of 1964

Closely following the Simkins decision, the Civil Rights Act of 1964 was passed by Congress and signed into law by President Lyndon Baines Johnson. Title VI of the Civil Rights Act prohibits federally-funded programs or activities from discriminating on the basis of race, color, or national origin. Federal agencies are responsible for enforcement of this law. In areas involving discrimination in health care, the Office for Civil Rights (OCR) of the Department of Health and Human Services (HHS) is responsible for enforcement. Title VI of the Act is the operative section that informs nondiscrimination in health care. It has three key elements (Civil Rights Act of 1964, Title VI):

1. It established a national priority against discrimination in the use of federal funds.
2. It authorized federal agencies to establish standards of nondiscrimination.
3. It provided for enforcement by withholding funds or "by any other means authorized by law."

Medicare and Medicaid are federal programs. The Civil Rights Act applies to practitioners and facilities that receive funds from those programs and is enforced by the Department of Health and Human Services Office for Civil Rights. The Act precludes discrimination on the basis of color, race, or national origin. Among other things, a recipient of federal funds may not engage in the following discriminatory acts (US Department of Health and Human Services, Office for Civil Rights, 2006b):

- Deny services, financial aid, or other benefits provided as a part of health and human services programs
- Provide a different service, financial aid, or other benefit, or provide them in a different manner from those provided to others under the program
- Segregate or separately treat individuals in any manner related to the receipt of any service, financial aid, or benefit

Since the Civil Rights Act of 1964 was passed, numerous other statutes and regulations have been created to address discrimination against ethnic minorities in health care. Included in those enforced by the OCR are the Hill-Burton Act and Executive Order No. 13,166, "Improving Access to Services for Persons with Limited English Proficiency" (US Commission on Civil Rights, 2004a).

Often legal cases that address ethnic and cultural issues arise through religious practices associated with the ethnic group. The Constitution's First Amendment, the right of freedom of religion, is interpreted by the Supreme Court to determine if certain ethnic practices are religious practices and therefore may not be impinged upon without a compelling governmental interest. The Goldman (Table 5.1) and Al-Khazraji (Table 5.2) cases that follow were decided by the Supreme Court and explore the scope of civil rights protections.

TABLE 5.1   Goldman v. Weinberger

GOLDMAN V. WEINBERGER, SECRETARY OF DEFENSE, ET AL. CERTIORARI TO THE UNITED STATES COURT OF APPEALS FOR THE DISTRICT OF COLUMBIA CIRCUIT

475 U.S. 503, No. 84-1097
Argued January 14, 1986
Decided March 25, 1986

Petitioner, an Orthodox Jew and ordained rabbi, was ordered not to wear a yarmulke while on duty and in uniform as a commissioned officer in the Air Force at March Air Force Base, pursuant to an Air Force regulation that provides that authorized headgear may be worn out of doors but that indoors "[h]eadgear [may] not be worn . . . except by armed security police in the performance of their duties." Petitioner then brought an action in Federal District Court, claiming that the application of the regulation to prevent him from wearing his yarmulke infringed upon his First Amendment freedom to exercise his religious beliefs. The District Court permanently enjoined the Air Force from enforcing the regulation against petitioner. The Court of Appeals reversed (*Goldman v. Weinberger,* 1986, p. 504).

The U.S. Supreme Court Held:

The First Amendment does not prohibit the challenged regulation from being applied to petitioner even though its effect is to restrict the wearing of the headgear required by his religious beliefs. That Amendment does not require the military to accommodate such practices as wearing a yarmulke in the face of its view that they would detract from the uniformity sought by dress regulations. Here, the Air Force has drawn the line essentially between religious apparel that is visible and that which is not, and the challenged regulation reasonably and evenhandedly regulates dress in the interest of the military's perceived need for uniformity. (*Goldman v. Weinberger,* 1986)

The Supreme Court has traditionally been deferential to the military in a vast array of matters. This case is an example of the Court's unwillingness to insert itself into military disciplinary matters.

Discussion

1. Do you agree with the Supreme Court's decision? Why?

2. Should the application of the First Amendment be limited when the military is involved? Why?

3. How does this decision impact other ethnic groups' religious beliefs?

TABLE 5.2   Saint Francis College v. Al-Khazraji

SAINT FRANCIS COLLEGE v. AL-KHAZRAJI

481 U.S. 604
Argued February 25, 1987
Decided May 18, 1987

Respondent professor, a United States citizen born in Iraq, filed suit in Federal District Court against petitioners, his former employer and its tenure committee, alleging that, by denying him tenure nearly three years before, they had discriminated against him on the basis of his Arabian race in violation of 42 U.S.C. 1981. The court . . . granted summary judgment for petitioners upon finding that 1981 does not reach discrimination claims based on Arabian ancestry. The Court of Appeals . . . reversed the District Court on the merits, holding that respondent had properly alleged racial discrimination in that, although Arabs are Caucasians under current racial classifications, Congress, when it passed what is now 1981, did not limit its protections to those who today would be considered members of a race different from the defendant's. The court said that, at a minimum, 1981 reaches discrimination directed against an individual because he or she is genetically part of an ethnically and physiognomically distinctive subgrouping of homo sapiens. Because the record was insufficient to determine whether respondent had been subjected to the sort of prejudice that 1981 would redress, the case was remanded. (*Saint Francis College v. Al-Khazraji*, 1987)

The U.S. Supreme Court Held:

A person of Arabian ancestry may be protected from racial discrimination under 1981. The Court of Appeals properly rejected petitioners' contention that, as a Caucasian, respondent cannot allege the type of discrimination that 1981 forbids since that section does not encompass claims of discrimination by one Caucasian against another. That position assumes that all those who might be deemed Caucasians today were thought to be of the same race when 1981 became law. In fact, 19th-century sources commonly described "race" in terms of particular ethnic groups, including Arabs, and do not support the claim that Arabs and other present-day "Caucasians" were then considered to be a single race. Moreover, 1981's legislative history indicates that Congress intended to protect identifiable classes of persons who are subjected to intentional discrimination solely because of their ancestry or ethnic characteristics. However, a distinctive physiognomy is not essential to qualify for 1981 protection. Thus, if respondent can prove that he was subjected to intentional discrimination based on the fact that he was born an Arab, rather than solely on the place or nation of his origin or his religion, he will have made out a 1981 case (*Saint Francis College v. Al-Khazraji*, 1987, p. 605).

Discussion

1. Do you agree with the Supreme Court's decision? Why?

2. What is the difference between the outcome in this case and the Goldberg case?

TABLE 5.2 *(Continued)*
3. Do you agree that people need protection of the law if they are part of "identifiable classes of persons who are subjected to intentional discrimination solely because of their ancestry or ethnic characteristics"?
4. How does this decision impact the delivery of health care to ethnic minorities?

The Hill-Burton Act: Recent Developments

The Hill-Burton Act has been amended a number of times since its inception. A recent amendment is entitled "Community Service Assurance under Title IV of the U.S. Public Health Service Act." It requires facilities to provide services to persons living within the service area without discrimination based on race, national origin, color, creed, or any other reason not related to the person's need for services. The subsequent HHS regulations set forth the requirements with which a Hill-Burton facility must comply, including (US Department of Health and Human Services, Office for Civil Rights, 2006b):

- A person residing in the Hill-Burton facility's service area has the right to medical treatment at the facility without regard to race, color, national origin, or creed.
- A Hill-Burton facility must post notices informing the public of its community service obligations in English and Spanish. If 10% or more of the households in the service area usually speak a language other than English or Spanish, the facility must translate the notice into that language and post it as well.
- A Hill-Burton facility may not deny emergency services to any person residing in the facility's service area on the grounds that the person is unable to pay for those services.
- A Hill-Burton facility may not adopt patient admission policies that have the effect of excluding persons on grounds of race, color, national origin, creed, or any other ground unrelated to the patient's need for the service or the availability of the needed service.

Accordingly, the Hill-Burton Act affirmatively requires nondiscriminatory care by recipients of their funds. Review Table 5.3 for a discussion of the process by which the Simkins case was decided.

TABLE 5.3   The Recognition of Rights

Simkins v. Moses H. Cone Memorial Hospital

Preston (1997) discussed how the Hill-Burton Act was instrumental in ending discrimination against black health care providers in the United States. He described how the process of challenging discrimination occurred. Jack Greenberg was an attorney working on civil rights actions for the NAACP in the 1960s with Thurgood Marshall, who was then an NAACP attorney and later became Solicitor General of the United States and a U.S. Supreme Court Justice. Greenberg was contacted by Dr. George Simkins, a Greensboro, North Carolina, dentist, for advice about discrimination against him in admitting his patients to a local hospital that was receiving Hill-Burton funds.

Greenberg recommended that Simkins apply for admitting privileges to the local hospitals. Moses H. Cone Memorial Hospital sent him an application and subsequently denied him privileges. The other two hospitals did not send applications. This discriminatory activity formed the basis of the case to challenge this activity. Other black physicians and dentists were recruited to join the case by requesting applications to the hospitals; all were denied. Along with the practitioners, patients were included as plaintiffs in the suit. One man was denied admission to one of the local hospitals for treatment of his ulcers.

As the case proceeded, the hospital's receipt of Hill-Burton funds became critical to success because it subjected the hospital to significant state and federal regulations, which included the stipulation that a state had to submit, for approval by the Surgeon General, a plan for hospital care that did not discriminate on the basis of race, creed, or color. If a separate-but-equal facility was built, the state agency had to submit a report enumerating the number of beds that were available for each racial group to the surgeon general. If the government was involved in hospitals using Hill-Burton funds, citizens were entitled to protection under the Fourteenth Amendment.

The local court found against Dr. Simkins and his colleagues, stating that the court did not have jurisdiction over civil rights activity cases. The Fourth Circuit of the U.S. Court of Appeals overruled the lower court, finding in favor of Dr. Simkins and granting the requested relief, the right to admit his patients to the local hospitals.

On March 2, 1964, the U.S. Supreme Court refused to review the Court of Appeals' decision, thereby upholding the Court of Appeals' ruling against the separate-but-equal provisions in the Hill-Burton program. Hospitals that were receiving Hill-Burton funds had to integrate (Watson, 1997).

Discussion

1. How has this case impacted the delivery of care to minorities in the United States since 1964?

2. Is there discrimination in the delivery of health care today, and, if so, how does this case apply to it?

Limited English Proficiency

On August 11, 2000, President Clinton signed Executive Order No. 13,166, entitled "Improving Access to Services for Persons with Limited English Proficiency." The purpose of the executive order was to improve access and eliminate language as a barrier to federally-assisted programs. All federal agencies were required to prepare a plan to improve access to their programs for limited English proficiency (LEP) persons (US Commission on Civil Rights, 2004b).

Subsequent HHS regulations promulgated for Medicare programs defined limited English proficient individuals as those who do not speak English as their primary language and who have a limited ability to read, write, speak, or understand English. Persons who meet the LEP definition may be eligible to receive language assistance in various programs that receive federal assistance (US Department of Health and Human Services, Office for Civil Rights, 2004).

A recipient of federal funds is required to take reasonable actions to ensure LEP persons have access to federally-funded programs. To determine if a provider is required to provide language assistance, a number of factors are assessed, including the number of LEP persons who are eligible for the program, the frequency in which an LEP person comes in contact with the program, the nature and importance of the program, and resources available and costs of services. If it is determined that language assistance is required, then a plan is required to identify LEP individuals in the program and develop that requisite assistance.

Culturally and Linguistically Appropriate Services (CLAS)

In compliance with Title VI and the LEP regulations, the HHS Office of Minority Health (OMH) has developed national standards entitled "National Standards for Culturally and Linguistically Appropriate Services in Health Care (CLAS)." The CLAS requirements are set out in Table 5.4. In promulgating these standards, OHM provided its rationale for preparing the standards and recommendations for their use.

OMH noted that the census data from 2000 reflected a significant increase in minority and foreign-born citizens. In fact, minority populations became the majority in California in 1999 (US Department of Health and Human Services, OPHS, Office of Minority Health, 2001). With these demographic changes came the challenge of patients who bring their cultural and language differences to their interactions with health care providers. It was determined that providing national standards for cultural and linguistically appropriate services would support a more comprehensive and consistent approach to cultural competence and improve access and quality of care as well as outcomes.

TABLE 5.4   National CLAS Standards

Culturally Competent Care

1. Health care organizations should ensure that patients/consumers receive from all staff members effective, understandable, and respectful care that is provided in a manner compatible with their cultural health beliefs and practices and preferred language.

2. Health care organizations should implement strategies to recruit, retain, and promote at all levels of the organization a diverse staff and leadership that are representative of the demographic characteristics of the service area.

3. Health care organizations should ensure that staff at all levels and across all disciplines receive ongoing education and training in culturally and linguistically appropriate service delivery.

Language Access Services

4. Health care organizations must offer and provide language assistance services, including bilingual staff and interpreter services, at no cost to each patient/consumer with limited English proficiency at all points of contact, in a timely manner, during all hours of operation.

5. Health care organizations must provide to patients/consumers in their preferred language both verbal offers and written notices informing them of their right to receive language assistance services.

6. Health care organizations must assure the competence of language assistance provided to limited English proficient patients/consumers by interpreters and bilingual staff. Family and friends should not be used to provide interpretation services (except on request by the patient/consumer).

7. Health care organizations must make available easily understood patient-related materials and post signage in the languages of the commonly encountered groups and/or groups represented in the service area.

Organizational Supports

8. Health care organizations should develop, implement, and promote a written strategic plan that outlines clear goals, policies, operational plans, and management accountability/ oversight mechanisms to provide culturally and linguistically appropriate services.

9. Health care organizations should conduct initial and ongoing organizational self-assessments of CLAS-related activities and are encouraged to integrate cultural and linguistic competence-related measures into their internal audits, performance improvement programs, and patient satisfaction assessments.

TABLE 5.4 *(Continued)*

Outcomes-Based Evaluations

10. Health care organizations should ensure that data about the individual patient's/consumer's race, ethnicity, and spoken and written language are collected in health records, integrated into the organization's management information systems, and periodically updated.

11. Health care organizations should maintain a current demographic, cultural, and epidemiological profile of the community as well as a needs assessment to accurately plan for and implement services that respond to the cultural and linguistic characteristics of the service area.

12. Health care organizations should develop participatory, collaborative partnerships with communities and utilize a variety of formal and informal mechanisms to facilitate community and patient/consumer involvement in designing and implementing CLAS-related activities.

13. Health care organizations should ensure that conflict and grievance resolution processes are culturally and linguistically sensitive and capable of identifying, preventing, and resolving cross-cultural conflicts or complaints by patients/consumers.

14. Health care organizations are encouraged to regularly make available to the public information about their progress and successful innovations in implementing the CLAS Standards and to provide public notice in their communities about the availability of this information.

Source: U.S. Department of Health and Human Services, Office of Minority Health. (2000). National Standards for Culturally and Linguistically Appropriate Services (CLAS) in Health Care. *Federal Register, 65*(247), 80865–80879.

The 14 CLAS standards are grouped into themes: culturally competent care, language access services, and organizational supports for cultural competence. Thereafter, the standards are characterized as mandates, guidelines, and recommendations. The mandated standards are numbers 4–7. Those standards must be met by all recipients of federal funds. Standard numbers 1–3 and 8–13 are guidelines, and they are recommended for adoption by both OMH and national accrediting agencies. Finally, the recommended standard, number 14, is suggested for voluntary adoption (US Department of Health and Human Services, OPHS, Office of Minority Health, 2001). These standards are intended to inform, guide, and facilitate practices regarding culturally and linguistically appropriate health care services.

Although the various aspects of cultural competence in health care will be discussed at length in later chapters, it is worth noting here that both federal and state governments have begun addressing the need for cultural competence through various

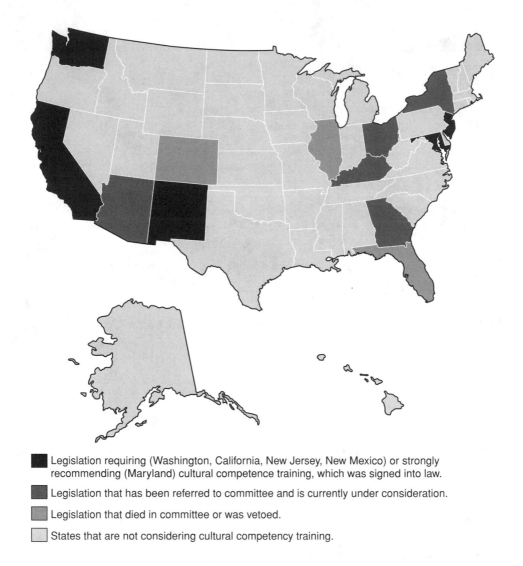

FIGURE 5.1   States proposing to implement cultural competency training.
Source: U.S. Department of Health and Human Services, Office of Minority Health. (2007, November 16). *Cultural competency legislation.*

standards and legislation. States are requiring cultural competence education in medical and nursing schools, and recent legislation in many states includes requiring cultural competency training for health care providers to receive licensure or relicensure. The map in Figure 5.1 indicates states that are proposing to implement cultural competency training.

PERSONAL HEALTH DECISIONS

Perhaps the area where law and cultural health issues intersect the most is in the area of personal health care decisions. How an individual approaches health care decisions is informed by his or her personal experiences as well as family, religious, and cultural influences. Different cultures approach how to undergo treatment, when to treat, and when to stop treatment differently. Even more importantly, who will make such decisions for a patient may differ from culture to culture.

Therefore, it is important to understand the legal construct that impacts health care decisions. The laws of all the states reflect an individual's Constitutional right to privacy and to make personal decisions free from outside influence. Consequently, the right to make health care decisions is personal to the patient involved, and no one else has the right to interfere. In cultures where family input is sought for such decisions, or a surrogate decision maker is used, this legal principle could create decision-making conflicts. A competent individual can always appoint someone else to make decisions for him or her, thus removing the conflict.

The more problematic situation is when the patient is unable to make his or her wishes known because of the patient's medical condition. In that situation it is important to have documents that were prepared in advance indicating who will make decisions for the person and what decisions are to be made that are consistent with the person's cultural beliefs. Health care powers of attorney are documents that appoint who will make decisions for the person if he or she is unable to decide. A living will documents what decisions and desires a person has about his or her care and end-of-life decisions, and it can, and should, include instructions respecting the person's cultural beliefs. Many states have combined these two documents into one advance health care document that covers all the various decisions. Whatever format is utilized in a particular state, the necessity of these documents remains. (See the Case Study later in this chapter.)

PRIVATE AND QUASI-GOVERNMENTAL REGULATORS

The Joint Commission, formerly the Joint Commission on Accreditation of Healthcare Organizations (JCAHO), is an independent, nonprofit organization that evaluates and accredits health care organizations in the United States. The Joint Commission has been setting the practice standards for health care organizations since 1951, with quality of care and safety being the primary goals. The Joint Commission accreditation is recognized as the national standard for health care organizations and is required for Medicare providers to maintain their status and receive Medicare reimbursement.

The Joint Commission has added standards related to culturally and linguistically appropriate health care services to its requirements for accreditation. Standards supporting the provision of care in a culturally- and language-appropriate manner include the following (The Joint Commission, 2007):

- Respecting the values and beliefs of the individual
- Providing appropriate communication, including interpretive services
- Providing appropriate informed consent
- Providing conducive end-of-life care
- Ensuring equality in the standard of care and staff competence

Accordingly, to maintain their status as Medicare providers and be eligible to treat Medicare patients and be reimbursed for those services, health care organizations must meet these standards.

ETHICAL CONSIDERATIONS

Ethics is concerned with moral conduct and judgment. It is a way of understanding moral principles. **Morality** involves traditions and beliefs about human conduct and right and wrong (Beauchamp & Childress, 2001). It includes our beliefs about what is the right or best thing to do and often includes religious, cultural, and family traditions. Often two characteristics emerge from these moral traditions: a consensus about what is right or wrong and an authority about the right thing to do, often a priest, a rabbi, or codes.

Ethical conduct involves complying with moral standards, and ethics is a process of attempting to negotiate a conflict between values and moral traditions. **Values** are personal beliefs about what is true or appropriate behavior. Not all values are moral values. When a conflict arises between moral traditions and personal values about what is right and wrong, ethics is utilized to reconcile the situation and assist in making the appropriate decision under the circumstances (Bioethics Consultation Group, 1992).

The legal system is a set of rules and regulations that are binding on the members of a society and set out what behavior is acceptable. They are subject to review and change as the society changes. The relationship between law and ethics significantly impacts health care decisions and cultural influences.

When law and ethics influence each other, society tends to benefit from the interaction because both reflect the effect of the other. When they exist separately, situations can arise where legal actions conflict with moral reasoning. Such a situation can give rise to an ethical action, such as civil disobedience. In situations where conflict exists within a society regarding a particular issue, law and ethics may only partially influence each other (Brent, 2001).

The relationship between health care and culture is greatly influenced by ethical principles. We see ethical principles reflected in laws and regulations, such as the Civil Rights Act or Hill-Burton Act, and in the actions of health care providers. The ethical principles that most impact cultural issues in health care are respect, autonomy, nonmaleficence, beneficence, and justice.

Respect is the underlying principle for all other ethical principles. It takes into account individuals' rights to make determinations about their health and to live or die with the consequences. Respect for others does not allow cultural, gender, religious, or racial differences to interfere with that individual right. Therefore, it forms the basis for all ethical practices. Respect is in evidence when the cultural heritage and practices of patients are considered in treatment even when the provider does not share that value.

Autonomy is the ethical principle that embodies the right of self-determination. It is the right to choose what happens to one's self and decision making. It is embodied in the concept of informed consent in health care, which is the right to be informed about recommended treatment prior to consent. Autonomy requires that certain conditions exist, including understanding; an absence of controlling influences, which is traditionally understood as liberty; and agency, which is the ability to act intentionally (Beauchamp & Childress, 2001).

For this ethical principle to be achieved, a patient must be informed in a manner that considers both cultural and language barriers to understanding. The CLAS and The Joint Commission standards discussed earlier are attempts to respect the ethical concept of autonomy.

In respect for autonomy, not only the right to choose is respected, but a right not to choose should be respected as well. Valuing a patient's right to defer decision-making to another person, or not to be informed about the extent of his or her condition, is as essential to the principle of autonomy as ensuring that a patient who desires autonomy is fully informed about his or her treatment options.

Understanding ethnic differences is imperative to properly apply this ethical principle. A UCLA research project studied ethnic differences related to disclosure of diagnosis and prognosis of a terminal disease and end-of-life decision-making. Their findings were summarized as follows:

> Korean Americans (47%) and Mexican Americans (65%) were significantly less likely than European Americans (87%) and African Americans (88%) to believe that a patient should be told the diagnosis of metastatic cancer. Korean Americans (35%) and Mexican Americans (48%) were less likely than African Americans (63%) to believe that a patient

should be told of a terminal prognosis and less likely to believe that the patient should make decisions about the use of life-supporting technology (28% and 41% vs. 60% and 65%). Korean Americans and Mexican Americans tended to believe that the family should make decisions about use of life support (Blackhall, Murphy, Frank, Michel, & Azen, 1995, p. 821).

Accordingly, the impact of ethnicity significantly affected the patient's attitude toward decision making related to terminal illness.

Another study investigated the manner in which disclosures related to risk and medical prognosis were received by Navajo patients. The investigators found that the medical concern for full disclosure conflicted with the Navajo belief that words, language, and thoughts shape reality and control events. Thus, the discussion of negative risks or negative outcomes could be interpreted as creating the very thing that is to be avoided. It was recommended that the use of a "positive ritual language" expected by the patient would be better received. Such a communication focuses on promotion and restoration of health rather than the possible negative outcomes (Caresse & Rhodes, 1995).

Consequently, it is imperative to autonomy that the patient's right to information and choice of treatment options also respects his or her right not to be told or to choose. Inquiring as to ethnic expectations before embarking on such discussions will promote patient comfort and culturally appropriate action.

Determining how to proceed in any particular situation may be difficult. Therefore, keeping in mind certain tenets will assist in maintaining respect for a patient's autonomy. Those tenets include (Beauchamp & Childress, 2001, p. 65):

1. tell the truth;
2. respect the privacy of others;
3. protect confidential information;
4. obtain consent for interventions with patient or surrogate;
5. when asked, help other[s] make important decisions.

Incorporated in autonomy are two other principles: **veracity** and **fidelity**. Veracity involves being truthful. It means providing necessary information in an honest way. Fidelity entails keeping one's promises or commitments. It requires not promising what one cannot do or control. Both of these principles are necessary for patients to be truly informed about their care.

Nonmaleficence is the principle that states that one should do no harm. Although simple in concept, it is often difficult in practice. In health care, actions can often cause harm, and very few treatment modalities are completely without risk of harm. Thus the practitioner must weigh the risks and benefits of any treatment.

However, it is the unknown harm that should be addressed in the cultural context. Practitioners should be aware that patients from cultures other than their own may perceive things as harmful that are not readily apparent. For example, physical examination of a female by a male practitioner is considered to be unacceptable in some cultures and can lead to serious consequences for the female patient. Making arrangements for a female examiner would evidence the ethical concept of nonmaleficence.

Beneficence is the principle that requires doing good or removing harm. It is often intertwined with nonmaleficence, but it is a distinct ethical construct. Beneficence is at work when balancing the risk, benefit, harm, and effectiveness of treatment. It requires that when harm is found, positive actions occur to remove or limit it. This ethical principle was at work when segregated hospitals were outlawed by the Civil Rights Act.

Justice is the ethical principle that holds that people should be treated equally and fairly. Justice requires that people not be treated differently because of their culture or ethnic background. Justice is also at issue when the allocation and distribution of limited health resources are discussed. Ensuring that health resources are available to all without regard to race or ethnicity is the theory of distributive justice. It is this ethical principle that is breached when care is denied or withheld on racial or ethnic grounds.

The fair opportunity rule of justice states that no one should receive social benefits based on undeserved advantages or be denied benefits on the basis of disadvantages (Beauchamp & Childress, 2001). Although this may seem fairly straightforward, it becomes difficult to manage when applied to the variances of social inequalities. The rule states that discrimination is not ethically justifiable on the basis of social status or ethnicity.

In health care distribution, the fair opportunity rule becomes apparent. Many studies indicate that racial- and gender-based discrimination has occurred in the utilization of limited health care resources. Beauchamp and Childress (2001) cite numerous studies wherein it was shown that women and African Americans had poorer access to care than white males, that African Americans had less access to coronary artery bypass and transplants, and that nonwhite populations constituted a greater percentage of dialysis patients and waited longer for transplants.

Such studies indicate that, as a society, the United States is not complying with the fair opportunity rule and needs to attend further to the principles of justice in the distribution of increasingly scarce health care resources.

Ethical principles are implicated in all areas of health care. However, when cultural issues are involved, special care needs to be exercised to ensure that these principles are applied in a manner that respects the cultural and ethnic influences of the situation.

The legal influences on cultural considerations in health care can provide protection for ethnic or cultural minorities or can place them at risk. The legal restrictions on cultural practices and the legal protections for cultural practices are important considerations when dealing with any cultural or ethnic group. Finally, the moral guidance of ethical principles should always guide action.

CHAPTER SUMMARY

There are numerous areas where cultural practices are impacted by legal and ethical principles. Common ethnic healing practices or use of ethnic remedies can, in some instances, violate laws regulating the practice of the healing arts.

The protection of ethnic minorities from discrimination in health care did not become codified until the 1960s as a result of intervention by the courts in discriminatory practices. Recently, we have seen the emergence of requirements by accrediting agencies for standards of cultural competence that respect the diversity within our society and provide for appropriate communication with those who do not speak English.

As we move into the future where the diversity of our nation increases, further efforts to ensure respect for cultural practices will evolve.

REVIEW

1. For the mandatory cultural competence standards, discuss policies a hospital could create to comply with those standards.
2. Choose three ethical principles and discuss how a health care provider could design his or her practice to respect those principles.
3. Discuss the factors you believe influenced the country to continue separate but equal hospitals.
4. Analyze the reasons you believe the government continues to monitor herbal remedies and traditional practitioners.

CASE STUDY

Mrs. Lee was a 49-year-old Chinese immigrant who spoke only Cantonese. She was admitted to the hospital with what was thought to be pneumonia but after testing was found to be lung cancer. While at the hospital, Mrs. Lee was constantly attended by her husband and children. One of her sons interpreted for her because she did not speak English.

During the course of the hospitalization, the son acted as the family spokesperson and began making the health care decisions. He would not discuss the diagnosis with the caregivers, and he did not want the doctors to speak with Mrs. Lee about her diagnosis. The doctors were concerned that they did not know what Mrs. Lee's wishes were because the family was interjecting itself between them and their patient.

When Mrs. Lee went home, she was treated by her family physician. The son attended every office visit and would not allow the doctor to discuss Mrs. Lee's diagnosis or to explore her desires regarding resuscitation. Mrs. Lee's condition deteriorated, and her cancer spread despite treatment. Eventually Mrs. Lee was admitted to the hospital with severe difficulty breathing. Her condition deteriorated quickly, and soon she became unable to respond. The family refused to discuss whether or not resuscitation should take place if her heart stopped. The doctor wrote an order not to resuscitate the patient and talked with Mr. Lee, who agreed to the order. The family continued to demand aggressive treatment for Mrs. Lee's deteriorating condition. The son demanded that his mother be placed on a respirator to prolong her life. When the doctors refused to do so, the son accused the doctors of not taking proper care of his mother and racial discrimination in their care. He threatened to sue the physicians if they did not comply with his wishes.

The physicians reviewed the care they had been providing to Mrs. Lee and held a family meeting to review the futility of further life-prolonging care and try to deal with the family's anger and hostility. The son continued to demand that all efforts to keep his mother alive be undertaken.

When Mrs. Lee finally stopped breathing, the family became distraught and demanded that she be resuscitated. Medications were administered to Mrs. Lee to placate the family, to no avail. When it became clear that Mrs. Lee was dead, the son accused the staff of being murderers.

There are several issues to consider about this case:

- What were the differences between the physicians' and family's view of what should be said to the patient and the family?
- What was the implication of the physicians not knowing the patient's wishes?
- What were the differences between the physicians' and family's view of withdrawal of care?
- How can the practitioners bridge these gaps and assist both the patient and family in dealing with the situation?
- Should treatment such as this be administered to a patient without the physicians ever determining what the patient herself wanted?
- How should the issue of medical futility be determined in this situation?

Source: Muller & Desmond. (1992).

GLOSSARY TERMS

Hill-Burton Act   autonomy
ethics   veracity
morality   fidelity
values   nonmaleficence
respect   justice

REFERENCES

Beauchamp, T., & Childress, J. (2001). *Principles of biomedical ethics* (5th ed.). New York: Oxford University Press.

Bioethics Consultation Group. (1992). *Forming a moral community*. Berkeley, CA: Author.

Blackhall, L., Murphy, S., Frank, G., Michel, V. & Azen, S. (1995). Ethnicity and attitudes toward patient autonomy. *Journal of the American Medical Association, 274*, 820–825.

Brent, N. (2001). *Nurses and the law* (2nd ed.). Philadelphia: W. B. Saunders.

Carresse, J., & Rhodes, L. (1995). Western bioethics on the Navajo reservation: Benefit or harm? *Journal of the American Medical Association, 274*, 826–829.

Center for Food Safety and Applied Nutrition. (2001, January 3). US Food and Drug Administration Publication. Retrieved June 15, 2008, from http://www.cfsan.fda.gov

Civil Rights Act of 1964, 42 USC 2000e, Title VI: 45 CFR 80.

Engelman Lado, M. (2001, Summer). Unfinished agenda: The need for civil rights litigation to address race discrimination and inequalities in health care delivery. *Texas Forum on Civil Liberties and Civil Rights, 6.1.*

Goldman v. Weinberger, Secretary of Defense, et al., 475 US 503 (1986).

Griswold v. Connecticut, 381 US 479 (1965).

Muller, J. H., & Desmond, B. (1992, September). Ethical dilemmas in a cross-cultural context: A Chinese example [Special issue]. In *Cross-cultural medicine: A decade later. The Western Journal of Medicine, 157*, 323–347.

People v. Lee Wah, 71 C. 80 (1886).

People v. Machado, 99 CA 702 (1929).

Plessy v. Ferguson, 163 US 537 (1896).

Preston, P. (1997). Hospitals and civil rights, 1945–1963: The case of Simkins v. Moses H. Cone Memorial Hospital. *Annals of Internal Medicine, 126*(11), 899–906.

Rhor, M. (2008, January 23). Folk medicines pose poison risk. *The San Francisco Chronicle*, p. A8.

Saint Francis College v. Al-Khazraji, 481 US 604 (1987).

Simkins v. Moses H. Cone Memorial Hospital, 323 F.2d 959 (1963).

The Joint Commission. (2007). *Requirements related to the provision of culturally and linguistically appropriate health care*. Retrieved July 10, 2008, from http://www.jointcommission.org/NR/rdonlyres/ 6941959E-D4BE-48D7-A2F8-A4834E84B263/0/JC_Standards_Document_2008.pdf.

US Commission on Civil Rights. (2004a, January 6). *Guidance to Federal Financial Assistance recipients regarding Title VI Prohibition Against National Origin Discrimination Affecting Limited English*

Proficient Persons. Retrieved March 25, 2009, from http://www.hhs.gov/ocr/civilrights/resources/specialtopics/lep/policyguidancedocument.html

US Commission on Civil Rights. (2004b, September). *Ten-year check-up: Have federal agencies responded to civil rights recommendations?* Retrieved July 23, 2008, from http://www.usccr.gov/pubs/10yr04/10yr04.pdf

US Department of Health and Human Services, Office of Minority Health. (2000). National Standards for Culturally and Linguistically Appropriate Services (CLAS) in Health Care. *Federal Register,* *65*(247), 80865–80879.

US Department of Health and Human Services, Office for Civil Rights. (2006a, June). *Your rights under the community service assurance provision of the Hill-Burton Act.* Retrieved May 22, 2008, from http://www.hhs.gov/ocr/civilrights/resources/factsheets/hillburton.pdf

US Department of Health and Human Services, Office for Civil Rights. (2006b, June). *Your rights under Title VI of the Civil Rights Act of 1964.* Retrieved May 22, 2008, from http.//www.hhs.gov/ocr/civilrights/resources/factsheets/yourrightsundertitleviofthecivilrightsact.pdf

US Department of Health and Human Services, OPHS, Office of Minority Health. (2001, March). *National standards for culturally and linguistically appropriate services in health care, final report.* Retrieved July 21, 2008, from www.omhrc.gov/assets/pdf/checked/finalreport.pdf

Watson, S. (1997). Race, ethnicity and hospital care: The need for racial and ethnic data. *Hospital Law,* *30,* 125.

Watson, S. (2001). Race, ethnicity and quality of care: Inequalities and incentives. *American Journal of Law and Medicine,* *27,* 203.

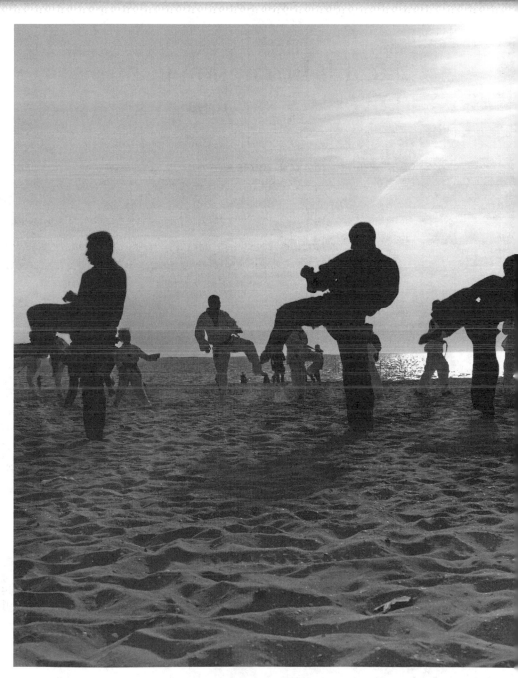

CHAPTER 6

Health Promotion in Diverse Societies

People who are Promotores(as) *have a gift for service and a noble and kind heart. We think about things and take care of people. We identify with the people and the needs of the community.*

—Mirian Perez, *Promotora*

There is a push, sometimes—"what's the recipe" or "what are the ten things you have to do in every multicultural community." My experience says that there is a contextualization that needs to happen.

—Zoe Cardoza Clayson

KEY CONCEPTS

- Fotonovela
- Digital divide
- Promotores
- Multicultural evaluation
- Reciprocity

CHAPTER OBJECTIVES

1. Describe the Health Belief and PRECEDE–PROCEED Models and how they can be utilized when working with diverse populations.
2. Explain at least three ways to deliver health information.
3. Identify at least four issues to consider when developing printed materials.
4. Describe at least three differences between traditional evaluation and multicultural evaluation.

Public health is focused on health promotion and disease and injury prevention through research, community intervention, and education. To accomplish these goals, health promotion activities need to be delivered within a cultural context. One-size-fits-all health promotion programs fail to take into consideration that there are unique ideals and goals regarding health and various ways to initiate health behavior change.

Health education and promotion programs for diverse populations are a challenge, but to be successful, the cultural dimensions of the target audience must be considered.

In this chapter we focus on program development, implementation, and evaluation. We begin with a discussion about models that can be used for developing a health promotion program. Then we discuss the development and delivery of your health message and multicultural evaluation. Program planning, implementation, and evaluation are the basis of any health promotion effort, but in this chapter we will pay special attention to considerations that need to be taken into account when working with diverse populations.

PROGRAM PLANNING FOR DIVERSE AUDIENCES

Interventions for promoting health and disease prevention in any population requires systematic planning. This organized effort requires an understanding of the culture of the target audience, because culture is a strong force in the determinants of health and behavior change. Although the overall steps to program development are the same, there are distinct factors that need to be taken into consideration when your audience is diverse. We begin with presenting models that can be used to create the frame for your program.

Planning Models

Models and theories are program-planning tools that assist with understanding the causes of behaviors, predicting behaviors, and evaluating the programs. Previous models focused more on the individual in isolation, but the more recent models take into consideration the social and physical environments.

Models are the starting place on which to build, and they can serve different purposes, which is why so many models exist. Promoting health in a multicultural setting requires using models that take the cultural context into consideration. There are numerous planning models, but only two are briefly described here, the Health Belief Model and the PRECEDE–PROCEED model, because an in-depth discussion of program planning models is not within the scope of this book.

Health Belief Model

The Health Belief Model (HBM) is a psychological model that attempts to explain and predict health behaviors by focusing on the attitudes and beliefs of individuals. The HBM was developed in the 1950s as part of an effort by social psychologists in the U.S. Public Health Service to explain the lack of public participation in health screening and prevention programs (e.g., a free and conveniently located tuberculosis screening project). Their focus was on increasing the use of preventive services, such as chest x-rays for tuberculosis screening and immunizations.

The developers assumed that people feared diseases and that health actions were motivated in relation to the degree of fear (perceived threat). They expected that if the potential benefits outweighed practical and psychological obstacles to taking action (net benefits), then action would occur. The Health Belief Model was one of the first models that adapted theory from the behavioral sciences to health problems, and it remains one of the most widely recognized conceptual frameworks of health behavior. The HBM has been adapted to explore a variety of long- and short-term health behaviors, including sexual risk behaviors and the transmission of HIV–AIDS. The key variables of the HBM are as follows:

- *Perceived threat.* Consists of two parts: perceived susceptibility and perceived severity of a health condition
- *Perceived susceptibility.* One's subjective perception of the risk of developing a particular health condition
- *Perceived severity.* Feelings about the seriousness of the consequences of developing a specific health condition
- *Perceived benefits.* Beliefs about the effectiveness of various actions that might reduce susceptibility and severity of a health condition
- *Perceived barriers.* Potential negative aspects from taking particular health actions, including physical, psychological, and financial demands
- *Cues to action.* Bodily or environmental events that trigger action
- *Self-efficacy.* The belief in being able to successfully execute the behavior required to produce the desired outcomes

It is important to note that a wide variety of demographic (i.e., age, gender, ethnicity, race), social and psychological (i.e., personality, social status, group pressure), and structural variables (i.e., prior experience with the disease, knowledge about the health condition) also may impact people's perceptions and then indirectly impact their health behaviors. Ways that these constructs can be applied are described in Table 6.1.

The Health Belief Model can be applied to multicultural health in several ways. For example, if a person has a fatalistic perception of how disease develops, the program planner would have to work with that ideology because that person's idea about perceived susceptibility would be very different than a person with a Western perspective.

TABLE 6.1	**Applications of the Health Belief Model**	
Concept	**Definition**	**Application**
Perceived susceptibility	One's opinion of chances of getting a condition.	Define population(s) at risk and the degree of risk. Personalize risk based on a person's features or behavior. Heighten perceived susceptibility if it is too low.
Perceived severity	One's opinion of how serious a condition and the condition that follows are as a result of the disease.	Explain the consequences of the risk and the condition.
Perceived benefits	One's opinion of the benefits of the action to reduce risk or seriousness of impact.	Clarify the positive effects to be expected from the behavior change.
Perceived barriers	One's opinion of the tangible and psychological costs of the advised action.	Identify and reduce barriers through reassurance, incentives, education, and assistance.
Cues to action	Strategies to activate change.	Provide how-to information, promote awareness, initiate media campaigns, write a newspaper or magazine article, provide reminders such as a postcard from a dentist or physician, obtain a friend's or family member's recommendation.
Self-efficacy	Confidence in one's ability to take action.	Provide training, guidance in performing action, and role modeling.

Source: Adapted from The Communication Initiative Network. (2003).

Precede–Proceed

The PRECEDE–PROCEED framework, illustrated in Figure 6.1, is an approach to planning that examines the factors that contribute to behavior change. PRECEDE is an acronym for **P**redisposing, **R**einforcing, and **E**nabling **C**onstructs in **E**ducational/**E**cological **D**iagnosis and **E**valuation, and PROCEED is an acronym for **P**olicy,

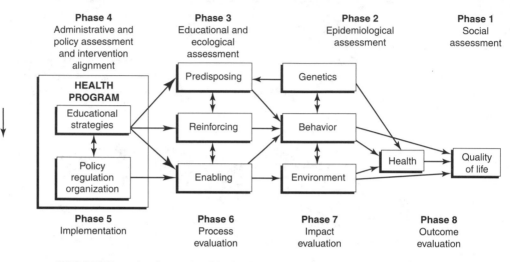

FIGURE 6.1   PRECEDE–PROCEED Model.
Source: Reprinted with permission from The Community Toolbox. (2007).

Regulatory, and **O**rganizational **C**onstructs in **E**ducational and **E**nvironmental **D**evelopment (McKenzie, Neiger, & Thackeray, 2009). These factors that contribute to behavior change are as follows:

- *Predisposing factors.* The individual's knowledge, attitudes, behavior, beliefs, and values before the intervention that affect their willingness to change
- *Enabling factors.* Factors in the environment or community of an individual that facilitate change
- *Reinforcing factors.* The positive or negative effects of adopting the behavior that influence continuing the behavior

The PRECEDE part of the model entails the planning steps that should occur prior to the intervention, and the PROCEED component includes the phases that should occur during and after the intervention. The eight phases of the framework are as follows:

- PRECEDE (the first four phases)
  - *Phase 1.* Social assessment
  - *Phase 2.* Epidemiological assessment

- *Phase 3.* Educational and ecological diagnosis
- *Phase 4.* Administrative and policy assessment and intervention alignment

- PROCEED (the second four phases)
  - *Phase 5.* Implementation
  - *Phase 6.* Process evaluation
  - *Phase 7.* Impact evaluation
  - *Phase 8.* Outcome evaluation

IMPLEMENTING YOUR HEALTH PROMOTION PROGRAM

Now that you have your framework for your health promotion program, you need to consider how you are going to deliver your message. There is a vast selection of ways to deliver your message (i.e., print materials, billboards, Internet, radio) and just as many options for settings (i.e., work sites, schools, barber shops, churches). But what message and what setting works best with difference cultures?

Public health programs are delivered to a wide audience, and you need to plan to deliver your program in a manner in which it will be well received and will promote behavior change. This entails considering the content of your message as well as how it is delivered. We begin this section with a discussion about health communication, which is about the content of your message. Then we move into how that message can be delivered.

Health Communication

The information in this section is adapted from *Making Health Communication Programs Work*, published by the U.S. Department of Health and Human Services (2001).

Almost all health promotion programs require communication, so it is an important component of program planning and delivery. Health communication encompasses the study and use of communication strategies to inform and influence individual and community decisions that enhance health. It links the domains of communication and health and is increasingly recognized as a necessary element of efforts to improve personal and public health. Health communication can contribute to all aspects of disease prevention and health promotion and is relevant in a number of contexts, including (1) health professional–patient relations, (2) individuals' exposure to, search for, and use of health information, (3) individuals' adherence to clinical recommendations and regimens, (4) the construction of public health messages and campaigns, (5) the dissemination of individual and population health risk information, that is, risk communication, (6) images of health in the mass media and the culture at large, (7) the education of consumers about how to gain access to the public health and health care systems, and (8) the development of telehealth applications.

Effective health communication can help raise awareness of health risks and solutions, provide the motivation and skills needed to reduce these risks, help them find support from other people in similar situations, and affect or reinforce attitudes. Health communication also can increase demand for appropriate health services and decrease demand for inappropriate health services. It can make available information to assist in making complex choices, such as selecting health plans, care providers, and treatments. For the community, health communication can be used to influence the public agenda, advocate for policies and programs, promote positive changes in the socioeconomic and physical environments, improve the delivery of public health and health care services, and encourage social norms that benefit health and quality of life.

The practice of health communication has contributed to health promotion and disease prevention in several areas. One is the improvement of interpersonal and group interactions in clinical situations (for example, provider–patient, provider–provider, and among members of a health care team) through the training of health professionals and patients in effective communication skills. Collaborative relationships are enhanced when all parties are capable of good communication.

Another area is the dissemination of health messages through public education campaigns that seek to change the social climate to encourage healthy behaviors, create awareness, change attitudes, and motivate individuals to adopt recommended behaviors. Campaigns traditionally have relied on mass communication (such as public service announcements on billboards, radio, and television) and educational messages in printed materials (such as pamphlets) to deliver health messages. Other campaigns have integrated mass media with community-based programs. Many campaigns have used social marketing techniques. Social marketing is the systematic application of marketing used to achieve specific behavioral goals for a social good. Table 6.2 provides a list of attributes of effective health communication.

Increasingly, health improvement activities are taking advantage of digital technologies, such as CD-ROMs and the World Wide Web (Web), that can target audiences, tailor messages, and engage people in interactive, ongoing exchanges about health. As a result, an emerging area is health communication to support community-centered prevention. Community-centered prevention shifts attention from individual- to group-level change and emphasizes the empowerment of individuals and communities to effect change on multiple levels.

The promotion of regular physical activity, healthy weight, good nutrition, and responsible sexual behavior requires a range of information, education, and advocacy

TABLE 6.2 Attributes of Effective Health Communication

- **Accuracy:** The content is valid and without errors of fact, interpretation, or judgment.

- **Availability:** The content (whether targeted message or other information) is delivered or placed where the audience can access it. Placement varies according to audience, message complexity, and purpose, ranging from interpersonal and social networks to billboards and mass transit signs to prime-time TV or radio, to public kiosks (print or electronic), to the Internet.

- **Balance:** Where appropriate, the content presents the benefits and risks of potential actions or recognizes different and valid perspectives on the issue.

- **Consistency:** The content remains internally consistent over time and also is consistent with information from other sources (the latter is a problem when other widely available content is not accurate or reliable).

- **Cultural competence:** The design, implementation, and evaluation process that accounts for special issues for select population groups (for example, ethnic, racial, and linguistic) and also educational levels and disability.

- **Evidence base:** Relevant scientific evidence that has undergone comprehensive review and rigorous analysis to formulate practice guidelines, performance measures, review criteria, and technology assessments for telehealth applications.

- **Reach:** The content gets to or is available to the largest possible number of people in the target population.

- **Reliability:** The source of the content is credible, and the content itself is kept up to date.

- **Repetition:** The delivery of/access to the content is continued or repeated over time, both to reinforce the impact with a given audience and to reach new generations.

- **Timeliness:** The content is provided or available when the audience is most receptive to, or in need of, the specific information.

- **Understandability:** The reading or language level and format (including multimedia) are appropriate for the specific audience.

Source: U.S. Department of Health and Human Services. (2001).

efforts, as does the reduction of tobacco use, substance abuse, injuries, and violence. For example, advocacy efforts to change prices and availability of tobacco and alcohol products have resulted in lower consumption levels. Effective counseling and patient education for behavior change require health care providers and patients to have good communication skills. Public information campaigns are used to promote increased fruit and vegetable consumption (such as the Fruits & Veggies—More Matters campaign), higher rates of preventive screening (such as mammograms and colonoscopies), higher rates of clinical preventive services (such as immunizations), and greater rates of adoption of risk-reducing behaviors (such as the Back to Sleep and *Buckle Up America!* campaigns).

Health communication alone, however, cannot change systemic problems related to health, such as poverty, environmental degradation, or lack of access to health care, but comprehensive health communication programs should include a systematic exploration of all the factors that contribute to health and the strategies that could be used to influence these factors. Well-designed health communication activities help individuals better understand their own and their communities' needs so that they can take appropriate actions to maximize health.

The environment for communicating about health has changed significantly. These changes include dramatic increases in the number of communication channels and the number of health issues vying for public attention, as well as consumer demands for more and better quality health information and the increased sophistication of marketing and sales techniques, such as direct-to-consumer advertising of prescription drugs and sales of medical devices and medications over the Internet. The expansion of communication channels and health issues on the public agenda increases competition for people's time and attention; at the same time, people have more opportunities to select information based on their personal interests and preferences. The trend toward commercialization of the Internet suggests that the marketing model of other mass media will be applied to emerging media, which has important consequences for the ability of noncommercial and public-health-oriented communications to stand out in a cluttered information environment.

Communication occurs in a variety of contexts (e.g., school, home, and work); through a variety of channels (e.g., interpersonal, small group, organizational, community, and mass media) with a variety of messages; and for a variety of reasons. In such an environment, people do not pay attention to all communications they receive but selectively attend to and purposefully seek out information. One of the main challenges in the design of effective health communication programs is to identify the optimal contexts, channels, content, and reasons that will motivate people to pay attention to and use health information.

A one-dimensional approach to health promotion, such as reliance on mass media campaigns or other single-component communication activities, has been shown to be insufficient to achieve program goals. Successful health promotion efforts increasingly rely on multidimensional interventions to reach diverse audiences about complex health concerns, and communication is integrated from the beginning with other components, such as community-based programs, policy changes, and improvements in services and the health delivery system. Research shows that health communication best supports health promotion when multiple communication channels are used to reach specific audience segments with information that is appropriate and relevant to them. An important factor in the design of multidimensional programs is to allot sufficient time for planning, implementation, and evaluation and sufficient money to support the many elements of the program. Public–private partnerships and collaborations can leverage resources to strengthen the impact of multidimensional efforts. Collaboration can have the added benefit of reducing message clutter and targeting health concerns that cannot be fully addressed by public resources or market incentives alone.

Research indicates that effective health promotion and communication initiatives adopt an audience-centered perspective, which means that promotion and communication activities reflect audiences' preferred formats, channels, and contexts. These considerations are particularly relevant for racial and ethnic populations, who may have different languages and sources of information. In these cases, public education campaigns must be conceptualized and developed by individuals with specific knowledge of the cultural characteristics, media habits, and language preferences of intended audiences. Direct translation of health information or health promotion materials should be avoided. Credible channels of communication need to be identified for each major group. Television and radio stations that serve specific racial and ethnic populations can be effective means to deliver health messages when care is taken to account for the language, culture, and socioeconomic situations of intended audiences.

An audience-centered perspective also reflects the realities of people's everyday lives and their current practices, attitudes, beliefs, and lifestyles. Some specific audience characteristics that are relevant include gender, age, education and income levels, ethnicity, sexual orientation, cultural beliefs and values, primary language(s), and physical and mental functioning. Additional considerations include their experience with the health care system, attitudes toward different types of health problems, and willingness to use certain types of health services. Particular attention should be paid to the needs of underserved audience members.

Targeting specific segments of a population and tailoring messages for individual use are two methods to make health promotion activities relevant to audiences. Examples include the targeted use of mass media messages for adolescent girls at increased risk of smoking, the tailoring of computer-generated nutritional information to help individuals reduce their fat intake and increase fruit and vegetable consumption, and a national telephone service for Spanish speakers to obtain AIDS information as well as counseling and referrals.

Interventions that account for the cultural practices and needs of specific populations have shown some success. For example, a breastfeeding promotion program for Navajo women that was based on investigations of their cultural beliefs about infant feeding practices showed increased rates of breastfeeding. Similarly, an intervention that used the **fotonovela**, a popular form of Latino mass media, to reach young people and their parents sought to improve parent–youth communication in Hispanic families and to influence the adolescents' attitudes about alcohol.

Advances in medical and consumer health informatics are changing the delivery of health information and services and are likely to have a growing impact on individual and community health. The convergence of media (computers, telephones, television, radio, video, print, and audio) and the emergence of the Internet create a nearly ubiquitous networked communication infrastructure. This infrastructure facilitates access to an increasing array of health information and health-related support services and extends the reach of health communication efforts. Delivery channels, such as the Internet, expand the choices available for health professionals to reach patients and consumers and for patients and consumers to interact with health professionals and with one another (e.g., in online support groups).

Compared to traditional mass media, interactive media may have several advantages for health communication efforts. These advantages include (1) improved access to personalized health information, (2) access to health information, support, and services on demand, (3) enhanced ability to distribute materials widely and update content or functions rapidly, (4) just-in-time expert decision support, and (5) more choices for consumers. The health impact of interactivity, customization, and enhanced multimedia is just beginning to be explored, and already interactive health communication technologies are being used to exchange information, facilitate informed decision making, promote healthy behaviors, enhance peer and emotional support, promote self-care, manage demand for health services, and support clinical care.

Widespread availability and use of interactive health communication and telehealth applications create at least two serious challenges. One is related to the risks associated with consumers' use of poor quality health information to make decisions. Concerns are growing about the Web making available large amounts of information that may be misleading, inaccurate, or inappropriate, which may put consumers at unnecessary risk. Although many health professionals agree that the Internet is a boon for consumers because they have easier access to much more information than before, professionals also are concerned that the poor quality of a lot of information on the Web will undermine informed decision making. These concerns are driving the development of a quality standards agenda to help health professionals and consumers find reliable Web sites and health information on the Internet. An expert panel convened by the U.S. Department of Health and Human Services describes high quality health information as accurate, current, valid, appropriate, intelligible, and free of bias.

The other challenge is related to the protection of privacy and confidentiality of personal health information, which are major issues for consumers, and these concerns are magnified when information is collected, stored, and made available online. As the availability and variety of interactive health applications grow, consumer confidence about developers' ability or intent to ensure privacy will be challenged. In the near future, personal health information will be collected during both clinical and nonclinical encounters in disparate settings, such as schools, mobile clinics, public places, and homes, and will be made available for administrative, financial, clinical, and research purposes. Although public health and health services research may require anonymous personal health information, policies and procedures to protect privacy will need to ensure a balance between confidentiality and appropriate access to personal health information.

The trend of rapidly expanding opportunities in health communication intersects with recent demands for more rigorous evaluation of all aspects of the health care and public health delivery systems and for evidence-based practices. Numerous studies of provider–patient communication support the connection among the quality of the provider–patient interaction, patient behavior, and health outcomes. As the knowledge base about provider–patient interactions increases, a need becomes apparent for the development of practice guidelines to promote better provider–patient communication. Additional evidence about the process of health information seeking and the role of health information in decision making also is needed. Health communication campaigns could benefit as well from more rigorous formative research and evaluation of outcomes. Expected outcomes should be an important consideration and central element of campaign design. Because health communication increasingly involves electronic media, new evaluation approaches are emerging. Given the critical role that communication plays in all aspects of public health and health care, health communication and outcomes research should become more tightly linked across all health communication domains.

Health-conscious consumers increasingly are proactive in seeking out health information. Individuals want information about prevention and wellness as much as about medical problems. Public health and the medical community share an interest in promoting—and sustaining—informed decisions for better health. Surveys suggest that people want to get health information from a professional and that counseling by health professionals can be effective both in reducing lifestyle risks and supporting self-management of chronic diseases like diabetes. However, diminished time in clinical visits and some clinicians' discomfort with open communication work against optimum information exchange. In addition, many people want information to be available when and where they need it most. Health information should be easily accessible, of good quality, and relevant for the needs of the person. The increasing use of the Internet as a source for health information will require greater awareness of the importance of the quality of information.

Often people with the greatest health burdens have the least access to information, communication technologies, health care, and supporting social services. Even the most carefully designed health communication programs will have limited impact if underserved communities lack access to crucial health professionals, services, and communication channels that are part of a health improvement project. Research indicates that even after targeted health communication interventions, low-education and low-income groups remain less knowledgeable and less likely to change behavior than higher education and income groups, which creates a knowledge gap and leaves some people chronically uninformed. With communication technologies, the disparity in access to electronic information resources is commonly referred to as the **digital divide**, which becomes more critical as the amount and variety of health resources available over the Internet increase and as people need more sophisticated skills to use electronic resources. Equitably distributed health communication resources and skills and a robust communication infrastructure can contribute to the closing of the digital divide and the overarching goal of *Healthy People 2010* to eliminate health disparities.

Even with access to information and services, disparities may still exist, because many people lack health literacy, which is increasingly vital to help people navigate a complex health care system and better manage their own health. Differences in the ability to read and understand materials related to personal health as well as navigate the health system appear to contribute to health disparities. People with low health literacy are more likely to report poor health, have an incomplete understanding of their health problems and treatment, and be at greater risk of hospitalization. The average annual health care costs of persons with very low literacy (reading at the grade two level or below) may be four times greater than for the general population. An estimated 75% of persons in the United States with chronic physical or mental health problems are in the limited literacy category. People with chronic conditions, such as asthma, hypertension, and diabetes, and with low reading skills have been found to have less knowledge of their conditions than people with higher reading skills.

Although the majority of people with marginal or low literacy are white native-born Americans, changing demographics suggest that low literacy is an increasing problem among certain racial and ethnic groups, non-English-speaking populations, and persons over age 65 years. One study of Medicare enrollees found that 34% of English speakers and 54% of Spanish speakers had inadequate or marginal health literacy. As the United States population ages, low health literacy among elderly people is potentially a large problem. Nearly half of the people in the elderly population have low reading skills, and reading ability appears to decline with age. A study of patients 60 years and older at a public hospital found that 81% could not read and understand basic materials such as prescription labels and appointments.

For health communication to contribute to the improvement of personal and community health stakeholders, including health professionals, researchers, public officials, and the lay public, must collaborate on a range of activities. These activities include (1) initiatives to build a robust health information system that provides equitable access, (2) development of high-quality, audience-appropriate information and support services for specific health problems and health-related decisions for all segments of the population, especially underserved persons, (3) training of health professionals in the science of communication and the use of communication technologies, (4) evaluation of interventions, and (5) promotion of a critical understanding and practice of effective health communication.

Health communication is a new focus area for *Healthy People 2010*. One of the objectives is to increase the proportion of households with access to the Internet at home. Although the proportion of people with access to the Internet has risen dramatically since 1995, many segments of the population lack access, such as low-income and rural households; persons with less education; and certain racial and ethnic groups, such as African Americans and Hispanics. Internet access rates vary considerably according to income. Barriers to Internet access include cost, lack of services in certain communities, limited literacy, lack of familiarity with different technologies, and, especially for people with disabilities, inaccessible formats that limit appropriate and effective technology use. Initiatives to promote universal access to the Internet will involve public and private sector stakeholders, particularly government agencies, and technology corporations.

Responses from the National Adult Literacy Survey indicate that approximately 90 million adults in the United States have inadequate or marginal literacy skills. Written information is not the only way to communicate about health, but a great deal of health education and promotion are organized around the use of print materials, usually written at the tenth grade level and above. These materials are of little use to people who have limited literacy skills. The result is that a very large segment of the population is denied the full benefits of health information and services.

Closing the gap in health literacy is an issue of fundamental fairness and equity and is essential to reduce health disparities. Public and private efforts need to occur in two areas: the development of appropriate written materials and improvement in skills of those persons with limited literacy. The knowledge exists to create effective, culturally and linguistically appropriate, plain language health communications.

Professional publications and federal documents provide the criteria to integrate and apply the principles of organization, writing style, layout, and design for effective communication. These criteria should be widely distributed and used. Many organizations, such as public and medical libraries; voluntary, professional, and community groups; and schools, could offer health literacy programs that target skill improvement for low-literacy and limited-English-proficient individuals. If appropriate materials exist and people receive the training to use them, then measurable improvements in health literacy for the least literate can occur.

With the rapidly growing volume of health information, advertising, products, and services available on World Wide Web sites, serious concerns arise regarding the accuracy, appropriateness, and potential health impact of these sites. People are using the Internet to look up information, purchase medications, consult remotely with providers, and maintain their personal health records. The potential for harm from inaccurate information, inferior quality goods, and inappropriate services is significant. Many initiatives are under way to identify appropriate and feasible approaches to evaluate online health sites. Professional associations are issuing guidelines and recommendations. Federal agencies, such as the Federal Trade Commission, are actively monitoring and sanctioning owners of Web sites that are false or misleading, and developers and purchasers of online health resources are being urged to adopt standards for quality assurance.

To allow users to evaluate the quality and appropriateness of Internet health resources, health-related Web sites should publicly disclose the following essential information about their site: (1) the identity of the developers and sponsors of the site (and how to contact them) and information about any potential conflicts of interest or biases, (2) the explicit purpose of the site, including any commercial purposes and advertising, (3) the original sources of the content on the site, (4) how the privacy and confidentiality of any personal information collected from users is protected, (5) how the site is evaluated, and (6) how the content is updated. An additional mark of quality, which should be present on a Web site, relates to the site's accessibility by all users. Contents of the site should be presented in a way that it can be used by people with disabilities and low-end technology.

Culture affects how people perceive and respond to health messages and materials, and it is related to how health behaviors and materials convey culture. Although it is important to acknowledge and understand the cultures within an intended audience, developing separate messages and materials for each cultural group is not always necessary or even advisable. For example, when print materials for a state program for low-income people depicted people of only one race, some intended audience members who were of that race felt singled out and said the materials suggested that only members of their racial group were poor. Careful intended audience research can help your program identify messages and images that resonate across groups—or identify situations in which different messages or images are likely to work best.

That being said, it does not mean that culture should be ignored. According to a Center for Substance Abuse Prevention *Technical Assistance Bulletin*, culturally sensitive communications:

1. Acknowledge culture as a predominant force in shaping behaviors, values, and institutions.
2. Understand and reflect the diversity within cultures. In designing messages that are culturally appropriate, the following dimensions are important:
   - *Primary cultural factors* linked to race, ethnicity, language, nationality, and religion
   - *Secondary cultural factors* linked to age, gender, sexual orientation, educational level, occupation, income level, and acculturation to mainstream society
3. Reflect and respect the attitudes and values of the intended audience; some examples of attitudes and values that are interrelated to culture include:
   - Whether the individual or the community is of primary importance
   - Accepted roles of men, women, and children
   - Preferred family structure (nuclear or extended)
   - Relative importance of folk wisdom, life experience, and value of common sense compared to formal-education-specific situations and advanced degrees
   - Ways that wealth is measured (material goods, personal relationships)
   - Relative value put on different age groups (youth versus elders)
   - Whether people are more comfortable with traditions or open to new ways
   - Favorite and forbidden foods
   - Body language, particularly whether touching or proximity is permitted in specific situations
   - Manner of dress and adornment
4. Refer to cultural groups using terms that members of the group prefer (e.g., many people resent the term "minority" or "nonwhite." Preferred terms are often based on nationality, such as Japanese or Lakota).
5. Substituting culturally specific images, spokespeople, language, or other executional detail is not sufficient unless the messages have been tested and found to resonate with the intended audience.
6. Use the language of the intended audience, carefully developed and tested with the involvement of the audience (US DHHS, 2001).

You may have a message that you want to target to a particular cultural group in which you need to take specific cultural factors into consideration. For example, say you have developed a suicide prevention hotline for Asian Americans, which provides services in a variety of Asian languages. You would not want to use a number in the hotline number that means death in any of the Asian cultures. Colors also have a wide variety of meanings in different cultures, so do your research. Also, some cultures do not respond well to health messages that try to induce change through fear, so be cautious of the images that you use. Of course, be sure to deliver your message in the appropriate language(s) and literacy levels.

DELIVERING YOUR HEALTH MESSAGE

There are copious ways to deliver your health message. Some methods have been shown to work better with specific cultures. For example, promotores(as) programs have been shown to be successful with the Hispanic population, and ethnic newspapers have been shown to work well with elder Asian Americans. It is important to look for model programs (also known as promising practices) when designing your implementation strategy. The following are a few types of interventions that you may not be familiar with that have been shown to be popular among certain ethnic groups, along with information about more traditional approaches.

Promotores

Promotores and promotoras are community members who promote health in their own communities. They provide leadership, peer education, and resources to support community empowerment (Migrant Health Promotion, 2005). As members of minority and underserved populations, they are in a unique position to build on strengths and to address unmet health needs in their communities. Promotores(as) integrate information about health and the health care system into the community's culture, language, and value system, thus reducing many of the barriers to health services. They provide peer education, support, and links to services. They also help make health care systems more responsive. With the appropriate resources, training, and support, promotores(as) improve the health of their communities by linking their neighbors to health care and social services, by educating their peers about disease and injury prevention, by working to make available services more accessible, and by mobilizing their communities to create positive change.

Organizations may refer to promotores(as) as "promotores(as) de salud," which literally means "health promoters." In English, most promotores(as) call themselves community health workers. There are many additional terms, including:

- Camp health aides
- Colonia health workers
- Lay health advisors
- Outreach workers
- Community health representatives
- Indigenous or village health workers

According to the National Community Health Advisor Study, approximately 600 programs collaborated with 12,500 promotores(as) in 1998, and the numbers continue to grow (Migrant Health Promotion, 2005).

Promotores(as) conduct outreach in places such as clients' homes, community centers, clinics, hospitals, schools, work sites, shelters, and farmworker labor camps. Many promotor(a) programs focus on serving the needs of specific ethnic or racial groups, and others focus on vulnerable segments of the population or prominent health problems. Although promotores(as) engage in a broad range of activities, they share a number of common roles. Promotores(as) provide the following (Migrant Health Promotion, 2005):

- A link between communities and health and human service agencies
- Informal counseling and support
- Culturally competent health education
- Advocacy
- Capacity building on individual and community levels
- First aid and emergency assistance

Promotores(as) effectively address many barriers to better health for underserved populations. Some of their accomplishments include (Migrant Health Promotion, 2005):

- Improving access to services
- Helping people understand the health and social service system
- Enhancing client and health provider communication
- Increasing appropriate rates of service utilization
- Decreasing costs for organizations and government programs
- Improving adherence to health recommendations
- Reducing the need for emergency and specialty services
- Improving overall community health status

Promotores(as) accomplish these and other outcomes by providing education and advocacy and building capacity in their communities (Migrant Health Promotion, 2005).

Fotonovelas

Fotonovelas are imaged-based interventions that have been very popular among Mexicans and Latin Americans. Fotonovelas also are known as "historietas," but technically the fotonovela is illustrated with photos and the historieta employs drawings; however the two terms often are used interchangeably (Independent Television Service, 2008). These comic books with complex perspectives and dark imagery have had a long history and far-reaching impact within the Latino and Chicano communities in the United States as well as Mexico and Latin America, where they continue to thrive in the popular culture (Independent Television Service, 2008).

In the United States, the fotonovela/historieta has a distinct manifestation in the Chicano/Latino community, providing a unique idiom through which the community addresses social concerns using a highly innovative visual language (Independent Television Service, 2008). Because of its popularity and flexibility, the fotonovela has been used in increasingly fresh ways by visual artists and writers to address important social issues within the Chicano/Latino community (Independent Television Service, 2008). Activists and religious groups also have turned to the form as an organizational tool for outreach and education, and to induce someone to convert to their own religious faith or political party. Fotonovelas are becoming more commonly used in public health as a way of delivering health information in a more creative manner. A representative from the Rural Women's Health Project (RWHP) stated, "RWHP fotonovelas reflect the struggles of communities in a positive light, incorporating role models who balance socio-cultural obstacles and disease prevention. The visual aspects of the novela are enticing and the style allows the reader to explore the health topics, increase self-identification and risk, and strengthen cultural identity" (Rural Women's Health Project, n.d.).

According to RWHP, the organization utilizes community actors and messages specific to the target community, and the fotonovelas successfully present health messages, document the work of communities, and unify them to both improve individual and community well-being. "The minimal text, popular language, and visuals of the fotonovelas allow them to be easily read by any community. These elements make fotonovelas an excellent educational tool for outreach workers, youth, and discussion groups" (Rural Women's Health Project, n.d.).

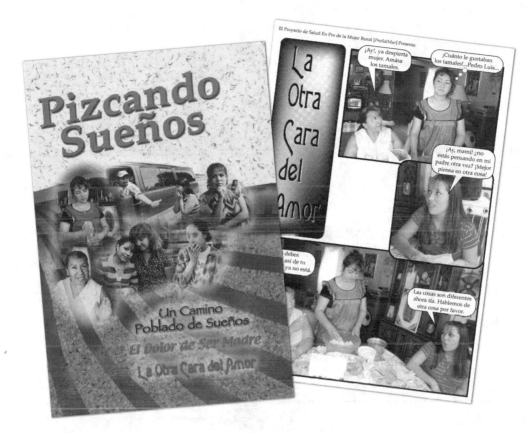

Source: Reprinted with permission from Rural Women's Health Project.

Printed Materials

Printed materials can be created in numerous forms, including newsletters, booklets, pamphlets, flyers, and newspapers. They can be placed on billboards, bathroom walls, and buses, or they can be inserted in envelopes with paychecks. Regardless of where they are, be sure that they are appropriate for your target audience.

Some issues to consider are literacy levels and language. You can check the literacy level by using the Fry Readability Graph (see Figure 6.2) or the Flesch-Kincaid Grade Level score, which is built into Microsoft Word.

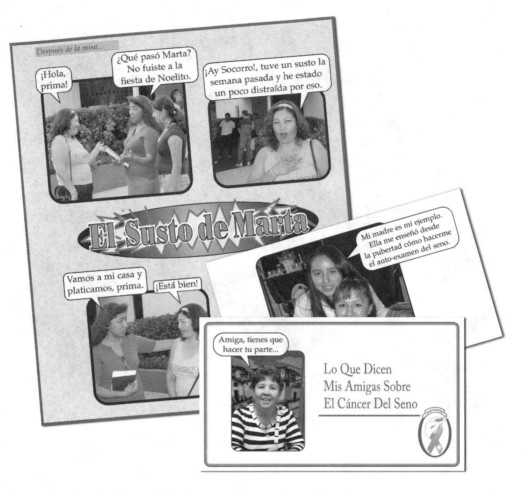

Source: Reprinted with permission from Rural Women's Health Project.

Fry Readability Graph

Directions for Use of the Fry Readability Graph

- Randomly select three 100-word passages from a book or an article.
- Plot the average number of syllables and the average number of sentences per 100 words on the graph to determine the grade level of the material.
- Choose more passages per book if great variability is observed and conclude that the book has uneven readability.
- Few books will fall into the solid black area, but when they do, grade level scores are invalid.

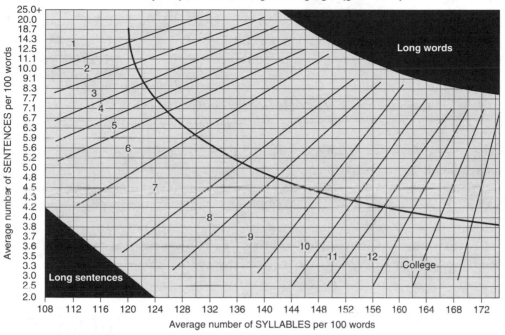

FIGURE 6.2 Fry Readability Graph.
Source: Discovery Education. (1995).

Additional Directions for Working Readability Graph

- Randomly select three sample passages and count exactly 100 words beginning with the beginning of a sentence. Don't count numbers. Do count proper nouns.
- Count the number of sentences in the hundred words, estimating length of the fraction of the last sentence to the nearest 1/10th.
- Count the total number of syllables in the 100-word passage. If you do not have a hand counter available, an easy way is to simply put a mark above every syllable over one in each word, then, when you get to the end of the passage, count the number of marks and add 100.
- Enter graph with average sentence length and number of syllables; plot dot where the two lines intersect. Area where dot is plotted will give you the approximate grade level.
- If a great deal of variability is found, putting more sample counts into the average is desirable (Discovery Education, 1995).

Flesch-Kincaid Grade Level Score in Microsoft Word

You also can check the readability level of a passage using the Flesch-Kincaid Grade Level score, which is built into the newer versions of Microsoft Word. In Word XP, to display readability statistics, use the following steps:

1. On the *Tools* menu, click *Options*, and click the *Spelling & Grammar* tab.
2. Select the *Show readability statistics* check box, and then click *OK*.
3. On the *Tools* menu, click *Spelling and Grammar*.

When Word finishes checking spelling and grammar, it displays information about the reading level of the document.

You also will want to consider visual readability. For example, fonts should be made larger and an appropriate amount of white space should be included when seniors are your target audience. Images are an important component of printed materials.

After you have delivered your message, you need to evaluate your program for several reasons, including determining its effectiveness.

EVALUATION IN A MULTICULTURAL SETTING

Effective program evaluation is a systematic way to improve and account for public health actions by involving procedures that are useful, feasible, ethical, and accurate. The Centers for Disease Control and Prevention (CDC) developed a framework to guide public health professionals in using program evaluations. It is a practical, non-prescriptive tool designed to summarize and organize the essential elements of program evaluation. The framework comprises steps in evaluation practice and standards for effective evaluation (see Figure 6.3).

The framework is composed of six steps that must be taken in any evaluation. They are starting points for tailoring an evaluation to a particular public health effort at a particular time. Because the steps are all interdependent, they might be encountered in a nonlinear sequence; however, an order exists for fulfilling each—earlier steps provide the foundation for subsequent progress. The steps are as follows (Centers for Disease Control and Prevention, 1999):

Step 1. Engage stakeholders.
Step 2. Describe the program.
Step 3. Focus the evaluation design.
Step 4. Gather credible evidence.
Step 5. Justify conclusions.
Step 6. Ensure, use, and share lessons learned.

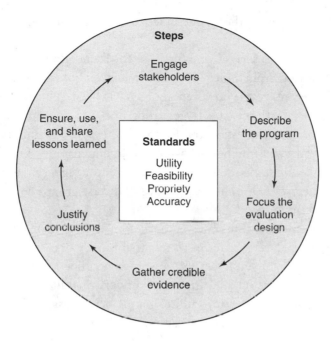

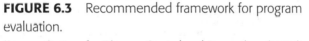

FIGURE 6.3   Recommended framework for program evaluation.

Source: Centers for Disease Control and Prevention. (1999).

Evaluation is a large subject and will not be covered in detail here because there are many other resources on the topic. For general information on public health evaluation, we suggest that you review the document "Framework for Program Evaluation in Public Health," which was developed by the Centers for Disease Control and Prevention. There are numerous other sources as well.

The focus of this section is to illuminate the differences between traditional evaluation and **multicultural evaluation** and to present strategies for making your program evaluation sensitive to diverse populations. The information in this section includes excerpts from a document produced by The California Endowment in 2005 titled *Commissioning Multicultural Evaluation: A Foundation Resource Guide* (Inouye, Yu, & Adefuin). Other resources from The California Endowment on the topic include *Voices from the Field: Health and Evaluation Leaders on Multicultural Evaluation* (2003), which offers different perspectives on multicultural evaluation and how to advance this approach in the health field, and *Multicultural Health Evaluation: An Annotated Bibliography*, which highlights key literature on the theory and practice of multicultural evaluation (Adefuin & Endo; 2003).

Evaluation has come to serve a vital function for foundations, policy makers, and programs as they rely on evaluation as a tool for management, strategic planning, and accountability. In recent years, however, there have been critical questions raised about how existing evaluation is still largely rooted in a Eurocentric worldview. Researchers are beginning to question the extent that existing evaluation frameworks and measures present valid findings across multiple dimensions of diversity, such as race, ethnicity, economic status, gender, sexual orientation, age, religion, disability, or immigration status. How can the cultural contexts of diverse groups be better integrated in evaluation theory and practice?

Multicultural evaluation integrates cultural considerations into its theory, measures, analysis, and practice. It requires conceptual frameworks that incorporate different worldviews and value systems, engages in data collection strategies that take into account potential cultural and linguistic barriers, includes a reexamination of established evaluation measures for cultural appropriateness, and/or incorporates creative strategies for ensuring culturally competent analysis and creative dissemination of findings to diverse audiences. Multicultural evaluation, like traditional evaluation, prioritizes impartial inquiry designed to provide information to decision makers and other parties interested in a particular program, policy, or intervention. In addition, multicultural evaluation aims to:

- Demystify issues of cultural difference so that relevant, culturally-based knowledge can be brought to bear in problem solving and strategic planning
- Distinguish the effects of race and ethnicity, immigrant status, age, socioeconomic factors, gender, sexual orientation, etc
- Build diverse community members' and target populations' capacities for self-assessing community needs, cultural resources, and solutions

As much as principles stand as a professional cornerstone to create standards of excellence, a widely adopted set of principles for multicultural evaluation has not yet been formalized within the evaluation field. At the same time, philanthropic leaders, scholars, evaluators, practitioners, and others are beginning to unite around a common set of principles for multicultural evaluation. A synthesis of some of the key principles includes:

- Inclusion in design and implementation
  - Multicultural evaluation is not imposed on diverse communities; communities understand and support the rationale for the research and agree with the methods used to answer key evaluation questions.

- Diverse beneficiary stakeholders are actively involved in all phases of the evaluation, including problem definition, development of research questions, methods chosen, data collection, analysis, and reporting.
- To the extent possible, multicultural evaluation empowers diverse communities to do self-evaluation through intentional capacity building in evaluation.
- Acknowledgment/infusion of multiple worldviews
  - Evaluators in multicultural evaluations have a genuine respect for communities that are being studied and seek deep understanding of different cultural contexts, practices, and paradigms of thinking.
  - Expert knowledge does not exclusively reside with the evaluator; the community being studied is assumed to know best their issues, strengths, and challenges.
  - The diversity of the communities being studied are represented in multicultural evaluation staffing and expertise whenever possible.
- Cultural and systems analysis
  - Multicultural evaluations take into account how historical and current social systems, institutions, and societal norms contribute to power and outcome disparities across different racial and ethnic communities.
  - Multicultural evaluations incorporate and trace impacts of factors related to racial, cultural, gender, religious, economic, and other differences.
  - Multicultural evaluation questions take a multilevel approach to understanding root causes and impact at the individual, interpersonal, institutional, cultural, system, and policy levels, rather than focusing the analysis solely on individual behavior.
- Appropriate measures of success
  - Measures of success in multicultural evaluations are discussed and/or collaboratively developed with those being evaluated.
  - Data collection instruments and outcome measures are tested for multicultural validity across populations that may be non-English speaking, less literate, or from a different culture.
  - Multicultural evaluation data collection methods and instruments accommodate different cultural contexts and consider alternative or nontraditional ways of collecting data.
- Relevance to diverse communities
  - Multicultural evaluations inform community decision-making and program design.
  - Findings from multicultural evaluations are co-owned with diverse communities and shared in culturally appropriate ways.

These principles align closely with the five guiding principles adopted in 1995 by the American Evaluation Association as quality standards of practice for the profession: (1) systematic inquiry, (2) competence, (3) integrity/honesty, (4) respect for people, and (5) responsibilities for general and public welfare. The guiding principles for multicultural evaluation, however, imply a higher threshold that takes into account these generally accepted standards of quality evaluation while overlaying explicit consideration of differences related to diversity in race and ethnicity, age, gender, sexual orientation, socioeconomic status, religion, disability, and/or immigrant status.

Multicultural evaluation is built from core elements of sound evaluation practices, such as data-based inquiry, valid and reliable measures, and impartial assessment. Multicultural evaluation also reflects characteristics of quality evaluations based on guidelines set forth by the American Evaluation Association, such as strongly respecting stakeholders' self-worth, considering perspectives of a full range of stakeholders, and (where feasible) providing benefit to those who contribute data. However, when the principles of multicultural evaluation are applied to all aspects of evaluation—from the evaluator; to design and planning; to data collection, analysis, reporting, and application of findings—the result is a significant shift in how evaluation is implemented. The characteristics of a multicultural evaluation are shown Table 6.3.

Traditional evaluation is based on a long history in which formally trained evaluators implement needs or impact assessments based on established measures of what is good practice. Multicultural evaluation is characterized by **reciprocity**. While still integrating their own expertise throughout the evaluation, the evaluator does not presume to understand the cultural context of diverse communities that are being studied. As a result, multicultural evaluation is characterized by a fundamental shift in how the evaluation is conceptualized and designed, how communities are engaged in the data collection and analysis, and how the findings from the evaluation are ultimately communicated and used.

Closely related to understanding the principles and characteristics of multicultural evaluation is defining the characteristics of evaluators that make them culturally competent. Articulating what those characteristics are, however, can be subjected to debate. Attributes of multicultural evaluators' competence do not lend themselves to a checklist or a formula. Rather, the multicultural knowledge, attitudes, and skill sets that evaluators bring to their work can best be viewed as evolving human skills that are developed over time. Some of the most often described characteristics are:

- *Experience in diverse communities.* Although an evaluator may not necessarily be from the same cultural background as the communities he or she is evaluating, cultural competence involves a broader world perspective, often gained from experience living or working with different cultural groups.

TABLE 6.3 Characteristics of a Multicultural Evaluation		
	Traditional Evaluation $\longrightarrow$	**Multicultural Evaluation**
Evaluator		
Where knowledge resides	Formally trained evaluators are the experts. $\longrightarrow$	Grantees, community members, and formally trained evaluators each have expertise. Each knows best their issues and strengths.
Evaluator role	Leader, judge, expert. $\longrightarrow$	Facilitator, translator, convener.
Design and planning	Evaluator presents design to commissioning entity for approval. $\longrightarrow$	Prioritizes developing rapport and trust with stakeholders to engage them in an inclusive planning process that infuses multiple worldviews.
Data collection	Conducted by evaluation professional. $\longrightarrow$	Conducted by all players. Facilitated by the evaluator, stakeholders are often trained in some collection methods and then implement them.
Data analysis	Results and their meaning are analyzed by evaluation professionals. $\longrightarrow$	Results and their meaning are derived with a focus on culture and system analysis.
Reporting	Written report, usually accompanied by brief presentation to commissioning entity. $\longrightarrow$	Jointly disseminated and presented in nontraditional formats. Results have relevance and utility to diverse communities.
Application of findings	Findings used as monitoring, judging device. $\longrightarrow$	Findings used to build capacity of community and community organizations.

Source: Inouye, Yu, and Adefuin. (2005).

- *Openness to learning about cultural complexities.* Culturally competent evaluators exhibit humility about what they think they already know and are open to in-depth understanding of the nuances and complexities of inter- and intracultural influences and variations.
- *Flexibility in evaluation design and practice.* Rather than coming in with prescriptive evaluation strategies, culturally competent evaluators realize limitations to established approaches and are willing to adapt to honor different cultural contexts.

- *Rapport and trust with diverse communities.* Culturally competent evaluators prioritize relationship building with diverse communities rather than viewing them solely as data sources. Relationships are viewed as mutually beneficial.
- *Acknowledgement of power differentials.* Culturally competent evaluators acknowledge the various power differentials possible in an evaluation, including those between the evaluator and those being evaluated, or between the commissioning entity (often a foundation) and those being evaluated.
- *Self-reflection for recognizing cultural biases.* Culturally competent evaluators take the time to become mindful of potential biases and prejudices and how they might be incorporated into their research.
- *Translation and mediation across diverse groups.* Culturally competent evaluators are skilled in translating jargon-laden evaluation findings to those who may not be trained in evaluation or have high levels of education, literacy, or English-language fluency. Likewise, evaluators also must be adept in communicating cultural paradigms and community voice back to funders.
- *Comprehension of historic and institutional oppression.* An understanding of oppression is critical for designing evaluations that integrate how historic and current social systems, institutions, and societal norms contribute to disparities among different communities.

The power imbalances that are inherent within both funder–grantee relationships and evaluator–community relationships require specific and explicit attention throughout the evaluation process. Understanding and implementing multicultural evaluation approaches is an ongoing process. A meaningful shift toward multicultural evaluation will be determined greatly by the individual and collective beliefs, experiences, and will of the people within the organization. Therefore, as with many personal or institutional journeys toward change, the path toward multicultural evaluation can be considered a progression along a continuum.

Table 6.4 maps the implementation of multicultural evaluation principles (outlined earlier) along a stepwise continuum. This continuum is adapted from the stages of cultural competency that were developed for the service delivery field. It assumes that the implementation of evaluation principles unfolds in four stages:

- *Cultural incompetence.* Diverse cultures are unacknowledged in evaluation.
- *Cultural blindness.* Awareness of diversity may exist but is not presumed to be a critical factor within evaluation design or implementation.
- *Cultural sensitivity.* Acknowledgement of cultural differences exists, and steps are taken to incorporate cultural considerations within existing evaluation models.

TABLE 6.4 **Continuum of Multicultural Evaluation (MCE)**				
MCE Principles	**Cultural Incompetence**	**Cultural Blindness**	**Cultural Sensitivity**	**Cultural Proficiency**
Inclusive design and implementation	Evaluation designed to be accountable to the board; community largely unaware evaluation is happening and is uninvolved in any aspect of the evaluation.	Communities may be involved in evaluation, but no consideration for representation of multiple and diverse community voices.	Recognizing different cultural contexts, evaluation gathers input from diverse communities, typically through one-time requests for feedback. Community members may feel that their input is tokenized.	Diverse communities are involved in meaningful ways from start to finish. Evaluation is accountable to *multiple* stakeholders, including grantees and community beneficiaries.
Acknowledgment and infusion of multiple world views	Funder assumptions and beliefs drive the evaluation; different perspectives and worldviews not acknowledged.	Mainstream values, beliefs, and perspectives drive evaluation; these are presumed to apply to diverse communities being studied.	Culturally competent evaluation strategies in place (i.e., translation of survey instruments; evaluators that reflect the diversity of community being studied; co-interpretation of findings). Evaluator still holds primary expertise.	Culturally competent evaluation strategies in place; evaluator approaches study with an intentional sense of humility; and expert knowledge is equally shared by evaluator and community being studied.
Cultural and systems analysis	Cultural and systemic power differences are not realized.	Cultural and systemic power differences are ignored.	Cultural and systemic power differences are acknowledged, but not analyzed.	In-depth analysis of cultural and systemic power influences on a community is incorporated into findings.

(Continues)

TABLE 6.4   Continuum of Multicultural Evaluation (MCE) (*Continued*)

MCE Principles	Cultural Incompetence	Cultural Blindness	Cultural Sensitivity	Cultural Proficiency
Appropriate measures of success	Evaluation does not consider the diversity of data sources not the relevance of methodology or measures.	Diversity may be acknowledged, but grantees and/or community success still judged using traditional methods and measures (often for the sake of "technical rigor").	Although traditional evaluation measures may still be used, additional strategies are in place to strengthen multicultural validity of findings (i.e., multimethod data collection, diversity considerations incorporated in analysis).	Validity of frameworks, tools, measures tested across *multiple* cultural groups, languages, and contexts; they are accordingly modified and/or new measures developed.
Relevance and utility to diverse community	Funder and/or evaluator priorities drive evaluation; results kept from communities because there is no recognition of their value to community or because it is assumed that they won't understand.	Results might be shared back but with no consideration of how they might be interpreted or used. Results are not useful because they are not rooted in multicultural analysis.	Results consider cultural context and are shared with community, but community may not feel ownership of results and dissemination because of their limited role in the evaluation.	Because of joint development, results are culturally relevant and used constructively for program improvement for diverse communities. There is consideration of how to share findings in culturally appropriate ways.

Source: Inouye, Yu, and Adefuin. (2005).

- *Cultural proficiency.* The way that evaluations are designed and implemented are fundamentally shifted to honor and capitalize upon the diverse cultural contexts in which target populations exist.

A true shift to a multicultural paradigm will take time. The extent to which some or all of the multicultural evaluation steps are incorporated into evaluation practice will determine if researchers and foundations are harbingers of the shifts that can revolutionize the evaluation world.

CHAPTER SUMMARY

When developing and delivering a health promotion program, there are additional considerations when the audience is a cultural group other than your own or composed of a diverse group. It is important that planners are sensitive and considerate of these differences to avoid wasting resources and possibly offending people.

In this chapter we covered models for program planning and ways to deliver and evaluate your program. The delivery method includes considering the content of your message as well as how it is disseminated. Some methods of delivery, such as promotores(as), work better with some cultural and ethnic groups than others. After the program is complete, evaluation is essential. You will want to be sure that your message is received as you intended and see what impact it has had on your target audience. We outlined some differences between traditional and multicultural evaluation, which should be considered.

REVIEW

1. What are the concepts of the Health Belief Model and PRECEDE–PROCEED?
2. What is health communication?
3. What are some issues to consider when using written communication?
4. How can you check the reading level of a document?
5. What are promotores(as) and fotonovelas?
6. How are traditional and multicultural evaluations different?

CASE STUDY

A study conducted by Kung, Chan, Chong, Pham, and Hsu-Hage (1997) was inspired by their identification of the problem that Asian migrant women have the lowest participation rate in breast screening services of all ethnic groups in Australia.

The researchers engaged in a project designed to increase awareness of the increasing incidence of breast cancer among Chinese women in Australia and to encourage women over 40 years of age to participate in breast screening. They began the study by conducting a survey to gather data about the patterns of Chinese women getting breast-screening services and to identify issues that may affect their attitudes toward breast cancer or participation in screening.

The overarching purpose of the study was to increase awareness about the rise in breast cancer among ethnic Chinese women in Australia through health promotion activities designed to encourage active participation in the breast-screening program. Factors associated with the Chinese women's low participation rate in breast screening services also were explored.

The researchers used a cross-sectional random survey, language-specific health promotion workshops (which incorporated videos in Cantonese and Mandarin that documented Chinese women's experience with breast screening), and mass media campaigns (in Cantonese and Mandarin, the most frequently spoken Chinese dialects in the Melbourne Chinese community). The target population was women of Chinese ethnicity aged 40 years and older.

The researchers determined that the major factors for the low participation rate were English language skills and the length of stay in Australia. Women who had inadequate English language skills or had newly arrived in Australia had greater difficulty accessing breast screening because of their lower knowledge base. For the government-funded "Breast Screen" to be effective, it is important to consider sociodemographic differences among populations at risk and to address the sociocultural barriers that affect access to the service. For ethnic Chinese, this may include appropriate use of a variety of ethnic media, provision of language-specific breast screening education programs, and the use of health service providers who speak Chinese dialects. This study supported the notion that the use of mass media and language-specific workshops are appropriate when health promotion is directed at ethnic populations.

Source: Kung, Chan, Chong, Pham, & Hsu-Hage. (1997).

GLOSSARY TERMS

fotonovela   multicultural evaluation
digital divide   reciprocity
promotores

REFERENCES

Adefuin, J. & Edo, T. (2003). *Multicultural health evaluation: An annotated bibliography*. Woodland Hills, CA: The california Endowment.

Centers for Disease Control and Prevention. (1999, September 17). Framework for public health and evaluation. *Morbidity and Mortality Weekly Report, 48*.

Discovery Education. (1995). *Kathy Schrock's guide for educators. Fry's readability graph*. Retrieved May 11, 2008, from http://school.discovery.com/schrockguide/fry/fry.html

Independent Television Service. (2008). *What is a foto-novela?* Retrieved May 10, 2008, from http://www.pbs.org/independentlens/fotonovelas2/what.html

Inouye, T. E., Yu, H. C., & Adefuin, J. (2005). The California Endowment. *Commissioning multicultural evaluation: A foundation resource guide*. Retrieved March 15, 2009, from http://www.spra.com/pdf/TCE-Multicultural-Evaluation.pdf

Kung, E. Y. L., Chan, A. C., Chong, Y. S., Pham, T., & Hsu-Hage, B. H. H. (1997). Promoting breast screen in Melbourne Chinese women using ethnic-specific health promotion strategies. *Internet Journal of Health Promotion*. Retrieved March 16, 2009, from http://rhpeo.net/ijhp-articles/1997/3/index.htm

McKenzie, J. F., Neiger, B. L., & Thackeray, R. (2009). *Planning, implementing, & evaluating health promotion programs: A primer*. San Francisco: Pearson/Benjamin Cummings.

Migrant Health Promotion. (2005). *Who are Promotores(as)?* Retrieved May 10, 2008, from http://www.migranthealth.org/our_programs/who_are_promotora.php

Office of Disease Prevention and Health Promotion. (n.d.). *Healthy People 2010. Health communication*. Retrieved April 22, 2008, from http://www.healthypeople.gov/Document/HTML/Volume1/11HealthCom.htm

Rural Women's Health Project. (n.d.). *What is a fotonovela?* Retrieved May 11, 2008, from http://www.rwhp.org/catalog_info/whatis.html

The California Endowment. (2003). *Voices from the field: Health and evaluation leaders on multicultural evaluation*. Retrieved May 11, 2008, from http://www.spra.com/pdf/VoicesBook.pdf

The Communication Initiative Network. (2003). *Health belief model*. Retrieved May 10, 2008, from http://www.comminit.com/en/node/27093

The Community Toolbox. (2007). *PRECEDE–PROCEED*. Retrieved May 10, 2008, from http://ctb.ku.edu/tools/sub_section_main_1008.htm

US Department of Health and Human Services. (2000). *Healthy People 2010: Understanding and improving health* (2nd ed). Washington, DC: US Government Printing Office.

US Department of Health and Human Services. (2001). *Making health communications programs work* (NIH Publication No. 04-5145). Bethesda, MD: Author.

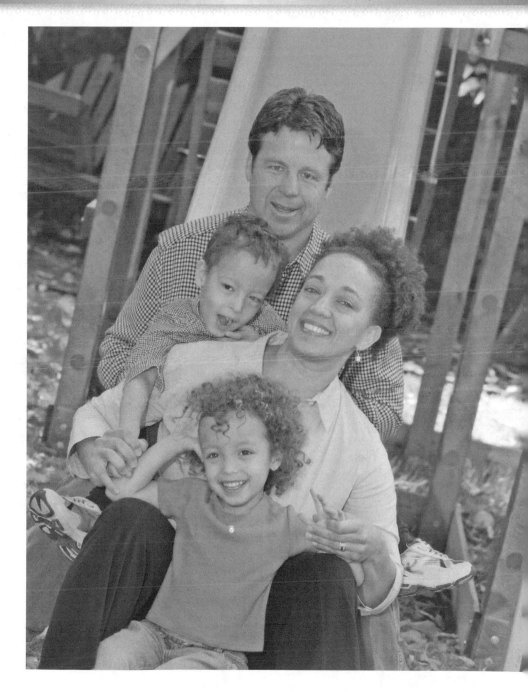

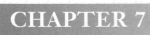

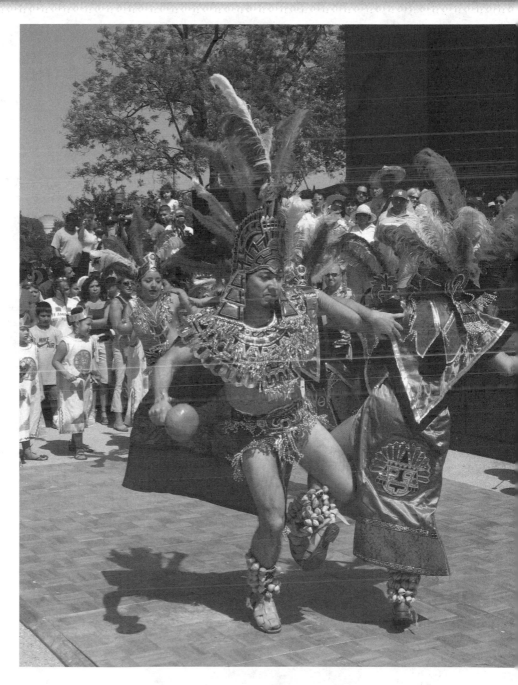

CHAPTER 7

Hispanic and Latino American Populations

Her days are slow, days of grinding dried snake into powder, of crushing wild bees to mix with white wine. And the townspeople come, hoping to be touched by her ointments, her hands, her prayers, her eyes. She listens to their stories, and she listens to the desert, always to the desert.

—Pat Mora

Preservation of one's own culture does not require contempt or disrespect for other cultures.

—Cesar Chavez

KEY CONCEPTS

- Empacho
- Santeria
- Espiritismo
- Orishas

CHAPTER OBJECTIVES

1. Provide an overview of the social and economic circumstances of Hispanics in the United States.
2. Provide an overview of Hispanic beliefs about the causes of illness.
3. Describe at least three unique diseases among Hispanics.
4. Describe Hispanics' health risk behaviors and common illnesses.
5. List at least six tips for working with Hispanic populations.

An unresolved debate is the use of the terms "Hispanic" and "Latino." Which is the politically correct term? Is there a difference? It depends on whom you ask. Some say it is a personal preference, and others argue that there are differences related to places of origin.

The argument against using the term "Hispanic" is that this term is based upon the Spanish word "hispano," which literally means "from Spain." Some people believe that the term "Hispanic" is incorrect because Hispanic American heritage goes further than just Spain. The Hispanic market is composed of people who come from as many as 20 different countries. The reason Hispanics speak Spanish is because of Spain's influence in history. Spaniards brought not only their language but also religion to different regions of the world. Most Hispanics are Catholic or Christian, and similar religions tend to translate into similar values. Therefore, the argument against this term is that Hispanics speak Spanish, but they are not all from Spain. What they do share is language and values.

The term "Latino" includes everyone from Latin America and therefore includes people from Brazil (who speak Portuguese). A commonality of Hispanics and Latinos is that they speak Spanish, yet the people in the largest country in South America do not speak Spanish. Brazil was colonized by Portugal and not by Spain, thus its inhabitants are of Portuguese descent. Brazilians speak Portuguese, which makes them Latin but not Hispanic. "Latino" also is not a genuine Spanish word, unlike "Hispanic." Some people believe that the term "Latino" is more derogatory than the word "Hispanic", because Latino refers to the Latin language of the Romans who conquered Spain.

In the United States, the term "Hispanic" gained acceptance after it was picked up by the government and used in forms and census to identify people with Spanish heritage. Hispanic is not a race but an ethnic distinction because Hispanics come from a variety of geographic regions and are not genetically related. The ethnic label "Hispanic" was the result of the desire to quantify the Spanish-speaking population for the U.S. Census Bureau. For years, the U.S. Census Bureau considered Hispanic to be a race. They changed that definition before the 1970 census, and in 1977 the U.S. racial classifications became American Indian, Alaskan Native, Asian or Pacific Islander, Black, and White. The government added ethnic classifications of "Hispanic Origin" and "Not of Hispanic Origin."

The term "Chicano" is a more exclusive term used solely in reference to people of Mexican descent and is used to describe only an American with Mexican heritage (Mexican American). Originally, "Chicano," which is an abbreviation of the word "Mexicano," was used by non-Hispanics as a racial slur. Around the 1950s, however, Mexican Americans adopted the word "Chicano." The word changed from a derogative to a source of confidence for Mexican Americans. Although the term "Chicano" is an old word, many elderly Hispanics of Mexican descent do not like it because the term had been used, long ago, as derogatory reference to Mexican people.

If you are trying to figure out how to refer to a group of people, the one concept on which most Hispanics and Latinos agree is that they prefer to be called by their immediate ethnic group. If you are referring to Mexican Americans, use that phrase instead of Hispanic or Latino. Because most Hispanics or Latinos in the United States are from Mexico and not Latin America, and "Hispanic" is the term more commonly used by the U.S. government, we will use the term "Hispanic" throughout this chapter unless the data source identifies the ethnic group differently.

HISTORY OF HISPANICS IN THE UNITED STATES

People often hold the misconception that Hispanics are a recent group to migrate to the United States. This erroneous perception is mostly due to the media attention given to Hispanic groups in the 1980s, when the census revealed that Hispanics were the fastest growing group in the United States. The reality is that Hispanics have a long history in the United States.

Mexican Americans were once concentrated in the states that formerly belonged to Mexico, primarily California, Arizona, New Mexico, Texas, and Colorado. Racial discrimination led to lynchings of Mexicans and Mexican Americans in the Southwest, which has long been overlooked in American history. Between 1848 and 1928, mobs lynched at least 597 Mexicans (Carigan, 2003). Mexicans were lynched at a rate of 27.4 per 100,000 of population between 1880 and 1930. This statistic is second only to that of the African American community during that period, which suffered an average of 37.1 per 100,000 population (Carigan, 2003). The Texas Rangers were an organized group known to brutally repress the Mexican American population in Texas. Historians estimate that hundreds, perhaps even thousands, of Mexicans and Mexican Americans were killed by the Texas Rangers (Carigan, 2003). Anti-Mexican mob violence and intimidation resulted in Mexicans being displaced from their lands, denied access to natural resources, and becoming politically disenfranchised. Mexican American identity has changed drastically over time. They have campaigned for voting rights, stood against educational and employment discrimination, and stood for economic and social advancement.

On the other side of the continent, many Cubans have desired to come to the United States because living in a socialist country under the dictatorship of Fidel and Raúl Castro has brought about inequality. These individuals seek more political freedom, a democratic form of government, and/or to live in a land of capitalism where there are fewer restrictions and more opportunities. To get to the United States, many Cubans turn to smugglers who charge high fees, or they may resort to making homemade boats and even rafts for the 90-mile journey from Cuba to Florida. Others fly to countries such as Mexico to enter the United States via that country. Not all are successful, and children and adults sometimes end up losing their lives in their efforts to reach American soil. In 1994 there was a wave of over 30,000 Cubans who tried to enter the United States. This caused the United States and Cuban governments to work out an immigration agreement. Cuba agreed to do a better job of patrolling their seas to prevent Cubans from leaving their country. If they were not successful in reaching Florida soil and were intercepted by the U.S. Coast Guard, which is responsible for overseeing America's seas and shores, the Cuban government also agreed that there would be no reprisal against the Cubans who were returned. However, in reality Cubans who are returned usually face some kind of punishment by the Cuban government, like imprisonment. The general rule is that when an individual reaches American soil, not American waters, they are allowed to remain in the United States. In 1994 the United States set a quota of 20,000 immigrant visas annually for Cubans, of which 5,000 come from a lottery system. One of the biggest incentives is that in a period of five years or less, Cuban immigrants may gain eligibility to apply for United States citizenship. However, there are some requirements as to who can apply for the lottery. The screening process is conducted to ensure that the prospective immigrants will not become a burden to the United States government. Lottery winners are entitled to bring their spouse and children younger than 21 years of age.

Puerto Rico is a territory of the United States. At the end of the Spanish-American War in 1898, the United States acquired Puerto Rico and has retained sovereignty ever since, and a large influx of Puerto Rican workers to the United States began. The Jones-Shafroth Act in 1917 made the move easier, because the U.S. Congress declared that all Puerto Ricans are U.S. citizens, enabling a migration free from all immigration barriers.

HISPANICS IN THE UNITED STATES

Hispanics are the fastest-growing major population group in the United States (New Century Foundation, 2006). According to the U.S. Census Bureau, they will account for one in four of the American population by 2050 (New Century Foundation, 2006). According to the 2006 U.S. Census Bureau population estimate, there are roughly 44.3 million Hispanics living in the United States (see Figure 7.1). This group represents almost 15% of the United States total population, and they experienced a 61% increase from 1990 to 2000 (U.S. Census Bureau, 2004). In 2004, among Hispanic

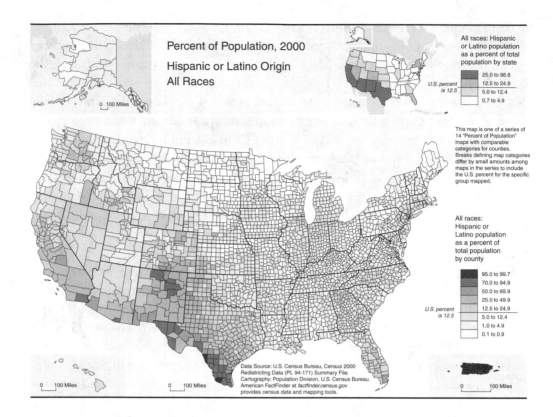

FIGURE 7.1   Percentage of population: Hispanic or Latino Origin, 2000.
Source: U.S. Census Bureau, Population Division (2008), http://www.census.gov/main/www/citation.html.

subgroups, Mexicans rank as the largest at 66%. The other 34% includes Central and South Americans (13%), Puerto Ricans (9.4%), and Cubans (3.9%); the remaining 7.5% are people of other Hispanic origins (U.S. Census Bureau, 2004).

States with the largest Hispanic populations are California (13 million) and Texas (8 million) (Office of Minority Health, 2008). The Hispanic population is younger than any other group. In 2000 the median age for Hispanics was 26.0 years, compared to 35.4 years for the total population (U.S. Census Bureau, 2004). Among Hispanics, Mexicans have the largest proportion of people under age 18 years (36%) (Office of Minority Health, 2008).

According to a 2006 U.S. Census Bureau report, 55% of Hispanics, in comparison to 85% of non-Hispanic Caucasians, have a high school diploma (Office of Minority

Health, 2008). Ten percent of Hispanics, in comparison to 24.6% of non-Hispanic Caucasians, have a bachelor's degree (Office of Minority Health, 2008). To some extent, Hispanics' low graduation rates reflect the language and cultural barriers faced by immigrants. United States–born Hispanics do better than foreign-born Hispanics, but according to a government survey of adults, even Hispanics who have been in the United States for more than three generations are twice as likely as whites and slightly more likely than blacks to report not having a high school diploma (U.S. Census Bureau, 2006 as cited in New Century Foundation, 2006). Hispanics who remain in school have lower test scores than whites (New Century Foundation, 2006). Hispanics are the least likely of the major population groups to attend college. In 2003, 28% of Hispanics aged 18 to 24 years were enrolled in college, compared to 38% of blacks and 52% of whites (New Century Foundation, 2006).

According to a 2004 U.S. Census Bureau report, 24.6% of Hispanics, in comparison to 13.4% of non-Hispanic Caucasians, work within service occupations; 16.8% of Hispanics, in comparison to 39.1% of Caucasians, work in managerial or professional occupations (Office of Minority Health, 2008). Casual day labor is some of the most difficult, badly compensated work in the United States, and it is done overwhelmingly by Hispanics. Of the estimated 118,000 day laborers in the country working on a given day, 59% are of Mexican and 28% are of Central American origin (New Century Foundation, 2006). Day laborers can earn about $15,000 if they work all year (Valenzuela, Theodore, Meléndez, & Gonzalez, 2006 as cited in New Century Foundation, 2006).

According to a 2004 study, 22.5% of Hispanics, in comparison to 8.2% of non-Hispanic Caucasians, were living at the poverty level (Office of Minority Health, 2008). Hispanics represented 14% of the total U.S. population but constituted 21.8% of the population living in poverty (Office of Minority Health, 2008). Fifty percent of Hispanic households use some form of welfare, which is the highest rate of any major population group (New Century Foundation, 2006).

It is significant to note that Hispanics have the highest health uninsured rates of any racial or ethnic group within the United States. In 2004 the Centers for Disease Control and Prevention reported that private insurance coverage among Hispanic subgroups varied as follows: 39.1% of Mexicans, 47.3% of Puerto Ricans, 57.9% of Cubans, and 45.1% of other Hispanic and Latino groups. Those without health insurance coverage varied among Hispanic subgroups: 37.6% of Mexicans, 20.4% of Puerto Ricans, 22.8% of Cubans, and 32.3% of other Hispanic or Latino groups (Office of Minority Health, 2008).

With regard to crime, Hispanics are 3.3 times more likely to be in prison than whites; they are 4.2 times more likely to be in prison for murder and 5.8 times more likely to be in prison for felony drug crimes (New Century Foundation, 2006). Young Hispanics are 19 times more likely than young whites (and slightly more likely than young blacks) to be in youth gangs (New Century Foundation, 2006). Hispanic incarceration rates are especially high for violent crimes, motor vehicle theft, and drug offenses (New Century Foundation, 2006). High drug offense rates reflect Mexico's role as an important source of drugs; 92% of the cocaine sold in the United States comes through Mexico, and it is our largest supplier of marijuana and second largest supplier of heroin (Placido, 2005 as cited in New Century Foundation, 2006). Hispanics are 2.9 times more likely to die from homicide than whites and are 3.4 times more likely than whites to die from gunshot wounds (New Century Foundation, 2006).

After they come to the United States, Mexicans retain longer and stronger attachments to their country of origin than do immigrants who have come greater distances. Thirty-three percent of citizens of Hispanic origin consider themselves to be Americans first (New Century Foundation, 2006). The rest consider themselves to be Hispanic/Latino or their former nationality first (New Century Foundation, 2006). Only 34% of Mexicans who are eligible for U.S. citizenship actually become Americans, the lowest figure for any national group (González, 2006 as cited in New Century Foundation, 2006). When they become citizens, Hispanics remain emotionally attached to their countries of origin.

With regard to their social structure, Hispanics tend to view the family as a primary source of support. Families are very close, broadly defined, and emotionally and financially supportive. Family often includes non-blood-related persons. Some non-Hispanics interpret these family characteristics as overinvolvement or dependence. The eldest male is typically the authority figure, and gender roles are traditional. Important decisions are made by the whole family, not the individual, because they tend to have a collectivist type of social structure. Elders should be shown respect, and they are viewed as authority figures within the community. Elders often provide child care for the grandchildren (Rhode Island Department of Health, n.d.).

Hispanics place higher value on individuals as opposed to institutions. They tend to trust and cooperate with individuals they know personally, and many dislike impersonal and formal structures. Hispanic customers may identify a health care worker by name rather than by job title or institution. In a professional situation, many Hispanics expect to be addressed formally (e.g., Mrs. Martinez), but also personally (e.g., How are your children?) (Rhode Island Department of Health, n.d.). The length of the social interaction is often viewed to be less important than the quality (Rhode Island Department of Health, n.d.).

With regard to communication, Hispanics tend to avoid conflict and criticism, because they prefer smooth social relations based on politeness and respect (Rhode Island Department of Health, n.d.). Overt disagreement is not considered to be appropriate behavior. Many Hispanics are characterized by warm, friendly, and affectionate relationships. Personal space is close and frequently shared with family members or close friends. Many Hispanics, particularly if they were not raised in the United States, may avoid direct eye contact with authority figures or in awkward situations. Many will nod affirmatively but not necessarily mean agreement. Silence may mean failure to understand and embarrassment about asking or disagreeing.

Modesty and privacy are important; therefore, health issues that are stigmatized should be discussed through an interpreter and not family members. Legally, family members should not be used as interpreters, but when one is used as interpreter, if the issue is personal, try to use a family member of the same gender. Sexuality issues are hard to discuss. Often the word for sex (*sexo*) is not even used; *tener relaciones* (to have relations) is used instead (Rhode Island Department of Health, n.d.).

BELIEFS ABOUT CAUSES OF HEALTH AND ILLNESS

Health is generally viewed by Hispanics as being and looking clean, being able to rest and sleep well, feeling good and happy, and having the ability to perform in one's expected role as mother, father, worker, etc. (Rhode Island Department of Health, n.d.). In Puerto Rico, the phrase *llenitos y limpios* (clean and not too thin) is used (Rhode Island Department of Health, n.d.). A person's well being depends upon a balance in emotional, physical, and social factors, and when they are not in balance, illness occurs. Some attribute physical illness to *los nervios*, believing that illness results from having experienced a strong emotional state. Thus, they try to prevent illness by avoiding intense rage, sadness, and other emotions (Rhode Island Department of Health, n.d.). Depression is not talked about openly.

There are many unique illnesses that Hispanics diagnose that are not part of the Western medical system. Some common illnesses and their causes are listed in Table 7.1.

Hispanic cultures view illnesses, treatments, and foods as having hot or cold properties, although how these are ascribed may vary by country. Some cultures consider health to be the product of balance among four body humours (blood and yellow bile are hot, phlegm and black bile are cold). One would balance a hot illness with cold medications and foods, etc. This might result in not following a doctor's advice to drink lots of fluids for a common cold, if one believes such drinks add more coldness to the body. Instead, hot liquids (tea, soup, broth) could be recommended

TABLE 7.1	Common Illnesses in the Hispanic Culture and Their Characteristics and Causes		
Illness	**Characteristics**	**Cause(s)**
Ataque de nervios (nervous attack)	Intense and brief expression of shock, anxiety, or sadness	Believed to be caused by family conflict or anger (e.g., screaming, kicking)
Bilis (bile rage)	Vomiting, diarrhea, headaches, dizziness, migraine, nightmares, loss of appetite, inability to urinate; brought on by livid rage and revenge fantasies	Believed to stem from bile pouring into bloodstream in response to strong emotion
Caida de la mollera (fallen fontanel)	Childhood condition characterized by irritability and diarrhea	Believed to be caused by abrupt withdrawal from the mother's breast
Empacho	Lack of appetite, stomachache, diarrhea, vomiting, constipation, cramps, or vomiting	Caused by poorly digested or uncooked food or overeating
Fatiga (shortness of breath or fatigue)	Asthma symptoms (especially in Puerto Rican usage) and fatigue	
Frio de la matriz (frozen womb)	Pelvic congestion and decreased libido believed to be caused by insufficient rest after childbirth	
Mal aire (bad air)	Cold air that is believed to cause respiratory infections and earaches	
Mal de ojo (evil eye)	Vomiting, fever, crying, restlessness	A hex cast on children, sometimes unconsciously, that is believed to be caused by the admiring gaze of someone more powerful
Mal puesto (sorcery)	Unnatural illness that is not easily explained	
Pasmo (cold or frozen face; lockjaw)	Temporary paralysis of the face or limbs or spasm of voluntary muscle	Exposure to cold air when body is overheated; caused by a sudden hot–cold imbalance
Susto (fright)	Anorexia, insomnia, hallucinations, depression, weakness, painful sensations	Traumatic experiences or shock

Sources: Adapted from Rhode Island Department of Health. (n.d.) and Juckett. (2005).

TABLE 7.2   Hot versus Cold Latino Diagnoses

Cold Conditions
- Cancer
- Colic
- Empacho (indigestion)
- Frio de la matriz (frozen womb)
- Headache
- Menstrual cramps
- Pneumonia
- Upper respiratory infections

Hot Conditions
- Bilis (bile, rage)
- Diabetes mellitus
- Gastroesophageal reflux or peptic ulcer
- Hypertension
- Mal de ojo (evil eye)
- Pregnancy
- Sore throat or infection
- Susto (soul loss)

Source: Juckett. (2005).

(Rhode Island Department of Health, n.d.). In Table 7.2 a list of hot and cold illnesses are provided.

Susto is illness that occurs from a frightful experience, and it is similar to anxiety in Western medicine. Symptoms include withdrawal from social interactions, listlessness, not sleeping well, and loss of appetite. Most people who believe in susto deem that anyone can get it; both adults and children can be affected. The soul leaves the body due to a frightening experience, and the body becomes susceptible to illness and disharmony. It can be caused by events such as the sudden, unexpected barking of a dog, tripping over an unnoticed object, having a nighttime encounter with a ghost who keeps your spirit from finding its way back into your body before you wake, or being in a social situation that causes you to have fear or anger, for example.

Mal de ojo, sometimes called "evil eye," is the illness that is a result of an envious glance from another individual. It mostly affects children. It has been defined as a hex caused by a gaze from a more powerful or stronger person looking at a weaker person (usually an infant or child but sometimes a woman). It may be someone from outside the family looking at the child with envy, or a stare from a powerful person who is admiring the child. It is usually caused inadvertently. Those affected may suffer symptoms including headaches, high fever, diarrhea, not sleeping well, increased fussiness, and weeping. It is not fully known what diseases in Western medicine correlate with mal de ojo; however, in severe cases the symptoms are similar to those of sepsis (the presence of pathogenic organisms or their toxins in the blood or tissues) and should warrant a medical evaluation. Cases of mal de ojo with frequent crying and no other symptoms are thought to be similar to colic.

Empacho describes stomach pains and cramps that are believed to be caused by a ball of food clinging to the stomach due to altered eating habits, eating spoiled food, overeating, and swallowing chewing gum. The disease state of empacho has often been defined as a perceived stomach or intestinal blockage. In most cases, it is not an actual obstruction but rather indigestion or gastroenteritis. Abdominal pain and bloating are symptoms of empacho. Some Hispanic populations also add nausea, vomiting, diarrhea, and lethargy as symptoms that may occur in some cases. It tends to occur more in young children, but people of all ages are susceptible. Empacho is considered to be a cold illness. Folk medicines used to treat empacho include greta (lead monoxide) and azarcón (lead tetroxide), which are dangerous and can cause lead poisoning. There have been case reports of deaths from these substances.

The ideology about illness and health is rooted in the fabric of the culture, and it is the fundamental element of traditional values. Even though the Mexican American culture utilizes Western medicine, they rely primarily on folk practitioners to treat traditional illnesses.

HEALING TRADITIONS

Some treatments for illness are provided by family members, but illness also may be treated by nonfamily members. Hispanic healing traditions include curanderismo in Mexico and much of Latin America, **Santeria** in Brazil and Cuba, and **Espiritismo** in Puerto Rico. Most of these traditions distinguish natural illnesses from supernatural illnesses. The healing traditions include a variety of methods as shown in Table 7.3.

Curanderos

A curandero (or curandera for a female) is a traditional folk healer or shaman who is dedicated to curing physical and/or spiritual illnesses. The curandero is often a

TABLE 7.3   Traditional Latino Diagnoses and Their Related Treatment Methods

Diagnosis	Traditional Treatment
Ataque de nervios (nervous attack)	No immediate treatment other than calming the patient
Bilis (bile, rage)	Herbs, including wormwood
Caida de la mollera (fallen fontanel)	Holding the child upside down or pushing up on the hard palate
Empacho (indigestion or blockage)	Treated by massaging the stomach and drinking purgative tea, or by azarcón or greta, medicines that have been implicated in some cases of lead poisoning
Fatiga (shortness of breath or fatigue)	Herbal treatments, including eucalyptus and mullein (gordolobo), steam inhalation
Frio de la matriz (frozen womb)	Damiana tea, rest
Mal aire (bad air)	Steam baths, hot compresses, stimulating herbal teas
Mal de ojo (evil eye)	The hex can be broken if the person responsible for the hex touches the child or if a healer passes an egg over the child's body
Mal puesto (sorcery)	Magic
Pasmo (cold or frozen face; lockjaw)	Massage
Susto (fright-induced soul loss)	Treatment may include a barrida (spiritualistic cleansing by sweeping the body with eggs, lemons, and bay leaves), herb tea, prayer; repeated until the patient improves

Source: Adapted from Juckett. (2005).

respected member of the community and is highly religious and spiritual. In Spanish the word curandero means healer. These healers often use herbs and other natural remedies to cure illnesses, but their primary method of healing is the supernatural because they believe that the cause of many illnesses are lost malevolent spirits, a lesson from God, or a curse. There are different types of curanderos/curanderas. Curanderos (traditional healers) use verbal charms or spells to produce a magic effect and herbs, sobadores practice manipulation, parteras are midwives, and abuelas (literally "grandmothers," although they are not necessarily related to the patient) provide initial care. Yerberos are primarily herbalists, and hueseros and sabaderos are bone/muscle therapists who emphasize physical ailments.

Curanderos treat ailments such as espanto (Spanish for shock), empacho (Spanish for surfeit, which means to feed in excess), susto (fright illness), mal aire (literally bad air), and mal de ojo (evil eye) with religious rituals, ceremonial cleansing, and prayers. Often curanderos contact certain spirits to aid them in their healing work. The remedies of the curanderos are often helpful but sometimes have negative effects on the health of their patients. For example, a common method of healing mollera caída, a condition in which an infant's fontanelle has sunken, is to hold the infant's feet with its head down and perform a ceremonial ritual. Some other traditional treatments, such as azarcón and greta (lead salts) and azogue (mercury), are also harmful because of their lead and mercury content. Other remedies are harmless. For example, a common method of treating mal de ojo (evil eye) is to rub an egg over the body of the sick to draw out the evil spirit that is causing the disease.

These methods of treating health problems often lead to conflict with modern medicine because doctors reject the curandero's healing as superstitious and worthless. As a result, curanderos have often experienced discrimination and been likened to witches by the medical profession and non-Hispanic communities. However, these remedies are important to the Hispanic culture, and disbelief may lead to insult, conflict, or the rejection of modern medicine. Other medical doctors, recognizing the benefits of the spiritual and emotional healing offered by curanderos, have begun to work in conjunction with them, supporting their use of rituals and ceremonies in the healing of the sick while insisting that patients receive modern medical attention as well.

Santeria

Santeria, also known as the "Way of the Saints," is an Afro-Caribbean religion based on beliefs of the Yoruba people in Nigeria, Africa. The traditions have been influenced by Roman Catholic beliefs. Santeria incorporates elements of several faiths and is therefore called a syncretic religion. It has grown beyond its Yoruba and Catholic origins to become a religion in its own right and a powerful symbol of the religious creativity of Afro-Cuban culture. For a long time, Santeria was a secretive underground religion, but it is becoming increasingly visible in the Americas. It was once considered to be a ghetto religion practiced only by the Caribbean poor and uneducated, but now Santeria has a growing following among middle-class professionals and other ethnic groups, such as whites, blacks, and Asian Americans.

Because of the history of secrecy, it is not known how many people follow Santeria. There is no central organization for this religion, and it is practiced in private, which makes it more difficult to determine the number of followers. There are no scriptures for this religion, and it is taught through word of mouth. The Santeria tradition is composed of a hierarchical structure according to priesthood level and authority.

Santeria practices include animal offerings, dance, and appeals for assistance sung to the **orishas**, which resemble the Catholic saints and are spirits that reflect one of the manifestations of Olodumare (God). Animal sacrifice also is a part of Santeria and is very controversial. Followers of Santeria point out that ritual slaughter is conducted in a safe and humane manner by the priests who are charged with the task. Furthermore, the animal is cooked and eaten afterwards by the community. In fact, chickens, a staple food of many African-descended and Creole cultures, are the most common sacrifice; the chicken's blood is offered to the orisha, and the meat is consumed by all.

Followers believe that orishas will help them in life, if they carry out the appropriate rituals, and enable them to achieve the destiny that God planned for them before they were born. This is very much a mutual relationship, because the orishas need to be worshipped by human beings if they are to continue to exist. In a Supreme Court case in 1993, Justice Kennedy said in his decision that:

> The Santeria faith teaches that every individual has a destiny from God, a destiny fulfilled with the aid and energy of the orishas. The basis of the Santeria religion is the nurture of a personal relation with the orishas, and one of the principal forms of devotion is an animal sacrifice. According to Santeria teaching, the orishas are powerful but not immortal. They depend for survival on the sacrifice. (*Church of Likumi Babalu Aye v. City of Hialeah*, 508 U.S. 520 (1993))

Drum music and dancing are a form of prayer and will sometimes induce a trance state in an initiated priest, who becomes possessed and will channel the orisha.

Espiritismo

Espiritismo is the Spanish word for "Spiritism." It is the belief in Latin America and the Caribbean that good and evil spirits can affect human life, such as one's health and luck. An opinion, doctrine, or principle (tenet) of Espiritismo is the belief in a supreme God who is the omnipotent creator of the universe. There also is a belief in a spirit world inhabited by discarnate spiritual beings who gradually evolve intellectually and morally.

Espiritismo has never had a single leader or epicenter of practice, so practice varies greatly between individuals and groups. Espiritismo has absorbed various practices from other religious and spiritual practices endemic to Latin America and the Caribbean, such as Roman Catholicism, curanderismo, Santeria, and voodoo.

A ritual associated with Espiritismo de Corzon, which is a form of Espiritismo that is practiced primarily in Cuba, is physically, mentally, and emotionally difficult. Those participating in the ritual stand in a circle holding hands while walking in a counterclockwise fashion (Olmos & Paravisini-Gebert, 2003). At the same time, they chant and beat the floor with their feet and swing their arms forcefully until they fall into a trance (Olmos & Paravisini-Gebert, 2003). The heavy breathing and stamping, which is heavily associated with chanting in African cults, serve one specific purpose (Olmos & Paravisini-Gebert, 2003). The noises create a hypnotic sound that leads the medium into a trance. Upon reaching this particular state of mind, the medium can contact the spirits for solutions to problems or aliments (Olmos & Paravisini-Gebert, 2003).

Puerto Rican Espiritismo shares many similarities in its origins to Cuban Espiritismo. Educated Puerto Ricans used Espiritismo as a way of justification in their mission to free the country from the grasp of Spanish colonialism (Olmos & Paravisini-Gebert, 2003). However, the religious movement encountered many setbacks in its early years in Puerto Rico. Those who were caught practicing it were punished by the government and ostracized by the Catholic Church (Olmos & Paravisini-Gebert, 2003). The movement, despite all the roadblocks, continued to spread in the country. The attempt to achieve spiritual communication through a medium was widely practiced all over the island.

BEHAVIORAL RISK FACTORS AND COMMON HEALTH PROBLEMS

The behaviors described here are linked to the common health problems that Hispanics face, but it is important to note that some of their illnesses are not related to behaviors. Their health problems are related to other social factors as well, such as poverty or lack of access to care.

Hispanics' typical diet is high in fiber with beans and grains (rice) as staple foods, and they rely on beans as a source of protein rather than meat. Leafy green vegetables and dairy are not a usual part of their diet (Rhode Island Department of Health, n.d.). Generally, Hispanics eat a lot of tropical fruits, fruit juices, and starchy root vegetables (e.g., potatoes, cassava, and plantains). The food pyramid for the traditional Latino diet can be found in Figure 7.2.

According to the 2003 to 2004 National Health and Examination Survey (American Health Association, n.d.), 73.1% of Mexican American males and 71.7% of Mexican

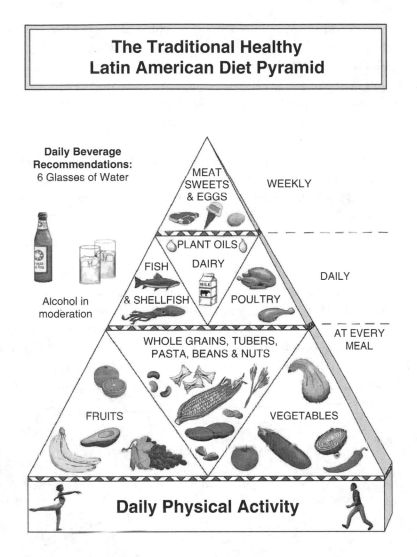

The Traditional Healthy
Latin American Diet Pyramid

Daily Beverage Recommendations:
6 Glasses of Water

WEEKLY

MEAT SWEETS & EGGS

PLANT OILS

FISH   DAIRY

DAILY

Alcohol in moderation

& SHELLFISH   POULTRY

AT EVERY MEAL

WHOLE GRAINS, TUBERS, PASTA, BEANS & NUTS

FRUITS   VEGETABLES

Daily Physical Activity

FIGURE 7.2   Food pyramid for traditional Latino diet.
Source: © 2000 Oldways Preservation & Exchange Trust. www.oldwayspt.org.
Reproduced with permission.

American females are overweight or obese, and of these, 27.3% of males and 38.4% of females are obese.

Hispanics have lower rates of smoking than most racial and ethnic groups. In 2005, 16.2% of Hispanics smoked (American Lung Association, 2007). There are significant variations in smoking rates among Hispanic subgroups. In 2005, 16.7% of Cuban Americans smoked, compared to 23.6% of Puerto Ricans, 21.2% of Mexican Americans, 14.3% percent of Dominicans, and 12.2% of Central and South Americans (American Lung Association, 2007).

Hispanic males have high rates of alcohol consumption. In 2000, 8.7% of Hispanics indicated excessive alcohol consumption. Excessive alcohol drinkers were defined as those who had more than 12 drinks of any type of alcoholic beverage in their lifetime and consumed more than 5 drinks on one occasion at least 12 times during the past 12 months, compared to 9.4% of non-Hispanic whites and 6.9% of non-Hispanic blacks (Centers for Disease Control and Prevention, n.d.). One possible explanation for the high drinking rate among males is the cultural ideology of machismo. Men strive to appear strong and masculine by drinking large amounts of alcohol.

There are substantial differences in drinking patterns among Hispanics. For example, Cuban Americans have lower rates of drinking than Mexican Americans and Puerto Ricans (Caetano, Clark, & Tam, 1998). Among Hispanics, those born in the United States were approximately three times more likely to engage in drinking and driving than those who were born elsewhere (Caetano & Clark, 1998). Hispanic men also had higher rates of having been arrested for driving under the influence of alcohol (19%), compared to white men (13%) and black men (11%) (Caetano & Clark, 1998).

QUICK FACTS

Cancer
- In 2004, Hispanic men were 13% less likely to have prostate cancer than non-Hispanic white men.
- In 2004, Hispanic women were 33% less likely to have breast cancer than non-Hispanic white women.
- Hispanic men and women have higher incidence and mortality rates for stomach and liver cancer.
- In 2003, Hispanic women were 2.2 times as likely as non-Hispanic white women to be diagnosed with cervical cancer.

Diabetes
- Mexican American adults were two times more likely than non-Hispanic white adults to have been diagnosed with diabetes by a physician.
- In 2002, Hispanics were 1.5 times as likely to start treatment for end-stage renal disease related to diabetes, compared to non-Hispanic white men.
- In 2004, Hispanics were 1.5 times as likely as non-Hispanic whites to die from diabetes.

Heart Disease
- In 2005, Hispanics were 10% less likely to have heart disease, compared to non-Hispanic whites.
- In 2004, Mexican American men were 30% less likely to die from heart disease, compared to non-Hispanic white men.
- Mexican American women were 1.3 times more likely than non-Hispanic white women to be obese.

HIV–AIDS
- Hispanics accounted for 18% of HIV–AIDS cases in 2005.
- Hispanic males had more than three times the AIDS rate than non-Hispanic white males.
- Hispanic females had more than five times the AIDS rate than non-Hispanic white females.
- Hispanic men were 2.6 times as likely to die from HIV AIDS than non Hispanic white men.
- Hispanic women were four times as likely to die from HIV–AIDS than non-Hispanic white women in 2004.

Immunization
- In 2005, Hispanic adults aged 65 years and older were 10% less likely to have received the influenza (flu) shot in the past 12 months, compared to non-Hispanic whites of the same age group.
- In 2005, Hispanic adults aged 65 years and older were 50% less likely to have ever received the pneumonia shot, compared to non-Hispanic white adults of the same age group.
- Although Hispanic children aged 19 to 35 months had comparable rates of immunization for hepatitis, influenza, MMR, and polio, they were slightly less likely to be fully immunized, compared to non-Hispanic white children.

Infant Mortality
- In 2004, infant mortality rates for Hispanic subpopulations ranged from 4.6 per 1,000 live births to 7.8 per 1,000 live births, compared to the non-Hispanic white infant mortality rate of 5.7 per 1,000 live births.
- In 2004, Puerto Ricans had 1.4 times the infant mortality rate of non-Hispanic whites.
- Puerto Rican infants were twice as likely to die from causes related to low birth weight, compared to non-Hispanic white infants.
- Mexican American mothers were 2.5 times as likely as non-Hispanic white mothers to begin prenatal care in the third trimester or not receive prenatal care at all.

Stroke
- In 2004, Hispanic men were 14% less likely to die from a stroke than non-Hispanic white men.
- In 2004, Hispanic women were 30% less likely to die from a stroke than non-Hispanic white women.

Source: Office of Minority Health. (2008).

CONSIDERATIONS FOR HEALTH PROMOTION AND PROGRAM PLANNING

The following are some concepts to consider when planning and implementing a health promotion program for this target audience.

- Preventive medicine is not a norm for most Hispanics. This behavior may be related to the Hispanic here-and-now orientation, as opposed to a future-planning orientation. It also is related to their fatalistic belief system.
- Some commonly known Hispanic sayings suggest that events in one's life result from luck, fate, or other powers beyond an individual's control. For example:
  - *Que será, será.* (What will be will be.)
  - *Que sea lo que Dios quiera.* (It's in God's hands.)
  - *Esta enfermedad es una prueba de Dios.* (This illness is a test of God.)
  - *De algo se tiene que morir uno.* (You have to die of something.)
- Persons with acute or chronic illness may regard themselves as innocent victims of malevolent forces. Severe illness may be attributed to God's design, bad behavior, or punishment. Genetic defects in a child may be attributed to the parents' actions.
- Consider sitting closer to Hispanic patients and clients than you would with people from other cultures.
- Be particularly aware of your nonverbal communication messages.
- Be aware that Hispanics often have higher exposure rates to environmental hazards due to living in urban environments, and males have high exposure due to their jobs.
- Family and friends may indulge patients, allowing them to be passive, which is an approach that may conflict with the Western view that active participation is required to prevent or heal much disease.
- Some Hispanic sayings support health promotion and illustrate the considerable status given to health and prevention:
  - *La salud es todo o casi todo.* (Health is everything, or almost everything.)
  - *Es mejor prevenir que curar.* (An ounce of prevention is worth a pound of cure.)
  - *Ayúdate que Dios te ayudará.* (Help yourself and God will help you.)
- "Helping yourself" may lead to placing responsibility for cure with the entire family. The challenge for health care professionals is to assess the amount of control patients believe they have over their health and to design interventions that build on traditional support systems.
- Vaccination is very important and adhered to for children.

- Western medicine is expected and preferred in case of severe illness, but some Hispanics also may use native healers, and the educator and provider should inquire about the utilization of other healers.
- Use appropriate titles to show respect, such as *señor* and *señorita*.
- A botanica is a resource store for herbs and other traditional remedies. Some Hispanics may go there before going to a physician or clinic. In many Latin American countries, pharmacists prescribe medications, and a wider range of medications is available over the counter. People may share medicines or write home for relatives to send them medications. Individuals may discontinue medication if it does not immediately alleviate symptoms or after their symptoms abate. Many Hispanics believe that taking too much medicine is harmful.
- When providing nutritional advice or education, use positive examples from Hispanic cultural foods.
- Consider suggesting family-based methods for increasing physical activity, such as dancing or walking with family members.
- If you have the patient's permission, involve the family members in the consultation because it may assist with increasing the listener's adherence to the recommendation(s).
- Consider using peer educators (promotoras) as community outreach workers for community-based efforts, because they have been shown to be successful with this community.
- Check for understanding and agreement, because Hispanics tend to avoid conflict and are hesitant to ask questions.
- Inquire about complementary and alternative treatments being used, because they are frequently utilized by Hispanics.
- Because of historic events, some Hispanics may distrust the health care system (many Puerto Rican women experienced involuntary sterilization and were adversely affected by birth control pill trials), view the health care system as an extension of a repressive government (Central Americans), or fear deportation, especially if they are not in the country legally.
- Some Hispanics confuse public health programs with welfare and avoid them due to stigma.

CHAPTER SUMMARY

Many people are not aware of the violent history of Hispanics in this country. Hispanics are the largest minority group in the United States, a group that is rapidly growing. They have strong ties to their country of origin, and many Hispanics, even after living here for a long period of time, do not view themselves as American. They have strong family ties and have held on to their cultural belief systems and practices. Hispanics have many unique features to their health belief systems and healing practices, and have types of healers that are not seen in other cultures, therefore, there are major differences that need to be considered when providing health care services to this population.

In this chapter, we have provided an overview of the history of Hispanics, including the fact that part of the United States previously belonged to Mexico. Many of the unique illnesses have been discussed, such as empacho and susto, along with treatment modalities, which include the treatment of hot and cold illnesses. Various types of healing systems have been discussed, such as curanderismo and Espiritismo. Common health behaviors and illnesses among this group have been explained, along with issues for consideration when developing health promotion and education efforts for this target population.

REVIEW

1. Explain the terms "Hispanic" and "Latino" and the reasons why they are not considered to be a race.
2. Provide an overview of the history of Hispanics in the United States.
3. Explain the socioeconomic conditions of Hispanics in the United States.
4. What are susto, empacho, and mal de ojo?
5. What are curanderismo, Santeria, and Espiritismo?
6. What are some of the common health risk behaviors and diseases among Hispanics in the United States?

CASE STUDY

This case focuses on a low-income, non-English speaking Latino patient and family. As you read through this story, pay special attention to issues involved in medical decision making, such as gender roles and values and interest in treatments outside of traditional Western medicine based on culturally constructed folk illness beliefs.

When Alejandro Flores was born, his parents were ecstatic and very proud. Alejandro was their first child born in the continental United States, in a world far away from their tradition and family in Puerto Rico. The Flores family had worked very hard to move to the northeast a year before Alejandro's birth, and they felt that his arrival helped connect them with their new home.

It is four years after Alejandro's birth, and the Flores family has grown even larger. There are now five children (three older than Alejandro and one 20-month-old baby) and Alejandro's grandmother living in the same apartment. Alejandro's mother, Señora Flores, takes care of her family as best she can, and she feels lucky to have her mother there to give her advice and a helping hand. Señor Flores works very hard as a custodian at a local school to provide his family with enough income. He has picked up a little English at work, but only Spanish is spoken at home.

Serious asthma problems run in the Flores family, and Alejandro is no exception. Although he looks healthy, Alejandro has had severe asthma for several years. When he was 2 years old, a series of awful wheezing episodes sent him to the hospital multiple times. His parents do their best to care for him, but they are both spread pretty thin and have limited time available. To help with all of Alejandro's asthma problems, the Flores family recently relocated to a new apartment that has air conditioning, and Sr. Flores has limited his smoking to outside on the patio. The family has two dogs, which could be a problem, but they just couldn't see getting rid of two loved members of their family.

Alejandro also takes a lot of medications for his asthma symptoms. His parents have been taught about asthma and have been given an asthma action plan—all in Spanish. They were told to call the clinic if at any time Alejandro's symptoms worsened. Despite these actions, Alejandro still continues to have heavy wheezing and a tight cough, especially at night.

With Alejandro continuing to have asthma problems, Sra. Flores became skeptical that the medications were not working. Under the guidance of her mother, she took Alejandro to an espiritista (in curandcrismo, the Mexican American healing system, an espiritista is a healer who serves as a medium for exorcisms and is adept at facilitating the help of benevolent spirits and removing malevolent spirits that surround the client). At the espiritista's advice, Sra. Flores stopped giving Alejandro all of the prescribed medications and began giving him an herbal tea that she believed, along with prayer, would take Alejandro's asthma symptoms completely away.

Alejandro and his parents attended their regularly scheduled visit to the clinic to see if the new medications were helping to control Alejandro's symptoms. This is the second visit since Alejandro's last hospitalization six months ago. Sra. Flores has not contacted anyone at the clinic about Alejandro's asthma getting worse, so the clinic staff assumes the best.

There are several issues to consider about this case:

- Why might Sra. Flores have chosen to consult an espiritista rather than call the clinic when Alejandro was not getting better?
- Do you think that traditional Latino gender roles might have some affect on this child and family's experience with the health care system?

- How might it be possible to incorporate alternative folk remedies with mainstream Western medicine in developing a treatment plan for Alejandro?

Source: Cross Cultural Health Care Case Studies. (n.d.).

MODEL PROGRAM

Sembrando Salud

Sembrando Salud is a culturally sensitive, community-based tobacco and alcohol-use prevention program in San Diego County, California, that is specifically adapted for migrant Hispanic adolescents and their families. The program is designed to improve parent–child communication skills as a way of developing and maintaining healthy decision making. Designed for youths 11 to 16 years old, the intervention consists of eight weekly two-hour sessions where adolescents meet in small groups. Sessions usually take place during the evenings at school or at other community-based organizations. Sessions are run by trained group leaders, all of whom are bilingual Mexican Americans. Group leaders are trained over 10 weekly sessions and are monitored throughout the intervention to ensure consistency and quality of program implementation.

The program interventions are a mix of interactive teaching methods, including videos, demonstrations, skill practice, group discussions led by a leader, and role-playing. All interventions include three central components: (1) information about the health effects of tobacco/alcohol use, (2) social influences on tobacco/alcohol use, and (3) training in refusal skills. Further, adolescents are exposed to how problems can be identified and analyzed, solutions can be generated, and decisions can be made, implemented, and evaluated. There is an additional emphasis on developing parental support for the healthy discussions and behaviors of adolescents through enhanced parent–child communications. Parental communication skills—such as listening, confirmation, and reassurance—also are developed. The program reinforces new behavioral skills, such as communicating with peers and adults and refusing alcohol and tobacco offers.

Evaluation

A randomized pretest–posttest control group study was implemented to determine whether the intervention held true to its design and affected parent–child communication. Schools within geographic regions were prerandomized to a treatment condition (tobacco and alcohol use prevention) or an attention-control condition (first aid/home safety). Each condition was designed to be equivalent in all respects (except for the content) and included eight weekly, two-hour sessions, with parents attending three of the eight sessions jointly with their adolescent. Each week was formatted into small-group evening sessions held on school grounds or at a neighborhood community agency.

Outcome

This culturally sensitive, family-based intervention for migrant Hispanic youth was found to be effective in increasing perceived parent–child communication in families with few children. Specifically, parents and children enrolled in the treatment condition reported greater improvements in communication than those in the attention-control condition. The intervention appeared to be more effective in smaller families, presumably because of the increased opportunity for parents to monitor and communicate with participating youths.

The study had notable limitations, so the results may not be generalized. First, the study targeted a hard-to-reach population, with 60% of those eligible not participating. This factor makes it difficult to generalize the findings to those who were not reached. Additional limitations include the short-term nature of the follow-up, which does not allow any determination of long-term effects, and reliance on self-report measures, which raises the concern that the promising results of the intervention are due to the desire of parents and their children to be presented in a positive light. That being said, it certainly is a noteworthy, promising practice.

Source: Office of Juvenile Justice and Delinquency Prevention. (n.d.).

GLOSSARY TERMS _____

empacho   orishas
Santeria   Espiritismo

REFERENCES _____

American Heart Association. (n.d.). *Statistical fact sheet—risk factors*. Retrieved March 31, 2008, from http://www.americanheart.org/downloadable/heart/1136820021462Overweight06.pdf

American Lung Association. (2007). *Smoking and Hispanics fact sheet*. Retrieved March 31, 2008, from http://www.lungusa.org/site/pp.asp?c=dvLUK9O0E&b=36002

Caetano, R., & Clark, C. L. (1998). Trends in alcohol-related problems among whites, blacks, and Hispanics: 1984–1995. *Alcoholism: Clinical and Experimental Research, 22,* 534–538.

Caetano, R., Clark, C. L., & Tam, T. (1998). *Alcohol consumption among racial/ethnic minorities.* Retrieved March 31, 2008, from http://www.hawaii.edu/hivandaids/Alcohol%20Consumption%20Among%20RacialEthnic%20Minorities%20%20%20%20%20Theory%20and%20Research.pdf

Carigan, W. D. (2003). The lynching of persons of Mexican origin or descent in the United States, 1848 to 1928. *Journal of Social History.* Retrieved March 28, 2008, from http://findarticles.com/p/articles/mi_m2005/is_2_37/ai_111897839/pg_1

Centers for Disease Control and Prevention. (n.d.). National Health interview surrey, 2000. Retrieved April 19, 2009, from http://www.cdc.gov/nchs/data/nhis/measure09.pdf.

Church of Likumi Babalu Aye v. City of Hialeah, 508 US 520 (1993).

Cross Cultural Health Care Case Studies. (n.d.). *The Case of Alejandro Flores.* Retrieved June 16, 2008, from http://support.mchtraining.net/national_ccce/case3/case.html

Juckett, G. (2005). Cross-cultural medicine. *American Family Physician.* Retrieved March 30, 2008, from http://www.aafp.org/afp/20051201/2267.html

New Century Foundation. (2006). *Hispanics: A statistical portrait.* Retrieved March 8, 2008, from http://www.amren.com/Reports/Hispanics/HispanicsReport.htm

Office of Juvenile Justice and Delinquency Prevention. (n.d.). *Programs guide. Sembrando Salud.* Retrieved January 16, 2008, from http://www.dsgonline.com/mpg2.5//TitleV_MPG_Table_Ind_Rec.asp?id=626

Office of Minority Health. (2008). *Hispanic/Latino profile.* Retrieved March 8, 2008, from http://www.omhrc.gov/templates/browse.aspx?lvl=2&lvlid=54

Oldways Preservation & Exchange Trust. Latino Nutrition Coalition. (n.d.). *Latin American diet food.* Retrieved March 17, 2008, from http://www.oldwayspt.org/

Olmos, M. F., & Paravisini-Gebert, L. (2003). *Creole religions of the Caribbean: An introduction from vodou and Santeria to obeah and Espiritismo.* New York: New York University Press.

Rhode Island Department of Health. (n.d.). *Latino/Hispanic culture & health.* Retrieved March 17, 2008, from http://www.health.ri.gov/chic/minority/lat_cul.php

US Census Bureau. (2004). *We the people: Hispanics in the United States.* Retrieved March 8, 2008, from http://www.census.gov/prod/2004pubs/censr-18.pdf

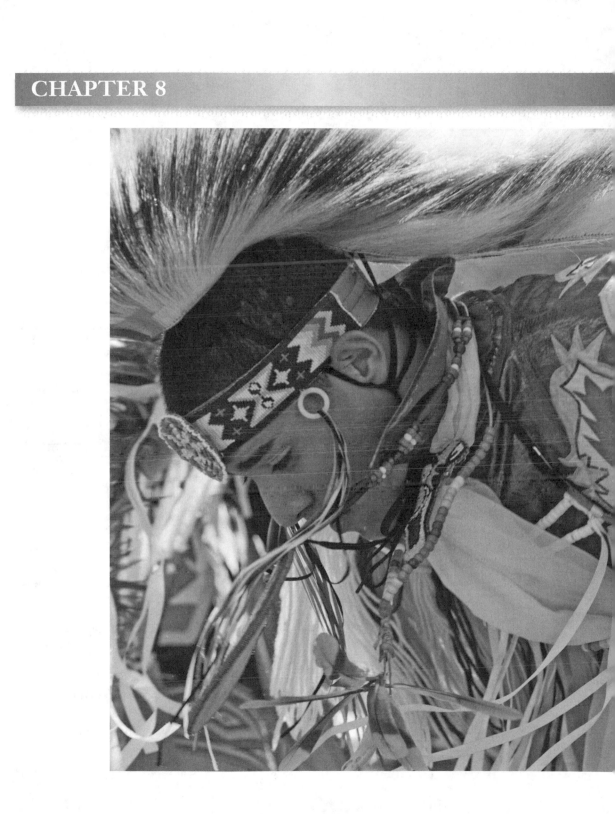

CHAPTER 8

American Indian and Alaska Native Populations

What we see as science, Indians see as magic. What we see as magic, they see as science. I don't find a hopeless contradiction. If we can appreciate each others views, we can see the whole picture more clearly.

—Hammerschlag (1988, p. 14)

Everything on the earth has a purpose, every disease an herb to cure it, and every person a mission. This is the Indian theory of existence.

—Mourning Dove Salish

KEY CONCEPTS

- Sweat lodges
- Talking circles
- Peyote
- Sand painting
- Medicine wheel
- Medicine bundle

CHAPTER OBJECTIVES

1. Provide an overview of the social and economic circumstances of American Indians and Alaska Natives in the United States.
2. Provide an overview of American Indian and Alaska Native beliefs about the causes of illness.
3. Describe at least three American Indian and Alaska Native healing practices.
4. Describe American Indian and Alaska Native health risk behaviors and common illnesses.
5. List at least six tips for working with American Indian and Alaska Native populations.

The terms "American Indian" and "Alaska Native" refer to people descended from any of the original peoples of North and South America (including Central America) and who maintain tribal affiliation or community attachment (US Census Bureau, 2002). There is a wide range of terms used to describe these groups, such as Native Indians, American Indians, Native American Indians, Indians, Indigenous, Aboriginal, Native Alaskans, and Original Americans. It is important to note that not all Native Americans come from the contiguous United States. Native Hawaiians, for example, also can be considered Native American, but it is not common to use such a designation. In this book we have chosen to use the same terminology as the 2000 United States census, which are American Indians and Alaska Natives, unless the data source uses other terms. Much of the data on these two groups have been gathered collectively, and when available, the data will be reported separately in this chapter.

The American Indian and Alaska Native populations are diverse, geographically dispersed, and economically disadvantaged (Management Sciences for Health, n.d.). Disease patterns among American Indians and Alaska Natives are associated with negative consequences of poverty, limited access to health services, and cultural dislocation (Management Sciences for Health, n.d.). Inadequate education, high rates of unemployment, discrimination, and cultural differences all contribute to unhealthy lifestyles and disparities in access to health care for many American Indian and Alaska Native people (Management Sciences for Health, n.d.).

American Indians and Alaska Natives also are very self-determined and proud people. In a special message on Indian affairs delivered on July 8, 1970, to Congress, President Richard Nixon declared:

> But the story of the Indian in America is something more than the record of the white man's frequent aggression, broken agreements, intermittent remorse and prolonged failure. It is a record of enormous contributions to this country—to its art and culture, to its strength and spirit, to its sense of history and its sense of purpose (President Nixon, July 8, 1970).

In this chapter we provide a brief history of American Indian and Alaska Native populations, information about their current status in the United States, their beliefs about the causes of illness and healing practices, behavioral risk factors, and the common health problems that they face. The first part of the chapter is focused on American Indians and the second section is about Alaska Natives, and then we combine the groups when we discuss key points to consider when working with these populations.

HISTORY OF AMERICAN INDIANS IN THE UNITED STATES

The American Indians are descendents of the first humans who migrated from Asia and Europe to North America about 30,000 years ago. Christopher Columbus "discovered" North America in 1492 during his voyage in search for the East Indies. He used the name "Indians" to describe the native people of the land.

The European invasion that began in the fifteenth century changed the lives of American Indians. In addition to the aggressive violence and wars against the American

Indians, new diseases, such as smallpox and measles, were introduced, and the indigenous Americans had no immunities to them. In addition, the Europeans' racism, genocide, and ethnocentrism prevented them from accepting the Indians as equals. The American Indians were viewed as a problem with the solution being to eradicate them through wars and to push any survivors westward.

In the nineteenth century, the westward expansion of the United States caused large numbers of American Indians to resettle farther west, often by force, almost always reluctantly. The United States Congress, under President Andrew Jackson, passed the Indian Removal Act of 1830, which authorized the president to conduct treaties to exchange American Indian land east of the Mississippi River for lands west of the river. As many as 100,000 Native Americans eventually relocated in the West as a result of this Indian Removal Act. In theory, relocation was supposed to be voluntary, but in practice great pressure was put on American Indian leaders to sign removal treaties. President Jackson told people to kill as many bison as possible to cut out the Plains Indian's main source of food (Kelman, 1999). At one point, there were fewer than 500 bison left in the Great Plains (Kelman, 1999).

Many steps were taken to "civilize" American Indians, such as not permitting them to speak their native language and creating Indian boarding schools. The Indian Citizenship Act of 1924 gave U.S. citizenship to American Indians, in part because of an interest by many to see them merged with the American mainstream and also because of the service of many Native American veterans in World War I.

AMERICAN INDIANS IN THE UNITED STATES

American Indians in the United States comprise a large number of distinct tribes. There are 561 federally recognized tribal governments in the United States. In addition, there are a number of tribes that are recognized by individual states but not by the federal government. The rights and benefits associated with state recognition vary from state to state. Being federally recognized is important to the tribes, because it describes the right of federally recognized tribes to govern themselves (called tribal sovereignty) and creates the existence of a government-to-government relationship with the United States. Thus, a tribe is not a ward of the government but an independent nation with the right to form its own government, enforce criminal and civil laws, levy taxes within its borders, establish its membership, and license and regulate activities. Nonrecognized tribes do not have these powers. Limitations on tribal powers of self-government include the same limitations applicable to states; for example, neither tribes nor states have the power to make war, engage in foreign relations, or

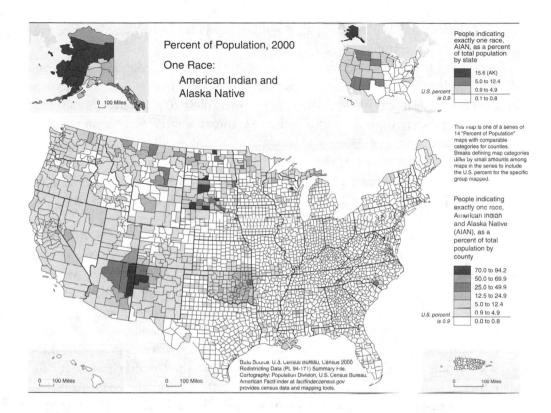

FIGURE 8.1 Percentage of population: American Indian and Alaska Native, 2000. Source. U.S. Census Bureau, Population Division (2008), http://www.census.gov/main/www/citation.html.

coin money (this includes paper currency). The federal government has a trust responsibility to protect tribal lands, assets, resources, and treaty rights. Others reasons why federal recognition is important is that the tribe has the right to label arts and crafts as Native American and apply for grants that are specifically reserved for American Indians.

According to the U.S. Census Bureau (2002), in 2000, 1.5% of the population reported being American Indian or Alaska Native. Forty-three percent live in the West, 31% in the South, 17% in the Midwest, and 9% in the Northeast (see Figure 8.1). California has the largest American Indian and Alaska Native population, followed by Oklahoma, Arizona, Texas, New Mexico, and New York (US Census Bureau, 2002). California and Oklahoma combined include about 25% of the total American Indian and Alaska Native population (US Census Bureau, 2002). As of 2000, the largest tribes in the United States by population were Cherokee, Navajo, Latin American, and Choctaw, respectively (US Census Bureau, 2002). As of 2006, of the 4.5 million

American Indians and Alaska Natives, 1.8 million lived on reservations or other trust lands (Office of Minority Health, 2008).

Seventy-six percent of American Indians and Alaska Natives aged 25 years and older have at least a high school diploma, and 14% aged 25 years and older have at least a bachelor's degree (Office of Minority Health, 2008). Slightly over 50,000 aged 25 years and older have at least an advanced graduate degree (i.e., master's, PhD, medical, or law) (Office of Minority Health, 2008). The median family income for American Indians and Alaska Natives is $33,627, with 26% of American Indians and Alaska Natives aged 16 years and older working in management and professional occupations. Twenty-five percent of American Indians and Alaska Natives live at the poverty level (Office of Minority Health, 2008).

In 2003, 45% of American Indians and Alaska Natives had private health insurance coverage, and 21.3% relied on Medicaid coverage (Office of Minority Health, 2008). Thirty percent had no health insurance coverage in 2005 (Office of Minority Health, 2008). The Indian Health Service (IHS), an agency within the U.S. Department of Health and Human Services, is responsible for providing federal health services to American Indians and Alaska Natives (Indian Health Service, 2007). The provision of health services to members of federally-recognized tribes grew out of the special government-to-government relationship between the federal government and Indian tribes. This relationship was established in 1787. The IHS is the principal federal health care provider and health advocate for Indian people, and its goal is to raise their health status to the highest possible level. The IHS currently provides health services to approximately 1.5 million American Indians and Alaska Natives. Approximately 57% of American Indians and Alaska Natives living in the United States rely on the Indian Health Service to provide access to health care services in 46 hospitals and over 600 other facilities (Indian Health Service, 2007).

Many of the American Indian and Alaska Native languages have become extinct since the invasion of the Europeans. Only eight indigenous languages of the continental United States currently have a population of speakers in the United States and Canada large enough to populate a medium-sized town (Rehling, n.d.). Navajo is the largest American Indian language still spoken, with about 149,000 speakers, followed by Cree, Ojibwa, Cherokee, Dakota, Apache, Blackfoot, and Choctaw (Rehling, n.d.).

American Indians believe in a Supreme Creator; most tribes also have lesser deities like Mary or Jesus figures and mediators between the spirit world and the earth (similar to saints in Christianity). They believe that people should try to maintain constant, daily harmony and contact with the Creator, follow all sacred teachings, and treat all life (people, animals, plants, rocks, rivers, rainbows, etc.) with respect.

American Indians are family-based people. American Indians are taught to respect their elders and obey their orders. The elders are seen as people with much knowledge and are considered to be the head of the household. After the elders, men are considered to be the leaders of the house. In addition to being the chiefs of the house, men also are viewed as the leaders of the tribe, protectors, and fighters. Traditionally, the men would go out and hunt to bring food for the whole community; as a result, they are still seen as the providers for the family.

Women are still viewed as the people who do all of the housework, gather materials, and take care of the home, and they teach the children the ways of the American Indians. The children have to learn the traditions of the tribe and community and have to respect the elders. The older family members keep an eye on the new generation to make sure that they are following traditions.

Besides believing in close family relations, American Indians also believe in living in a community. Many different tribes live together in one community. To be a member of the community, a person does not need to be from the same tribe or even have blood relations with anyone from the community. As many as 80 different tribes can live together in one community (West Virginia Division of Culture and History, 2008). The elders are in charge of teaching and guiding the community in the ways of the tribes and have the responsibility to pass on their history orally. They also teach the community the traditional ways of the tribe. They show the new generation how to make traditional arts and crafts and show them the traditional rituals.

One of the rituals is storytelling or experiencing stories through songs or other performances. Songs play an important part of the American Indians' lives. The songs the American Indians execute are usually ancestral songs that tell the story of the ancestors and of hardships they had to face. Many of the songs are related to nature and hunting. The songs are considered to be the property of the person who dreamt it or of the community after that person passes away. If someone wants to reenact the song, they must obtain special permission from the community.

Music and dance are often linked together in performances. Everyone who attends the performance has to take part in it one way or another. The American Indians believe that even witnessing a performance is considered having participated in the performance. The dances are a way the American Indians express themselves and what surrounds them. The dances are done to celebrate an occasion and to promote unity and togetherness. During the dance, the dancers make lots of noise and wear certain kinds of clothes, depending on the event. For example, they might dress up as animals or like spirits to honor them.

With regard to their dietary practices, American Indians believe that certain foods are sacred. For example, some American Indians believe the Great Spirit

Hashtali gave the American Indians corn as a present, so it is considered to be sacred. Corn is used quite frequently for meals because it can be easily grown and does not require a lot of work. The American Indians use corn to make flour and bread, and it can be eaten as is or dried. Another sacred food is blood soup, which is made from a mixture of blood and corn flour cooked in broth. Blood soup may be used as a sacred meal during the nighttime Holy Smoke ceremony of the Sioux, which is a celebration of Mother Earth that involves the use of the peace pipe (Advameg, 2007). Wolves and coyotes are the only animals that are not hunted for food, because they are regarded as teachers or pathfinders and held as sacred by all tribes (Advameg, 2007). At marriage ceremonies, the bride and groom exchange food instead of rings (Advameg, 2007). The groom brings venison or some other meat to indicate his intention to provide for the household, and the bride provides corn or bean bread to symbolize her willingness to care for and provide nourishment for the household (Advameg, 2007).

American Indian diets and food practices have changed possibly more than any other ethnic group in the United States. Although the current diet of American Indians may vary by tribe and by personal traits such as age, it closely resembles that of the U.S. white population. There is no statistically significant difference in the overall diet quality of American Indians and the rest of the U.S. population, but the majority of American Indians do consume too much fat (62% of their diet is fat) (Advameg, 2007). On any given day, only 21% of American Indians eat the recommended amount of fruit, 34% eat the amount of vegetables that are recommended, 24% eat the recommended amount of grains, and 27% consume the recommended amount of dairy products (Advameg, 2007). American Indians also are four times more likely to report not having enough to eat than other U.S. households (Advameg, 2007).

The U.S. Department of Agriculture (USDA) food guide for American Indians can be found in Figure 8.2. The bald eagle is shown on the pyramid because almost all American Indians attach special significance to the eagle and its feathers. Images of eagles and their feathers are used on many tribal logos as symbols of the American Indians. To be given an eagle feather is the highest honor that can be awarded within indigenous cultures. Bald and golden eagles (and their feathers) are highly revered and considered to be sacred within American Indian traditions, culture, and religion. They represent honesty, truth, strength, courage, wisdom, power, and freedom. Because these birds roam the sky, they are believed to have a special connection to God. According to traditional American Indian beliefs, the Creator made all the birds of the sky when the world was new. Of all the birds, the Creator chose the eagle to be the leader . . . the Master of the Sky. The eagle is considered to be a messenger to God (American Eagle Foundation, n.d.).

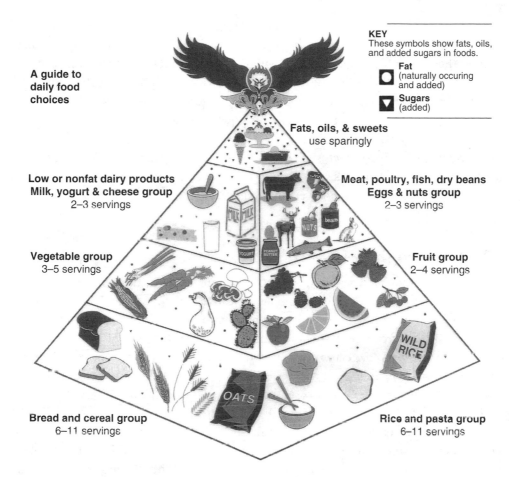

KEY
These symbols show fats, oils, and added sugars in foods.

□ **Fat** (naturally occuring and added)

▼ **Sugars** (added)

A guide to daily food choices

Fats, oils, & sweets
use sparingly

Low or nonfat dairy products
Milk, yogurt & cheese group
2–3 servings

Meat, poultry, fish, dry beans
Eggs & nuts group
2–3 servings

Vegetable group
3–5 servings

Fruit group
2–4 servings

Bread and cereal group
6–11 servings

Rice and pasta group
6–11 servings

FIGURE 8.2 Native American food guide.
Source: CANFIT, Berkeley, CA. For more information, call 510-644-1533 or info@canfit.org. Used with permission.

BELIEFS ABOUT CAUSES OF HEALTH AND ILLNESS AMONG AMERICAN INDIANS

To American Indians, health is a continual process of staying strong spiritually, mentally, and physically. This strength keeps away or overcomes the forces that cause illness. People must stay in harmony with themselves, other people, their natural environment, and their Creator. Adhering to traditional and tribal beliefs and obeying tribal religious codes is another part of staying healthy because violating tribal tenets or laws has consequences like physical or mental illness, disability, ongoing bad luck, or trauma. The violation must be set right before harmony and health can be restored. American Indians believe illness is the price to be paid either for something that happened in the past or for something that will happen in the future; therefore, each person is responsible for his or her health. Illness is not looked upon as abnormal.

This group does not believe in biomedicine or germ theory, because they believe illness is caused by personal responsibility, qualities, and spirits (Spector, 2004). There are three distinct causes of illness to trigger patient suffering: (1) by a hostile spirit thrusting a foreign object, such as a sharp stone, insect, or a tangled thread, into the person; (2) by the patient's soul leaving the body on its own accord; (3) and by the patient's soul being stolen away by enemy spirits (Haas, 2007).

HEALING TRADITIONS AMONG AMERICAN INDIANS

Most American Indian tribes have healing traditions that are not based on Western science and are related to their beliefs about the causation of illness and disease. Therefore, many healing traditions and rituals focus on harmony, and the overall purpose is to bring participants into harmony with themselves, their tribe, and all of life. Healing occurs when someone is restored to harmony and connected to universal powers. Traditional healing is holistic. It focuses on the person, not the illness, so the process does not focus on symptoms or diseases, because it addresses the total individual.

Traditional healing practices are still used frequently. Marbella, Harris, Diehr, Ignace, and Ignace (1998) conducted semistructured interviews in an urban setting to gain an understanding of the prevalence, utilization patterns, and practice implications of the use of Native American healers together with the use of physicians. Thirty tribal affiliations were represented. These researchers found that 38% of the patients see a healer, and of those who do not, 86% would consider seeing one in the future. Most patients reported seeing a healer for spiritual reasons. Among those seeing healers, the most frequently mentioned were spiritual healers (50.9%), herbalists (42.1%), and medicine men (28.1%). These percentages add up to more than 100% because some patients reported seeing more than one type of healer (Marbella et al., 1998). More than a third of the patients seeing healers received different advice from their physicians and healers. The patients rate their healer's advice higher than their physician's advice 61.4% of the time. Only 14.8% of the patients seeing healers tell their physician about their use of healers (Marbella et al., 1998).

In the following section we discuss **sweat lodges**, **talking circles**, plants and herbs, healing ceremonies, and types and practices of healers. The information has been divided into these categories to help organize the information for the reader, but the categories are arbitrary to some extent. For example, healers use plants and herbs, but we have put them into separate categories for educational purposes.

Sweat Lodges

Sweat lodges are used for healing and balancing. American Indians consider sweat lodges to be a good way to clean one's body and sweat out illness or disease (Bonvillain, 1997). Hot stones covered in water are placed in a small, confined, dark enclosure, creating a steam bath. The stones, considered by American Indians to be their oldest living relatives, are usually lava rocks that do not break when heated. Sweating removes toxins from the body, stimulates the endocrine glands, and makes the heart pump more blood. American Indians believe that sweat lodges also bring balance and health to spirit, mind, and body. They use sweat lodges in many ways, such as before spiritual undertakings, to bring clarity to a problem, to call upon helpful spirits, and to reconnect with the Great Spirit.

Even the building of a sweat lodge is sacred and symbolic. As shown in Figure 8.3, willow saplings are bent and tied together to form a square with four sides, which

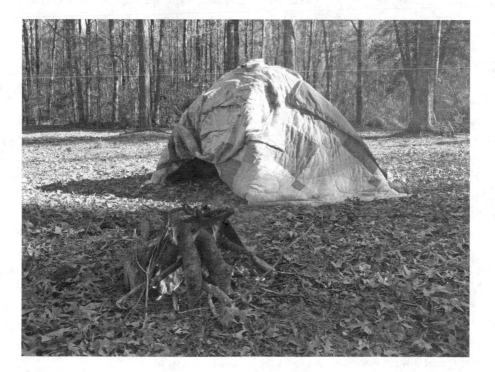

FIGURE 8.3 Sweat lodge.
Source: Courtesy of Kirk Shoemaker.

represents the sacred four directions. There usually is a single entryway that faces either west or east. The connected poles create a frame that looks like an over-turned basket, which symbolically represents items such as the womb or arch of the sky. In some tribes there are 28 poles, which represent either the ribs of a woman, a female bear or turtle, or the lunar cycle. The framework is covered in the skins of buffalo or other animals that represent the animal world. The interior of sweat lodges can be created out of many different materials depending on what is available to the community. The interior can be made out of furs, grasses, or various types of bark from trees. A small pit, or alter, is dug in the center of the lodge for the stones. A branch that represents the tree of life is placed in the middle of the alter and is surrounded by small stones. Antlers to move the hot stones and a medicine pipe are placed near the alter.

Before the sweat lodge is used, "The One Who Pours the Water" purifies the surrounding area by smearing it with sacred herbs to ensure that positive spirits will be present. A stone tender stays outside the lodge, heating stones and passing them inside when summoned by The One Who Pours the Water. One heated stone is not used; it is left for the spirits to sweat with and honors the spirits who have come to the ceremony.

Talking Circles

Talking circles are highly regarded among American Indian people, because they reflect the circle of life. To American Indians, the circle represents that all life is cyclical in nature, such as the changing of the seasons, the phases of the moon, the shape of the world, and the shape of the universe. All parts in the circle are equal.

Traditionally, the group gathers in a circle, and the facilitators provide a list of general but important questions for discussion. These questions may be used as a guide for discussion, but they also are useful to facilitate opportunities for casual, informal conversation and storytelling. The group passes around what is called a "talking feather." Whoever has the feather states what is on his or her mind but has not been said. When that person is finished talking, the feather is handed to the next person in a clockwise direction, and the next person says what has been left unsaid. The person who holds the feather cannot be interrupted. Traditionally, an eagle feather, which is a sacred symbol, was passed around the circle. Sometimes other objects are used. Today the practice is so ingrained in the behavior of Indian people that it is not always necessary to use an object in the circle.

Plants and Herbs

American Indians use herbs to purify the spirit and bring balance to people who are unhealthy in spirit, mind, or body. They learned about the healing powers of herbs by watching sick animals. They use a wide variety of plants and herbs for healing. In fact, there are so many that books have been written on them. A few of the herbs will be covered here, but describing all of them is beyond the focus of this book.

One plant they use is sage, which is believed to protect against bad spirits and to draw them out of the body or the soul. American Indians use sage for many purposes, such as to heal problems of the stomach, colon, nasal passages, kidneys, liver, lungs, pores of the skin, bones, and sex organs; to heal burns and scrapes; as an antiseptic for allergies, colds, and fever; as a gargle for sore throat; and as a tea to calm the nerves. Cedar, a tall evergreen tree, is a milder medicine than sage. It is combined with sage and sweetgrass, a plant that grows in damp environments like marshes or near water, to make a powerful mixture used in sacred ceremonies. Cedar fruit and leaves are boiled and then drank to heal coughs. For head colds, cedar is burned and inhaled. Some of the other herbs that are used include acacia, prickly pear, saw palmetto, sunflower, yerba mansa, cliffrose, and cayenne.

Tobacco, often smoked in medicine pipes, is one of the most sacred plants to American Indians, and it is used in some way in nearly every cure. It is smoked pure and is not mixed with chemicals. When American Indians smoke sacred tobacco and other herbs, their breath, which they consider to be the source of life, becomes visible. When smoke is released, it rises up to the Great Spirit carrying prayers. People who share a pipe are acknowledging that they share the same breath. There are many different types of medicine pipes; some are for war, sun, and marriage, and there are tribal, personal, ceremonial, and social pipes. The pipe itself, made of wood with a soft pithy center, is symbolic, and some are shaped like animals. The bowl represents the female aspect of the Great Spirit–Mother Earth. The stem represents the male aspect of the Great Spirit–Father Sky. Together, the bowl and stem represent the union that brings forth life. The bowl in which tobacco is burned also symbolizes all that changes. The stem signifies all that is unchanging. Smoking the pipe is a central component in all ceremonies because it unites the two worlds of spirit and matter.

Another important plant that is used is peyote, which is a hallucinogenic drug. **Peyote** is a spineless, dome-shaped cactus (*Lophophora williamsii*) that is native to Mexico and the southwest United States. It has buttonlike tubercles that are chewed fresh or dry. Peyote has a history of ritual religious and medicinal use among certain indigenous American Indian tribes going back thousands of years. Peyote is legal only on Indian reservations because of its spiritual and healing properties (Bonvillain, 1997). It is viewed by American Indians as an agent that allows one to encounter spirits and receive visions or messages from spirits or Gods. American Indians also believe that peyote "can be used to make a person throw up and thus this would expel the illness from the body" (Bonvillain, 1997).

Healing Ceremonies

Ceremonies are used to help groups of people return to harmony, and they are not used for individual healing. The ceremonies used by the tribes vary, and there are differences in the way they practice medicine.

For example, the Navajo heal through their **sand painting**, see Figure 8.4. Sitting on the floor of a house, the medicine person begins painting at sunrise using ground colored rocks and minerals. The paintings depict the gods, elements of the heavens, and religious objects. After the painting which includes complex forms and designs in great detail, is completed, the patient is placed in the center of the painting. The healing

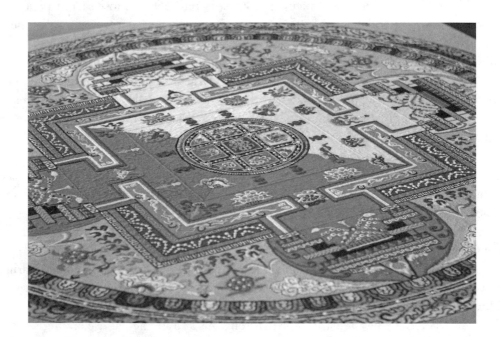

FIGURE 8.4   Sand painting.
Source: © Bestweb/ShutterStock, Inc.

ceremony, which includes rituals and chants, is performed. Before sunset, the medicine person destroys the painting. The sands are sent to the desert and scattered on the four winds.

The Iroquois practice medicine through their False Faces, a religious society. Each spring and fall, when most illnesses occur, society members wear strange and distorted masks to drive illness and disease away from the tribe. Wearing these masks and ragged clothes and carrying rattles made from tortoise shells, they perform a dance. After the dance, society members go from house to house to rid the community of evil.

Some tribes use medicine wheels, see Figure 8.5. The medicine wheel's large circle measures 213 feet around. The 28 spokes radiating from its center represent the number of days in the lunar cycle. A medicine wheel is a metaphor or symbol that represents the circle of life and the individual journey each person must take to find his or her own path. Within the medicine wheel are the four cardinal directions and the four sacred colors. The wheel is typically separated into four sections, which represent the north, south, east, and west. The Mother Earth is below the wheel and the Father Sky is above it. The south (white) represents fire and passion, and the animals that are

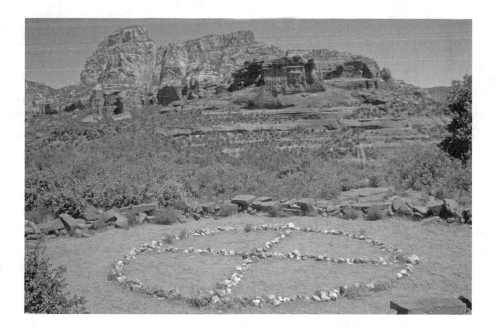

FIGURE 8.5 Medicine wheel.
Source: © Dana White/PhotoEdit, Inc.

associated with it, such as the eagle and lion, represent pride, strength, and courage. The north (blue) represents air and flight and is associated with winged animals that fly, such as the owl and hummingbird. The west (black) is associated with water and emotions and is associated with animals that work in teams and prepare for winter, such as the snake (because it sheds its skin) and the beaver. The east (red) is linked to the earth and wisdom and is related to animals that have layers of fat to sustain them during the winter, such as the buffalo. The wheel helps American Indians to see exactly where they are and in which areas they need to develop to realize and fulfill their potential. They see that people are all connected to one another, and by showing the intricacies of the interwoven threads of life, they can envision their role in life. It helps them understand that without their part in the tapestry, the bigger picture is not as it should be. It is a model to be used to view self, society, or anything that one could ever think of looking into.

Healers

Medicine men are prominent healers in the American Indian community. Medicine men can be male or female. They have knowledge about the interrelationships of human beings, the earth, the universe, plants, animals, the sun, the moon, and the stars (Spector, 2004). These healers are in tune with the way human beings interact with the world around them, and they are able to use their environment to help provide treatment. A healer is held in high regard because it has taken him or her many years of training and apprenticeship to be able to heal the community. Many American Indians first consult a medicine man before seeking other health professionals because of their belief that the treatment they receive from the traditional healer is better than treatment from health care establishments (Spector, 2004).

Medicine men have power that other members of the tribe do not have. Their power comes from visions that lead them into studying medicine or by being born into a family with many generations of medicine people. In many tribes, both men and women can serve as medicine people, but in some, like the Yurok in California, only women can be medicine people. Some medicine people are also shamans (holy men and women). A shaman is a healer who goes on a "soul journey" or a "soul flight" to the spirit world, aided by the power of songs, drums, rattles, and other objects, to communicate with spirits then performs a healing ceremony (Haas, 2007). All medicine people are considered to be learned and are respected members of the tribe.

Medicine people have naturalistic skills. Some medicine people specialize in areas like herbal medicine, bone setting, midwifery, or counseling. Often the medicine man cures people simply because they believe in him or her (placebo effect). Medicine people bring hope, understanding, and confidence to patients, which are often as powerful as modern medicine could have been. They work in the unseen world of good and bad spirits to restore harmony and health.

American Indians believe that they are related to all forms of life. Medicine people make medicine tools out of materials from nature, including fur, skins, bone, crystals, shells, roots, and feathers. They use these tools to evoke the spirit of what the tool has been made of, which helps strengthen their inner powers. For example, a medicine drum is made of wood and animal skins. When medicine people play the drum, they can call up the assistance of the spirits of the tree and the animal from which the drum was made.

Medicine people keep their medicine tools in a **medicine bundle**, see Figure 8.6. This is a large piece of cloth or hide that they tie securely with a thong, piece of yarn, or string. The contents of the medicine bundle are sacred. Each medicine person may own or share different medicine bundles: one's own, the tribe's, and bundles for special purposes, like seeking visions, hunting, or protection in battle. Some are passed down from one generation to the next. Personal medicine bundles are private, and asking about another person's medical tools is forbidden. Some medicine bundles are small enough to be worn around the neck. Medicine bundles that belong to tribes are often called the "grandmothers", because they have the power to nourish and nurture the tribe and promote continued well-being. Tribal medicine bundles grow stronger with each passing year.

Tribes carefully guard the knowledge of their medicine people. Members of the tribe who want to become medicine people must first serve a long apprenticeship with an experienced medicine person. In many tribes, medicine men cannot charge for their services. Gifts, however, are expected. Some tribes do require payment and have set lists of standard gifts. Nearly all tribes recognize tobacco as a gift of respect.

One way medicine men help heal the community is by using various forms of plants and herbal remedies. Medicine men spend many years during their apprenticeship in mastering the uses of plants and herbal remedies to be able to cure disease (Bonvillain, 1997). They know which various plants or teas cure different illnesses. For example, one type of plant medicine men used during the 1500s to cure scurvy, caused by a deficiency of vitamin C, was white pine or hemlock (Bonvillain, 1997). Hemlock is an excellent source of vitamin C, according to Frankis (2006). The most widely used plant in healing the American Indian community is tobacco. Tobacco has many useful purposes, such as treating burns, earaches, stomach cramps, and inflammation (Bonvillain, 1997).

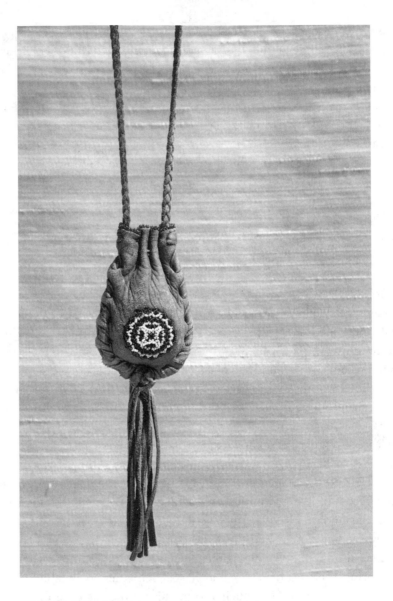

FIGURE 8.6   Medicine bundle.
Source: © Khumina/ShutterStock, Inc.

Certain people in each tribe are recognized as healers. They receive special teachings. Healing traditions are passed from one generation to the next through visions, stories, and dreams. Healing does not follow written guidelines. Healers work differently with each person they help. They use their herbs, ceremony, and power in the best way for each individual. Healing might involve sweat lodges, talking circles, ceremonial smoking of tobacco, herbalism, animal spirits, or vision quests. Each tribe uses its own techniques. The techniques by themselves are not considered to be "traditional healing." They are only steps toward becoming whole, balanced, and connected.

BEHAVIORAL RISK FACTORS AND COMMON HEALTH PROBLEMS AMONG AMERICAN INDIANS

The major behavioral health risk factors for American Indians are seat belt nonuse, cigarette smoking, heavy drinking, sedentary lifestyles, being overweight or obese, and lack of preventive behaviors, such as health screenings. These risk factors have led to American Indians' disproportionately high mortality from alcoholism, tuberculosis, diabetes, injuries, suicide, heart disease, stroke, cancer, lung disease, and homicide. The leading causes of death among American Indians and Alaska Natives in 2003 were as follows (National Center for Health Statistics, 2006):

- Diseases of the heart
- Malignant neoplasms
- Unintentional injuries
- Diabetes mellitus
- Chronic liver disease and cirrhosis
- Cerebrovascular diseases
- Chronic lower respiratory disease
- Influenza and pneumonia
- Suicide
- Nephritis, nephrotic syndrome, and nephrosis

It is important to note that these behavioral risk factors and common health problems in American Indians vary greatly among the tribes and regions. For example, Denny, Holtzman, and Cobb (2003) found that the prevalence of current cigarette smoking ranged from 21.2% in the Southwest to 44.1% in the Northern Plains, and the awareness of diabetes was lower in Alaska than in other regions. Therefore, it is important for health care professionals to gather data about the specific tribe and geographic region prior to developing any individual or community-based interventions.

American Indians have a high risk of motor vehicle deaths and injuries, which is caused by several factors. One factor is that they have the lowest rate of using seat belts in the nation. The other reason is their high rate of drinking and driving.

Denny et al. (2003) defined cigarette smoking as the respondent having ever smoked more than or equal to 100 cigarettes in his or her life and currently smoking.

These researchers found that cigarette smoking was highest in the Northern Plains (44.1%) and Alaska (39.0%) and lowest in the Southwest (21.2%). American Indian and Alaska Native respondents were more likely to report cigarette smoking (32.2%) than respondents of other racial and ethnic groups (22.3%) (Denny et al., 2003). The lands of American Indians do not impose taxes, and they do not have laws that prevent the sale of alcohol and tobacco products to minors. Because of this, the young population easily uses alcohol and tobacco products. American Indians believe that tobacco is sacred, and it is therefore more often used in ceremonies.

Diabetes also has become a problem within the American Indian community. American Indians and Alaska Natives are 2.2 times as likely to have diabetes as non-Hispanic whites (American Diabetes Association, n.d.). As illustrated in Figure 8.7, among other ethnicities, American Indians have the highest rate of diabetes.

The American Indian population has suffered from many suicide deaths. American Indian and Alaska Native males in the 15- to 24-year-old age group have the highest suicide rate, 27.99 per 100,000, compared to white (17.54 per 100,000), black

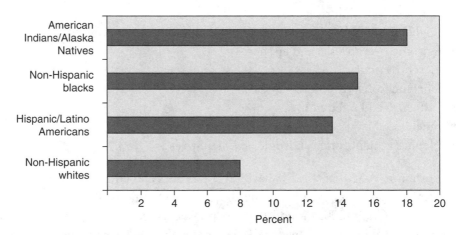

Footnote: For American Indians/Alaska Natives, the estimate of total prevalence was calculated using the estimate of diagnosed diabetes from the 2003 outpatient database of the Indian Health Service and the estimate of undiagnosed diabetes from the 1999-2002 National Health and Nutrition Examination Survey. For the other groups, 1999-2002 NHANES estimates of total prevalence (both diagnosed and undiagnosed) were projected to year 2006.

FIGURE 8.7 Estimated age-adjusted total prevalence of diabetes in people aged 20 years or older, by race/ethnicity: United States, 2005.
Source: Centers for Disease Control and Prevention. (2006).

(12.8 per 100,000), and Asian and Pacific Islander (8.96 per 100,000) males of the same age (Suicide Prevention Resource Center, n.d.). Suicide was the leading cause of death for American Indians and Alaska Natives between the ages of 10 and 34 years (Suicide Prevention Resource Center, n.d.).

QUICK FACTS

Cancer
- In 2002, American Indian/Alaska Native men were 30% less likely to have prostate cancer as non-Hispanic white men.
- In 2002, American Indian/Alaska Native women were 30% less likely to have breast cancer as non-Hispanic white women.
- American Indian/Alaska Native men were twice as likely to be diagnosed with stomach and liver cancers as white men.
- American Indian women were 20% more likely to die from cervical cancer, compared to white women.

Diabetes
- American Indian/Alaska Native adults were 2.3 times as likely as white adults to be diagnosed with diabetes.
- American Indians/Alaska Natives were twice as likely as non-Hispanic whites to die from diabetes in 2003.
- American Indian/Alaska Native adults were 1.6 times as likely as white adults to be obese.
- American Indian/Alaska Native adults were 1.3 times as likely as white adults to have high blood pressure.

Heart Disease
- American Indian/Alaska Native adults are 1.2 times as likely as white adults to have heart disease.
- American Indian/Alaska Native adults are 1.4 times as likely as white adults to be current cigarette smokers.
- American Indian/Alaska Native adults are 1.6 times as likely as white adults to be obese.
- American Indian/Alaska Native adults are 1.3 times as likely as white adults to have high blood pressure.

HIV–AIDS
- American Indian/Alaska Natives have a 40% higher AIDS rate than their non-Hispanic white counterparts.
- American Indian/Alaska Native men have a 10% higher AIDS rate, compared to non-Hispanic white men.
- American Indian/Alaska Native women have three times the AIDS rate of non-Hispanic white women.

(Continues)

Immunization
- In 2005, American Indian/Alaska Native children aged 19 to 35 months received the recommended doses of vaccines for measles, mumps, rubella, Hib-Imune, polio, and chicken pox at the same rate as non-Hispanic white children.
- In 2005, American Indian/Alaska Native adults aged 18 to 64 years were slightly more likely than their non-Hispanic white counterparts to have received the influenza (flu) shot in the past 12 months.

Infant Mortality
- American Indians/Alaska Natives have 1.5 times the infant mortality rate as non-Hispanic whites.
- American Indian/Alaska Native babies are 2.2 times as likely as non-Hispanic white babies to die from sudden infant death syndrome (SIDS), and they are 1.4 times as likely to die from complications related to low birth weight or congenital malformations, compared to non-Hispanic whites babies.
- American Indian/Alaska Native infants are 3.6 times as likely as non-Hispanic white infants to have mothers who began prenatal care in the third trimester or did not receive prenatal care at all.

Stroke
- In general, American Indian/Alaska Native adults are 60% more likely to have a stroke than their white adult counterparts.
- American Indian/Alaska Native women have twice the rate of stroke as white women.
- American Indian/Alaska Native adults are more likely to be obese than white adults, and they are more likely to have high blood pressure, compared to white adults.

Source: Office of Minority Health. (2008).

HISTORY OF ALASKA NATIVES IN THE UNITED STATES

The natives of Alaska are one of the oldest civilizations, and they have experienced numerous conflicts in relation to land possession and redistribution. Alaska Natives were living on their land when Russians arrived to make their claims on the land. After years of Russian rule, Alaska was purchased by the United States in 1867. In 1906 the Homestead Act established land to the following individuals: "Indian or Eskimo of full or mixed blood who resides in and is a native of said district, and who is the head of a family, or is 21 years of age; and the land so allotted shall be deemed the homestead of the allotted and his heirs in perpetuity, and shall be inalienable and non-taxable until otherwise provided by Congress" (Alaska Native Heritage Center, 2000). This act was the first to establish land for Alaska Natives, but it left out many tribes.

Discrimination and segregation was prevalent in Alaska, especially between Alaska Natives and whites (Russians and Americans). In 1945, Alaska passed a law that ended legal segregation, and this marked the start of a new beginning. According to the Alaska Native Claims Settlement Act of 1971, 40 million acres of land and nearly a billion dollars was awarded to Alaska Natives.

ALASKA NATIVES IN THE UNITED STATES

Alaska Natives include people from villages or tribes such as Aleut, Inupiat, Yupik, Eskimo, and Athabaskan peoples. Today Alaska Natives face difficulty in conforming to the American culture. Many natives have been forced to live outside their accustomed villages due to a lack of resources. As a result, some native families have been affected by these demographic changes. Alaska Natives who choose to move to the city no longer hunt or fish and are adopting unhealthy American food standards. These types of changes may contribute to some of the health disparities that Alaska Natives face. Even though Alaska Natives have faced a turbulent past, traditional Alaska Native culture can still be seen within their social environment.

There are many different languages that Alaska Natives use to communicate. The Alaska Native Language Center currently reports 20 known native languages. However, this organization also reports that many languages will go extinct by the next generation (Palca, 2002). Unfortunately, because there is a variety of languages, it is difficult to accommodate all of them in the public education system. Cultural and linguistic differences are one of the root causes of why Alaska's education system is failing its native students.

Villages consist of mostly related families; however, if residents are not related, they are still treated as one big family. Alaska Natives typically develop close-knit relationships with one another. Village members watch out for one another, and food is always shared when an animal is caught. Alaska Natives believe that if a person shares his or her food, the person will catch more animals in the future. When a young male experiences his first kill, it is tradition for him to give the entire kill to the elders, who are highly respected and are needed to pass on traditions from generation to generation. The tradition of sharing and giving is a major part of Native Alaskan culture.

Hunting, fishing, and gathering are the way of life in rural Alaska (Alexandria, 1994). Native Alaskans' diet mainly consists of fish, deer, moose, whale, seal, caribou, duck, walrus, and sea lion. Alaska Natives consume about 40% protein in their daily diet. They typically suffer some deficiencies in their diet, such as calcium, vitamin D, and vitamin C (Nobmann, Byers, Lanier, Hankin, & Jackson, 1992). However, there are some plants that can be eaten to make up for the deficiency if they grow in the surrounding environment. Usually, the men do the strenuous hunting, and the women gather berries and plants that will aid in nutrition. Women also prepare and store the food after it is gathered. The common methods for food preparation have caused the highest rates of *Clostridium botulinum* outbreaks in the world (Shaffer, Wainwright, Middaugh, & Tauxe, 1990). Currently, prevention efforts are in place to stop the growth of the toxic bacteria, which is also found naturally in the soil.

Religion was never a big part of life in a native village. Currently, the main religions of Alaska include Russian Orthodox and Christianity. However, years ago Native Alaskans were focused on survival instead of organized religion.

BELIEFS ABOUT CAUSES OF HEALTH AND ILLNESS AMONG ALASKA NATIVES

Despite the fact that some Alaska Natives are nonreligious, traditional natives believe that the cause of illness is derived from spirits (Alexandria, 1994). To get rid of an illness, a shaman is needed to remove the ill spirit and restore health. Healing ceremonies can take place in public, and the shaman encourages village members to participate to get rid of the bad spirit that is causing the illness. In addition, some shamans have medical skills, such as treating burns with fat, cleaning wounds with urine, amputating frozen gangrenous limbs, and setting broken bones. Traditional natives believe that shamans have the ability to fly and reach the heavens.

Currently, beliefs about the causes of illness are beginning to shift. Alaska Natives noticed that they were less likely to get sick when they traveled in small nomadic bands. However, when Alaska Natives began to settle, they noticed that people were more likely to become ill and die. As a result, they have begun to lean toward the germ theory. Shamans are still used today, because it is often difficult to reach health care clinics. In some instances, both a shaman and Western medicine are used in combination to treat illness.

HEALING TRADITIONS AMONG ALASKA NATIVES

There are many ancient traditions for healing that are used by Alaska Natives.

> Alaska Native traditional healing practices are rooted in a 10,000 year history and are re-emerging today as an holistic healing approach for individuals and communities. These methods are often used in combination with western-based medical therapies for the purpose of health promotion, disease prevention, pain reduction and enhancement of psychological wellness. (Corral, 2007)

Alaska Native traditional healing may indeed be pairing up with Western medicine in some regions of Alaska where that is plausible, and there are some specific examples of this phenomenon. For example, Alaska Natives refer to traditional healers as "traditional healers" and "tribal doctors." Though they may sound as if they are one of the same, there is one very important distinction: Traditional healers are members of the communities who learn the traditional healing methods by observing other traditional healers over a number of years. Formal standardized training or apprenticeship does not exist. Tribal doctors are similar to traditional healers in the sense that they are very knowledgeable about native traditional healing modalities. The difference is that tribal doctors go through some sort of formal standardized training, and they most often work under the supervison of or in alliance with physicians. This alliance that tribal doctors have formed with physicians clearly demonstrates the connection between Native Alaskan traditional healing modalities and Western medicine (Corral, 2007).

Despite the emergence of a complementary relationship between Alaskan traditional healing and Western medicine, traditional healing practices are quite distinguishable when compared to the Western medicine mode of treatment.

> While allopathic medicine focuses on identifying and treating a specific diagnosis, traditional healing strives to restore the patient's sense of natural balance and harmony with self, community and culture. Traditional healing attempts to nurture the mind–body–spirit connection, and to actively involve the patient in finding renewed commitment to lifelong health and wellness. (Corral, 2007)

Medicinal plants, such as roots, berries, leaves, and flowers, have historically been used as healing agents throughout Alaska's many regions. These medicinal plants are used in numerous ways to heal everything from the common cold, flesh wounds, and mouth sores, to promoting healthy pregnancy, to many other applications (Corral, 2007). A common medicinal plant that is widely used in Alaska and British Columbia for treating a variety of ailments, including arthritis, fever, and diabetes, is known as Devil's Club (*Oplopanax horridus* [OH]). According to Tai and colleagues (2006), ethanolic extract of OH has antiproliferative (meaning that it prevents the spread and growth of cells) effects on several types of cancer cells, and it has strong antioxidant activity. The medicinal plants are aimed more at healing the bodily ailments, but other traditional healing modalities are also focused on the spirit and the mind.

Drumming, dancing, and singing are known to be very powerful sources of healing among Alaska Natives. The ceremonies incorporate music, movement, and drum rhythms to penetrate the people involved and aid them in fully expressing emotion, increasing physical energy, making a strong connection with life and one another, and promoting happiness. This also helps to promote overall well-being and a sense of love among the community. These ceremonies can be used to prevent drug and alcohol abuse, domestic violence, and suicide, which are some of the most prevalent problems among Alaska Natives (Corral, 2007).

BEHAVIORAL RISK FACTORS AND COMMON HEALTH PROBLEMS AMONG ALASKA NATIVES

Unfortunately, many of the issues that Alaska Natives struggle with are due to unhealthy and risky behaviors. The top behavioral risk factors are alcohol consumption, smoking and chewing tobacco, drug use, inadequate exercise, obese body weight, unhealthy diet, violence, and suicide.

Alcohol has caused health problems and behavioral issues in many societies, but Alaska Natives have been struck much harder than most. There are many theories as to why alcohol is such a major issue in Alaska, but one study conducted by the National Center for American Indian and Alaska Native Mental Health Research goes back to the beginning. According to this study, alcohol was not a part of Alaska's culture until it was introduced by the Russians, who used it to abuse the natives and take advantage of them. Alcohol quickly became a problem in small villages, spreading like wildfire. The immediate effect was an increase in spouse abuse and neglect of daily chores. This behavior led to shame and guilt, which was often dealt with by more drinking. This behavior is learned by the children in the home, and the cycle continues. The average starting age for drinking is now at around 9 years old (Seale, Shellenberger, & Spence, 2006). Seale et al. (2006) sum up the cultural effects in this statement: "The stress, confusion, and depression caused by the dramatic cultural changes of the twentieth century were described as a major influence on alcohol consumption" (p. 11). The traditional culture for many Alaska Natives is gone, and they are left to live with limited resources for success. Without adequate health education and easy access to medical or mental health care, it has become a difficult task to fight a problem of alcohol abuse.

Alcohol abuse has been linked to many health problems, both directly and indirectly. One deadly health outcome associated with alcohol is suicide, which is the fourth leading cause of death among Alaska Natives (Alaska Native Epidemiology Center, 2007). "Suicide is a particularly critical problem among male Alaska Natives, who are 14 to 40 times more likely to commit suicide than any other United States male in the same age group" (Seale, et al., 2006, p. 2).

Another behavioral risk factor that is extremely prevalent among Alaska Natives is the use of tobacco. Smoking and/or chewing tobacco is practiced by half of all

Alaska Natives older than the age of 12 years. "Of those patients who were screened for tobacco use during 2006, 46% were smokers. Fifty-nine percent used some form of tobacco" (Alaska Native Epidemiology Center, 2007, p. 30).

Obesity is a problem among Alaska Natives. Twenty-three percent of U.S. whites are obese, compared to 31% of Alaska Natives (Alaska Native Epidemiology Center, 2007). In addition, Alaska Native adults get less than half the amount of some sort of physical activity as that of U.S. whites: 25% and 51%, respectively (Alaska Native Epidemiology Center, 2007).

Like all cultural groups in the United States, Alaska Natives suffer from many health problems that greatly affect their way of life. These health problems result in an overall lower life expectancy. The 10 leading causes of death for Alaska Natives between 1989 and 1998 in order of frequency were cancer, unintentional injuries, heart disease, suicide, cerebrovascular disease, chronic obstructive pulmonary disease, pneumonia and influenza, homicide and legal intervention, chronic liver disease, and diabetes (Lanier, Ehrsam, & Sandidge, 2002).

Unintentional injuries and suicides are ranked second and fourth among Alaska Natives, and both of these health disparities are preventable. "Unintentional injuries are the leading cause of death in children and young adults and are responsible for the greatest number of years of life lost in Alaska" (Alaska Department of Health & Social Services, 2002, p. 4). The high rate of alcohol abuse among Alaska Natives contributes to the toll of injuries (Alaska Department of Health & Social Services, 2002). Some of the other contributing factors to the high rate of unintentional injuries are the prevalence of guns in homes, no laws that require helmets, and inadequate seat belt laws. "Firearm death rates for Alaska Natives are more than four times the national rate" (Alaska Department of Health & Social Services, 2002, p. 4). "Guns are readily available in many homes in Alaska due to recreational and subsistence hunting" (Alaska Department of Health & Social Services, 2002, p. 4). In Alaska there are no laws that require people to wear helmets while they are riding a motorcycle, snowmobile, all-terrain vehicle (ATV), or bicycle (Alaska Department of Health & Social Services, 2002). The absence of these laws is very unfortunate because the use of a helmet could reduce the death rate. "The state of Alaska does have a seat belt law, but police officers are not allowed to issue a citation unless they have another reason to pull over the vehicle" (Alaska Department of Health & Social Services, 2002, p. 6). Unfortunately, these laws are not very proactive in combating the problems that Alaska Natives face.

Mental health problems contribute to the accident and suicide rates as well. "Estimates project about 10 percent of Alaska's children and youths (age 5 to 18) have severe emotional disturbances, and 6.2 percent of Alaska's adult population under age 55 suffer from severe mental illness" (Alaska Department of Health & Social Services,

2002, p. 4). "Together, accidents and suicides accounted for about 72 percent of all deaths in the 15–34 age group" (Alaska Department of Health & Social Services, 2002, p. 6). It is awful that there is such a high prevalence of mental health problems among Alaska Natives, and yet 175 villages in Alaska have no local mental health services other than the occasional itinerant provider (Alaska Department of Health & Social Services, 2002). "Around 90 percent of all people who kill themselves have a mental or substance abuse disorder or a combination of disorders" (Alaska Department of Health & Social Services, 2002, p. 5).

CONSIDERATIONS FOR HEALTH PROMOTION AND PROGRAM PLANNING

The following are some concepts to consider when planning and implementing a health promotion program for this target audience.

- Native peoples use their tribal names when referring to themselves, so it is advised that health care professionals ask individuals or groups how they prefer to be addressed.
- Recognize that there are varying degrees of acculturation levels, so health care professionals need to assess where the patient or client is on the continuum of acculturation.
- Recognize that there is great diversity among the tribes, so do not make assumptions.
- Holistic thinking is common and should be used to identify appropriate and acceptable prevention and treatment plans.
- Try to accommodate complementary and alternative forms of healing.
- Do not be surprised or offended by a hand shake that is softer or gentler than you are accustomed to.
- Be patient with silence, and give the listener time to reflect on what you said prior to responding.
- Prolonged eye contact should be avoided, because it is viewed as being disrespectful.
- Work with the families and remember that elders are respected.
- Do not encourage or try to reward competitive behavior, because cooperation is valued by these cultures.
- Do not appear to be in a hurry, because it may give a negative impression of you.
- Do not interrupt the person who is speaking, because it is considered to be extremely rude.

- Keep nonverbal communication to a minimum.
- With the exception of a hand shake, touch is not usually acceptable.
- Remember that listening is more valued than speaking.
- Be aware that suspicion and mistrust may exist.
- When developing community programs, involve the community members.
- Be aware of superstitions such as unlucky and lucky numbers and colors.
- Consider the incorporation of talking circles into your program.

CHAPTER SUMMARY

American Indians and Alaska Natives have a history of being conquered by other nations, having foreign cultures impose upon their way of life, and being the victims of discrimination. Fortunately, they have been able to hold on to their traditional culture in many ways. They continue to express their traditional values within their villages by maintaining close-knit families and using traditional healing modalities to prevent and heal illness. Unfortunately, both groups experience major health disparities, such as high incidence of suicide, alcoholism, cancer, unintentional injuries, diabetes, and mental illness. Through quality and culturally-sensitive health promotion programs, perhaps one day American Indians and Alaska Natives will experience better health and gain access to quality health care.

In this chapter we discussed the challenges that these populations encountered historically. We learned that these populations do not believe in the germ theory as the cause of disease, although some Alaska Natives are adopting this belief system. We learned about their various approaches to healing, such as sweat baths and ceremonies, and their common behaviors, risk factors, and illnesses. General tips for working with these populations were provided, but we caution that there is a vast amount of diversity within these groups, so it is important not to generalize.

REVIEW

1. Describe the histories of American Indians and Alaska Natives in the United States.
2. According to American Indian and Alaska Native beliefs, how is illness caused?
3. What are sweat lodges, talking circles, and medicine wheels?
4. Describe some plants and herbs that are used for healing.
5. Describe what medicine men are and their approach to healing.

CASE STUDY

Don is a 45-year-old, full-blood Indian who is married and has five children. The family lives in a small, rural community on a large reservation in New Mexico. Don was sent to boarding school for high school, and then he served in the war. He recently was treated through Veterans Affairs (VA), which is where he participated in a posttraumatic stress disorder (PTSD) support group. Don suffers from alcoholism. It began soon after his initial patrols in the war, which involved heavy combat and, ultimately, physical injury. He exhibits the hallmark symptoms of PTSD, including flashbacks, nightmares, intrusive thoughts on an almost daily basis, marked hypervigilance, irritability, and avoidant behavior.

Don is fluent in English and his native language, which is spoken in his home. He is the descendant of a family of traditional healers. Consequently, the community expected him to assume a leadership role in its cultural and spiritual life. However, boarding school interrupted his early participation in important aspects of local ceremonial life. His participation was further delayed by military service and then forestalled by his alcoholism. During boarding school, Don was frequently harassed by non-Indian staff members for speaking his native language, for wearing his hair long, and for running away. Afraid of similar ridicule while in the service, he seldom shared his personal background with fellow infantrymen. Don was the target of racism and was called "Chief" and "blanket ass."

Some 10 years after his return from the war, Don began cycling through several periods of treatment for his alcoholism in tribal residential programs. It was not until one month after he began treatment for his alcoholism at a local VA facility that a provisional diagnosis of PTSD was made. Upon completing that treatment, he transferred to an inpatient unit that specialized in combat-related trauma. Don left the unit against medical advice, sober but still experiencing significant symptoms.

Don's tribal members frequently refer to PTSD as the "wounded spirit." His community has long recognized the consequences of being a warrior, and indeed, a ceremony has evolved over many generations to prevent as well as treat the underlying causes of these symptoms. Within this tribal worldview, combat-related trauma upsets the balance that underpins someone's personal, physical, mental, emotional, and spiritual health. Don did not participate in these and other tribal ceremonies until after he was diagnosed at the VA with PTSD. His sobriety has been aided by involvement in the Native American Church, with its reinforcement of his decision to remain sober and its support for positive life changes.

Though Don has a great deal of work ahead of him, he feels that he is now ready to participate in the tribe's major ceremonial intended to bless and purify its warriors. His family, once alienated but now reunited, is excited about that process.

There are several issues to consider about this case:

- What cultural issues exist in this scenario?
- How did Don's culture help and hinder his situation?
- Are there steps that could have been taken to help prevent Don's alcohol problem?

Source: Adapted from National Alliance on Mental Illness. (2003).

MODEL PROGRAM

American Indian Life Skills Development

The American Indian Life Skills Development curriculum is a school-based, culturally-tailored, suicide-prevention curriculum for American Indian adolescents. Tailored to American Indian norms, values, beliefs, and attitudes, the curriculum is designed to build self-esteem, identify emotions and stress, increase communication and problem-solving skills, and recognize and eliminate self-destructive behavior, including substance abuse. The curriculum provides American Indian adolescents with information on suicide and suicide-intervention training and helps them set personal and community goals.

Each lesson in the curriculum contains standard skills training techniques for providing information about the helpful or harmful effects of certain behaviors, modeling of target skills, experimental activities, behavior rehearsal for skill acquisition, and feedback for skills refinement. The curriculum can be delivered three times a week over 30 weeks during the school year or as an after-school program.

Evaluation

The research design was nonrandom, quasi-experimental with two conditions: an intervention and a no-intervention condition. A multimethod approach was used to assess the effectiveness of the curriculum. It included a pretest and posttest self-report survey of risk factors associated with suicide, behavioral observations of suicide intervention skills targeted in the curriculum judged by two American Indian graduate students, and peer ratings of classmates' skills and abilities relevant to suicide intervention. Freshman students enrolled in a required language arts class were eligible for the study, and juniors were included to increase the sample size. Sophomores were expressly excluded because of their participation in a program pilot test the previous year. Sixty-nine students were assigned to the intervention condition, and 59 students were assigned to the no-intervention condition. The sample was 64% female and 36% male. A pretest indicated that 81% of the sample was in the moderate to severe range on the Suicide Probability Scale. Forty percent of students reported that a relative or friend had committed suicide, and 18% reported having personally attempted suicide. Moreover, 79% of those students who attempted suicide in the past had attempted two times or more, 70% had tried within six months of the pretest, 17% had required medical attention, and 22% had informed no one about the attempt. Posttests were conducted eight months after the pretest.

Outcome

Overall, the evaluation produced evidence to suggest the curriculum succeeded in creating a healthier psychological profile. Students exposed to the curriculum scored better (lower) than the no-intervention group at posttest on suicide probability and hopelessness, and the intervention group showed greater ability to perform problem-solving and suicide intervention skills in a behavioral assessment. However, the evaluators noted potential threats to validity because of the coexistence of the two groups throughout the intervention.

Source: Helping America's Youth. (n.d.).

GLOSSARY TERMS

sweat lodges

talking circles

peyote

shaman

medicine bundle

REFERENCES

Advameg. (2007). *Diet of Native Americans.* Retrieved March 9, 2008, from http://www.faqs.org/nutrition/Met-Obe/Native-Americans-Diet-of.html

Alaska Department of Health & Social Services. (2002). *Healthy Alaskans 2010, volume 1: Targets for improved health.* Retrieved February 7, 2008, from http://www.hss.state.ak.us/dph/targets/ha2010/volume_1.htm

Alaska Native Epidemiology Center. (2007). Regional health profile for Yukon-Kuskokwim Health Corp. Retrieved February 12, 2008, from http://www.anthc.org/cs/chs/epi/upload/Regional_Health_Profile_YKHC_0707.pdf

Alaska Native Heritage Center. (2000). *Information about Alaska Native cultures.* Retrieved February 16, 2008, from http://www.akhistorycourse.org/articles/article.php?artID=195

Alexandria, V. (1994). *People of the ice and snow.* Richmond, VA: Time Life.

American Diabetes Association. (n.d.). *Total prevalence of diabetes and pre-diabetes.* Retrieved February 7, 2008, from http://www.diabetes.org/diabetes-statistics/prevalence.jsp

American Eagle Foundation. (n.d.). *American eagle & Native American Indian*. Retrieved March 10, 2008, from http://www.eagles.org/native_american.htm

Bonvillain, N. (1997). *Native American medicine*. Philadelphia: Chelsea House.

Centers for Disease Control and Prevention. (2006). *National diabetes fact sheet*. Retrieved December 1, 2006, from http://www.cdc.gov/diabetes/pubs/estimates05.htm#prev4

Corral, K. (2007). *Alaska Native traditional healing*. Retrieved February 2, 2008, from http://altmed.creighton.edu/AKNative

Denny, C. H., Holtzman, D., & Cobb, N. (2003). Surveillance for health behaviors of American Indians and Alaska Natives: Findings from the behavioral risk factor surveillance system, 1997–2000. *Morbidity and Mortality Weekly Report, 52*(SS07), 1–13. Retrieved March 16, 2008, from http://www.cdc.gov/mmwr/preview/mmwrhtml/ss5207a1.htm

Frankis, M. P. (2006). *Picea sitchensis (Bongard)*. Retrieved February 14, 2008, from http://www.conifers.org/pi/pic/sitchensis.htm

Haas, M. J. (2007). *Shaman song*. Retrieved February 2, 2008, from http://www.shamansong.com/gpage.html3.html

Hammerschlag, C. A. (1988). *The dancing healers: A doctor's journey of healing with Native Americans*. San Francisco: Harper.

Helping America's Youth. (n.d.). *American Indian life skills development*. Retrieved October 31, 2008, from http://guide.helpingamericasyouth.gov/programdetail.cfm?id=635

Indian Health Service. (2007). *Indian health service introduction*. Retrieved March 13, 2008, from http://www.ihs.gov/PublicInfo/PublicAffairs/Welcome_Info/IHSintro.asp

Kelman, S. (1999). *American government*. New York: Holt Rinehart & Winston.

Lanier, A. P., Ehrsam, G., & Sandidge, J. (2002). Alaska Native mortality. Retrieved March 25, 2008, from http://surveillance.cancer.gov/documents/disparities/native/ANMortality.pdf

Management Sciences for Health. (n.d.). *American Indians & Alaska Natives: Health disparities overview*. Retrieved March 3, 2008, from http://erc.msh.org/mainpage.cfm?file=7.3.0.htm&module=provider&language=English#readmoe

Marbella, A. M, Harris, M. C., Diehr, S., Ignace, G., & Ignace, G. (1998). Use of Native American healers among Native American patients in an urban Native American health center. *Archives of Family Medicine, 7*, 182–185.

National Alliance on Mental Illness. (2003). American Indian and Alaska Native. Retrieved on March 18, 2009, from http://www.nami.org/Content/ContentGroups/Multicultural_Support1/CDResourceManual.pdf

National Center for Health Statistics. (2006). *Health, United States, 2005*. Retrieved March 17, 2008, from http://www.ncbi.nlm.nih.gov/books/bv.fcgi?rid=healthus05.table.379

Nixon, President Richard. (1970). *Special Message on Indian Affairs*. Retrieved from http://www.undeclaredutes.net/pdf/nixonmessage.pdf

Nobmann, E. D., Byers, T., Lanier, A. P., Hankin, J. H., & Jackson, M. Y. (1992). The diet of Alaska Native adults: 1987–1988. *American Journal of Clinical Nutrition, 55*, 1024–1032.

Office of Minority Health. (2008). *American Indian/Alaska Native profile*. Retrieved March 8, 2008, from http://www.omhrc.gov/templates/browse.aspx?lvl=2&lvlid=52

Palca, J. (2002). *Saving Alaska's native languages*. Retrieved February 9, 2008, from http://www.npr.org/programs/morning/features/2002/mar/alaska/

Rehling, J. (n.d.). *Native American languages*. Retrieved March 8, 2008, from http://www.cogsci.indiana. edu/farg/rehling/nativeAm/ling.html

Seale, J., Shellenberger, S., & Spence, J. (2006). Alcohol problems in Alaska Natives: Lessons from the Inuit. *American Indian and Alaska Native Mental Health Research: The Journal of the National Center*, *13*(1), 1–31. Retrieved February 18, 2008, from Academic Search Premier database.

Shaffer, N., Wainwright, R. B., Middaugh, J. P., & Tauxe, R. V. (1990). Botulism among Alaska Natives: The role of changing food preparation and consumption practices. *The Western Journal of Medicine*, *153*, 390–393.

Spector, R. E. (2004). *Cultural diversity in health and illness*. Upper Saddle River, NJ: Pearson Education.

Suicide Prevention Resource Center. (n.d.). *Suicide among American Indians/Alaska Natives*. Retrieved February 7, 2008, from http://www.sprc.org/library/ai.an.facts.pdf

Tai, J., Cheung, S., Cheah, S., Chan, E., & Hasman, D. (2006, November 24). In vitro anti-proliferative and anti-oxidant studies on Devil's Club *Oplopanax horridus*. *Journal of Ethnopharmacology*, *108*(2), 228–235.

US Census Bureau. (2002). *The American Indian and Alaska Native population: 2000*. Retrieved March 4, 2008, from http://www.census.gov/prod/2002pubs/c2kbr01-15.pdf

US Census Bureau. (2008). *Population density of the United States, and selected maps of race and Hispanic origin: 2000*. Retrieved November 9, 2008, from http://www.census.gov/population/www/censusdata/2000maps.html

US Department of Agriculture. (2007). *Ethnic/cultural food guide pyramid*. Retrieved March 7, 2008, from http://fnic.nal.usda.gov/nal_display/index.php?info_center=4&tax_level=3&tax_subject=256&topic_id=1348&level3_id=5732

West Virginia Division of Culture and History. (2008). *Native American communities in West Virginia*. Retrieved February 5, 2008, from http://www.wvculture.org/arts/ethnic/native.html

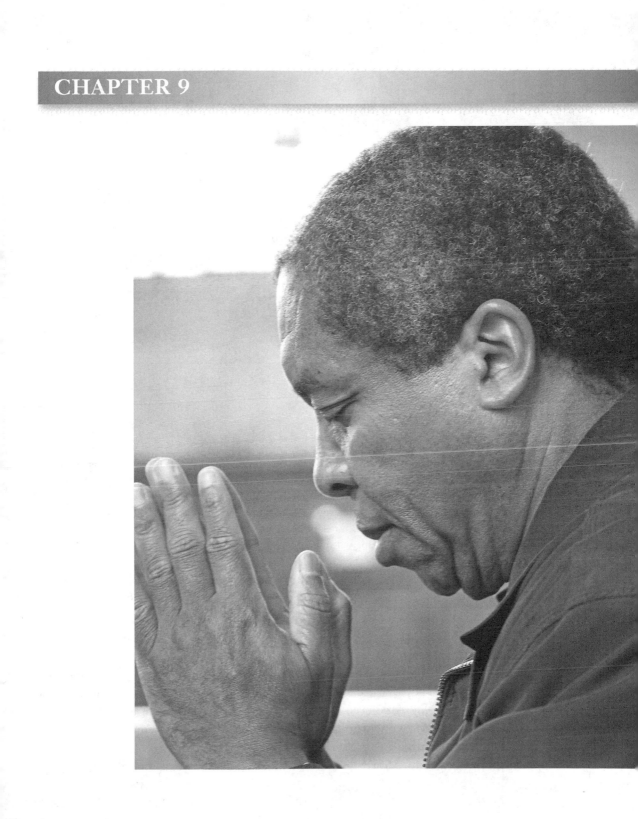

CHAPTER 9

African American Populations

I have a dream that my four little children will one day live in a nation where they will not be judged by the color of their skin, but by the content of their character.

—Martin Luther King, Jr.

If I'd known I was going to live this long, I'd have taken better care of myself.

—Eubie Blake

KEY CONCEPTS

- Tuskegee study
- Voodoo
- Candomblé

CHAPTER OBJECTIVES

1. Provide an overview of the social and economic circumstances of African Americans in the United States.
2. Provide an overview of African American beliefs about the causes of illness.
3. Describe at least three African American healing practices.
4. Describe African American health risk behaviors and common illnesses.
5. List at least six tips for working with African American populations.

The term "black people" usually refers to humans with dark skin color, so the term has been used to categorize a number of diverse populations into one common group. Some definitions of the term include only people of relatively recent sub-Saharan African descent. Others extend the term to any of the populations characterized by dark skin color, a definition that also includes certain populations in geographic regions such as South Asia and Southeast Asia. African Americans are defined as people who have origins in any of the black racial groups in Africa. Historically identified by a number of terms (Negro, colored, black) over the decades, the current politically correct term to refer to anyone who has roots in any of the African countries is African American. This term also is preferable to the younger members (aged 30 years and younger) of this group. However, older members (aged 60 years and older) may still prefer to be called Negro or colored, and middle-aged members (aged 30 to 60 years) may prefer to be called black. It is acceptable to ask African Americans what ethnic term they personally prefer (Nobles & Goddard, 1990). In the literature the terms "African American" and "black" are used. The term "black" incorporates a broader population. For example, black Caribbean Islanders fall within the category of black but not African American. In this chapter, we focus on African Americans, but when we refer to research, the term used in the original source is used.

In this chapter we discuss the unique history of African Americans, which includes forced migration. This history plays a role in the following parts of the chapter, which includes a discussion about their current position within the United States, beliefs about the causes of illness and how to treat it, health behaviors, and common health problems. Then we move into a discussion about how to create a successful community health program taking these factors into consideration.

HISTORY OF AFRICAN AMERICANS IN THE UNITED STATES

The slave trade, which was called the "transatlantic slave trade," was the forced migration of Africans to the New World, which occurred in or around the Atlantic Ocean (The New York Public Library, 2007). It lasted from the sixteenth century to the nineteenth century, and an estimated 12 million men, women, and children were forced to migrate to the United States from their homeland of Africa. The majority of the ancestors of African Americans came from a part of Africa bounded by the Senegal River in the north and by Angola in the south. This area was also called the area of catchment, which is the known area from which the slaves were taken (Perry, 1998). Africans were taken by force, made to be slaves, and shipped to other countries against their will (Perry, 1998). Under these circumstances it is very unlikely that families stayed intact. With the influx of Africans to America came a new culture and a new way of life for the future generations of African Americans.

African indentured and enslaved laborers assisted with the European colonial expansion in North America as they cleared the land, erected shelters, and constructed forts. They raised subsistence crops, gathered lumber, raised cattle and hogs, and harvested exports that supported the colonial economies. People of African descent, free and bound, helped defend the colonies against Indians and against other European colonial powers' attempts at territorial expansion. After the British colonies established territorial dominance along the Atlantic coast, people of African descent— many second and third generation Americans, some free or near-free indentured servants, and some bound in slavery—involved themselves in the politics of revolution.

They fought in the wars of rebellion and participated in the birth and growth of the United States.

Even though African Americans made these great contributions to North America, they faced horrific acts and mistreatment, sexual assault, lynching, and other forms of violent acts and discrimination. During the time of slavery, slave overseers were authorized to whip and brutalize noncompliant slaves. Each state had laws (known as slave codes) that defined the status of slaves and the rights of masters; the codes gave slave owners near-absolute power over the rights of their human property. These codes indemnified or even required the use of violence and were condemned by people who opposed slavery as being evil. In addition to physical abuse and murder, slaves were at constant risk of losing members of their families if their owners decided to trade them for profit, punishment, or to pay debts. A few slaves retaliated by murdering owners and overseers, burning barns, killing horses, or staging work slowdowns. After slavery and the Civil War ended, black codes were used to regulate the freedoms of former slaves. The black codes outraged people in the North because it seemed that the South was creating a form of quasi-slavery to evade the results of the war. After winning the 1866 elections, the Republicans put the South under military rule. The new governments repealed all the black codes, and they were never reenacted. Even with the changes in laws, African Americans still faced unequal treatment and discrimination, which continues into the present day.

AFRICAN AMERICANS IN THE UNITED STATES

African Americans constitute almost 13% of the American population (Centers for Disease Control and Prevention [CDC], 2008), and they live throughout America but are mostly concentrated in southern states (see Figure 9.1). In 2006, the 10 states with the largest black populations were New York, Florida, Texas, Georgia, California, Illinois, North Carolina, Maryland, Virginia, and Michigan (Office of Minority Health, 2008). African Americans are the second largest minority population, following the Hispanic/Latino population. At the time of the 2000 census, 58% of African Americans lived in urban areas (CDC, 2008).

With many African Americans living in urban cities, overcrowding in some urban areas has added to the stress for many residents. These areas tend to be surrounded by the symptoms of poverty, high crime, and inadequate housing (Walker, 1996). In fact, murder is the leading cause of death among young African American males (Campinha-Bacote, 1998). These impoverished neighborhoods often lack adequate health care institutions, such as hospitals, clinics, and pharmacies.

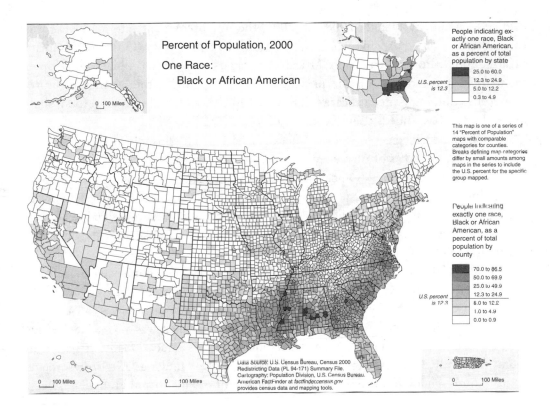

FIGURE 9.1 Percentage of population: Black or African American, 2000.
Source: U.S. Census Bureau, Population Division (2008), http://www.census.gov/main/www/citation.html.

African Americans have to contend with higher poverty levels. In 2006, the U.S. Census Bureau reported that 20% of African Americans, in comparison to 8% of non-Hispanic Caucasians, were living at or below the poverty level (Office of Minority Health, 2008). This represents a large number of single African American women with children. The effect of poverty on one's health is extensive. In this country the poor are more likely to be sick, compared to those with higher incomes who live longer and healthier lives (Office of Minority Health, 2008). Poverty itself is a hardship because it is related to marital stress and dissolution, health problems, low educational attainment, deficits in psychological functioning, and crime. According to a U.S. Census Bureau report (2006), the average African American family's median income was $31,969, in comparison to $52,423 for non-Hispanic Caucasian families

(Office of Minority Health, 2008). In 2006, the unemployment rate for blacks was twice that for non-Hispanic whites (8% and 4%, respectively) (Office of Minority Health, 2008). Poverty confronts African Americans with daily problems and forces them to be concerned with the present necessities of life rather than the future. Sometimes obtaining medical care has to wait while money is allocated to food, shelter, and other basic needs (Leininger, 1995).

A lower percentage of African Americans have health insurance coverage than whites. In 2006, 17.3% of African Americans, in comparison to 12% of non-Hispanic Caucasians, were uninsured (Office of Minority Health, 2008). In 2004, 55% of African Americans, in comparison to 78% of non-Hispanic Caucasians, used employer-sponsored health insurance (Office of Minority Health, 2008). Also in 2004, 24.6% of African Americans, in comparison to 7.9% of non-Hispanic Caucasians, relied on public health insurance (Office of Minority Health, 2008).

In 2004, 74% of blacks received a high school diploma, compared to 81% of non-Hispanic whites (Office of Minority Health, 2008). The percentage of all white adults over the age of 25 years in 2003 who held a graduate degree was 9.8%, compared to the percentage of all African American adults, which was 5.3% (US Census Bureau, 2006). Even when African Americans progress educationally, it has been found that only 47% who are college graduates earn as much as Anglo-Americans who are high school graduates only (US Department of Health and Human Services, 2000).

Most African American children live in a single-parent household. Sixty-eight percent of African American births are to unmarried parents, compared to whites (29%) and Hispanics (44%) (Christopher, 2006). Sixty-two percent of all African American households are headed by a single parent, compared to 27% of white and 35% of Hispanic households, and 61% of black children live in low-income families (Christopher, 2006).

Because of the high percentage of female-headed households in the African American community, when women are unable to handle various situations they usually rely on grandmothers, mothers, aunts, and godmothers to provide assistance (Campinha-Bacote, 1998). Large, extended family networks are the norm for most African Americans. It is not uncommon to have children grow up in the same household as their grandparents and around the comer from several aunts, uncles, and cousins (Ladner & Gourdine, 1992). This is in keeping with the tradition of the matriarchal lineage in many African villages and the fact that in slavery times many fathers were taken away from the family and sold (Ladner & Gourdine, 1992).

African American people have a deep reliance on faith. Spirituality plays a major role in African American culture and is often expressed through religious practices and activities. The black church has been a cornerstone in the African American community, serving as an organizing place and stabilizing entity. It has been noted that health screening programs may best be initiated through community and church activities where the entire family is usually present (Jennings, 1996 as cited in Fields, 2001).

In general, there is a mistrust of the health care system by most African Americans. This mistrust has been fueled by incidences, such as the **Tuskegee study**, in which the U.S. Public Health Service conducted a study from 1932 to 1972 on hundreds of black men with syphilis. The men were not treated with antibiotics that would have cured the disease, and indeed, most of them died (Clarke-Tasker, 1993). The scientific and medical communities reacted with shock after the study was exposed; however, most African Americans universally saw the study as a blatant act of genocide perpetrated against blacks by whites. As a result, many people in the African American community believe that health care professionals simply do not value their lives.

The number of African American health care professionals is low, which further compounds the issues of mistrust in the African American community. In 1999 only 3.6% of all physicians and 4.9% of registered nurses were African American (U.S. Department of Health and Human Services, n.d.). These numbers are not in proportion to the overall African American population.

The distrust in the medical system is not a paranoid reaction. Research shows that blacks commonly receive disrespect in health care settings (Welch, 2003). Many blacks experience adverse encounters due to negative assumptions and images (Welch, 2003). The most common assumption is related to women's sexual promiscuity (Welch, 2003). Consider the experience of Betty, a 40-year-old black woman who works in health care. Here she describes her experience with a health care provider during a visit for a Pap smear:

> I went to this doctor. I had an infection. . . . She said, "How many sex partners do you have?" I said "Gulp" and just looked at her. . . . She said, "Oh, you don't know how many". . . . I felt like I was a little piece of garbage. I was just . . . stereotyped: "There was a little black woman who's out havin' all of these men who comes in here with an infection. . . ." (Welch, 2003)

Subtle insults and comments make blacks feel inferior in health care settings. This mistrust is what leads African Americans to rely on traditional healing methods or to not seek care until it can no longer be avoided.

African Americans experience discrimination in other areas outside of the health care system as well. People who are constantly treated unfairly tend to have more stress, which can lead to emotional, physical, and behavioral problems. When people face discrimination during adolescence, they tend to have behavioral problems that lead to antisocial behavior. Teens can feel out of place among their peers, and because they choose not to talk about it, they act out their frustration that they keep inside. They may engage in aggressive and/or illegal acts, such as fighting and shoplifting. As a young teen, one may feel that there is nowhere to turn, which pushes one to consider suicide. Often when adults go through depression because of racial discrimination, they develop abnormal behaviors, such as being irritable and hostile toward others for no reason, having insomnia, and discriminating against others around them. Growing up around discrimination usually causes adolescents to have a hard time concentrating in school and achieving their goals. As adults it can lead to low self-esteem because they become less satisfied with their lives, thinking that every other race is better than theirs. Sometimes when people have had some kind of interaction with racial discrimination, they tend to think the world is out to get them. Everywhere they go, they think there's racial discrimination, even when there isn't any sign of discrimination. Physically, there are many effects of racial discrimination. It causes stress, which can lead to problems such as high blood pressure and a weakened immune system. Another physical effect of racial discrimination is obesity and diabetes. Due to racial discrimination, many unhealthy behaviors arise, such as smoking, drinking, drug use, and binge eating. Another unhealthy behavior is that someone experiencing racial discrimination can verbally abuse someone or be very discriminating toward other people outside of their race. People who experience racial discrimination are usually from lower socioeconomic status (SES). This is partially a result of discrimination that occurs when seeking employment and in the work place.

BELIEFS ABOUT CAUSES OF HEALTH AND ILLNESS

Many low-income blacks traditionally separate illnesses into two categories: natural and unnatural illnesses (Welch, 2003). *Natural illness* occurs as a result of God's will or when a person comes into unhealthy contact with the forces of nature, such as exposure to cold or impurities in the air, food, or water. Natural illness also can occur as a punishment for sins (Welch, 2003). Cures for natural illness include an antidote or other logical protective actions. *Unnatural illness*, on the other hand, is considered to be the result of evil influences that alter God's intended plan (Welch, 2003). These illnesses are often founded on a belief in witchcraft, in which individuals exist who possess power to mobilize the forces of good and evil. The use of voodoo healers among Haitians and other West Indian blacks is an example. Treatment or cures for unnatural illness can be found in religion, magic, amulets, and herbs. Many of these beliefs are African in origin, and aspects of them may be seen among African Americans of all backgrounds (Welch, 2003).

Many African Americans believe that health is a gift from God; illness is a result of something that was not pleasing to God (Sadler & Huff, 2007). African Americans have historically believed that illness may be due to their failure to live according to God's will. Some African Americans even believe that illness comes directly from Satan (Roberson, 1985 as cited in Fields, 2001). Although most African American communities rely on religion and their relationship with God as a main reason for illness, some community members do not. As with any community, it is difficult to truly determine how the African American community perceives the cause of disease, illness, or injury because no two African Americans are alike.

Like all cultures, there are many different beliefs from the past that continue to the present. Many of the beliefs are not supported by medical research. For example, some African American beliefs and traditions surrounding pregnancy and birth include the following (Moore, 2007):

- A pregnant woman is not supposed to hold her hands up over her head. It is believed she will strangle the baby.
- A pregnant woman should not cross her legs when sitting. This will cause hemorrhoids.
- A pregnant woman should indulge her food cravings or the baby will have unpleasant physical or personality traits that match the characteristics of the food.
- Babies are not named until it is known if they will survive. It is believed that spirits of the dead cannot see and therefore cannot harm a child who does not have a name.
- The placenta has a spirit of its own and must be secretly buried where it will never be disturbed and negatively affect the child.
- A small portion of the umbilical cord is wrapped in paper and put away to ensure the newborn will not get colic.
- Talismans are used for protection and to connect the child to ancestral powers and the spirits of nature.

- New mothers are to rest and be cared for in the initial four to eight weeks after birth, assisted by their family and the community.
- Henna body art is used during the postpartum period. The henna beautification lifts the new mother's spirits, wards off depression, and signifies the mother's new and higher social status.

HEALING TRADITIONS

African American healing traditions encompass a variety of beliefs and practices. Some of them were brought through slavery and ancestral roots. The ancestral roots from West Africa brought many herbal and spiritual healing techniques. Types of healers that African Americans use include faith or spiritual healers. African American healers may choose to use rituals, charms, and/or herbs. Today, African Americans can choose if they want to be seen by a biomedical doctor or a traditional healer. Although they have the freedom to choose their practitioner, certain factors can affect their choice, such as trust, access to care, insurance, as well as other socioeconomic factors.

Prayer is the most common treatment for illness among people who believe that illness is caused by God's will. Roberson (1985 as cited in Fields, 2001) stated that spiritual beliefs form a foundation for the health belief systems of African Americans. Instead of going to the doctor when they are ill, some African Americans will pray for their actions that caused them to get sick, giving God a chance to make them healthy before having to seek the help of Western medicine (University of Washington Medical Center, 2007).

Herbs and remedies are another important aspect of the healing traditions of African Americans. Most home remedies are learned from caregivers, such as mothers or grandmothers (Warner, 2005). Some herbs and remedies that are used include the following (Ansorge, 1999; Spector, 2004; Warner, 2005):

- St. John's wort is used for scrapes, strains, and burns. Today it is known for being a mild treatment for depression.
- Petals from an African plant called okra are used to cure boils.
- Wild yam is used to cure indigestion.
- Rectified turpentine with sugar is used to treat a cough.
- Nine drops of turpentine nine days after intercourse may act as a contraceptive.
- Sugar and turpentine are used to get rid of worms.
- Dried snake ground up and brewed as tea is used to treat blemishes.

- Cool baths, isopropyl alcohol (topically), warming the feet, and cool drinks or Popsicles are used to treat fever.
- Catnip, senna extract, chamomile, cigarette smoke, and walking are used to treat colic.
- Whiskey, pennies, eggs, and ice cubes or popsicles alleviate teething.

In addition, another type of remedy that African Americans commonly use is wearing bad-smelling objects, such as bags containing gum resin or asafetida (rotten flesh), around the neck. Although this traditional method does not have any healing properties, it is said to ward off infectious disease (Ansorge, 1999).

The goal of treatment for unnatural illness is to remove evil spirits from the body. Traditional healers, who are usually women, are consulted. These women possess knowledge regarding the use of herbs and roots as well as mystical voodoolike powers. Some African Americans who believe that they have been hexed will often seek out a voodoo-type healer in addition to or instead of a licensed medical provider (Leininger, 1995 as cited in Fields, 2001).

Voodoo (from *vodoun*, meaning spirit) originated in Africa nearly 10,000 years ago (Dakwar, 2004). Although its origins remain mysterious and elusive, scholars are fairly certain that its birthplace was somewhere in West Africa. It is recognized as one of the world's oldest religions (Dakwar, 2004). Voodoo was brought to this country in 1724 with the arrival of slaves from the West African coast (Spector, 2004). Historian Sharla Fett identified four themes that link the medical practices of Southern slaves to those of the West and Central African cultures. The four themes include beliefs that medicine posses a spiritual force, preparing medicine brings the healer closer to spiritual power, healing maintains relationships between the living and the world of ancestors, and power can be used for healing and harming (Savitt, 2002). Voodoo is divided into two types: white magic and black magic. White magic is known to be harmless and includes the use of powders and oils that are pleasantly scented. On the other hand, black magic is quite rare but dangerous and includes the use of oils and powders with a foul and vile odor (Spector, 2004). The practice involves candle-lit rituals and spiritual ceremonies, most commonly held by women. Chest pain, luck, success, attracting money, and evil intentions are just a few examples of reasons why people practice voodoo (Spector, 2004). Today, it is most commonly practiced in areas of the South and in Northern cities with large populations of African Americans (Ansorge, 1999).

During the nineteenth and twentieth centuries, voodoo suffered persecution in both America and the Caribbean (Dakwar, 2004). The practice of voodoo was made illegal, and the spiritual tools of voodoo—fetishes, rods, and sculptures—were confiscated and destroyed (Dakwar, 2004). Simultaneously, a campaign to discredit and disparage voodoo in the public eye began; this led to the popular understanding of voodoo as malicious, dark, foolish, primitive, dangerous, and violent, which continues to this day. Today, voodoo is practiced by millions of people in Africa, America, and the Caribbean (Dakwar, 2004).

Santeria, which was described in Chapter 7, also is practiced by African Americans. In fact, the religion is based on the West African religions that were brought to the New World by slaves, who were imported to the Caribbean to work the sugar plantations. These slaves carried with them their own religious traditions, including a tradition of possession trance for communicating with the ancestors and deities, the use of animal sacrifice, and the practice of sacred drumming and dance. Those slaves who landed in the Caribbean and Central and South America were nominally converted to Catholicism. However, they were able to preserve some of their traditions by fusing together various Yoruban beliefs and rituals with elements from the surrounding Catholic culture. In Cuba this religious tradition has evolved into what we know today as Santeria, the Way of the Saints. Today, hundreds of thousands of Americans participate in this ancient religion. Many are of Hispanic and Caribbean descent, but as the religion moves out of the inner cities and into the suburbs, a growing number of followers are of African American and European American heritage.

Another religion tied to the days of slavery is **Candomblé**, which was developed in Brazil by enslaved Africans who attempted to recreate their culture on the other side of the ocean. The rituals involve animal sacrifices, healing, dancing, drumming, and the possession of participants by orishas, which are religious deities that are said to represent human characteristics such as bravery, love, and honor. Today, Candomblé is widely practiced in Brazil, but because of its secrecy it is unknown how widespread it is in the United States.

Attempts at spiritual healing may be concealed from Western health care providers to avoid the stigma attached to such practices, which may be labeled as devil worshipping or mumbo jumbo by mainstream European American culture (Welch, 2003). When such medical or health-related information is revealed, providers should place it in its proper cultural context.

BEHAVIORAL RISK FACTORS AND COMMON HEALTH PROBLEMS

Some of the adverse behaviors that particularly affect the African American community are drug use, smoking, nutritional habits, and limited physical activity. The consumption and trafficking of drugs such as alcohol and cocaine in the African American community is market driven and stimulated by unemployment, poverty, despair, alienation, depression, hopelessness, and dependency (addiction). Alcoholism is the most significant social and health problem within the African American population. Studies have shown that 60% of homicides in the African American community are alcohol related (Hill, 2007). Despite years of protest from African Americans, their communities are still plastered with billboards that have messages about alcohol. African American youth continue to be shown more alcohol advertisements than any other youth group in the United States (Hill, 2007).

With regard to smoking, African Americans smoke approximately 35% fewer cigarettes per day than do whites (Ellis, 2005). They are not considered to be heavy smokers. In fact, the average African American adult smokes significantly fewer cigarettes than the average white adult. However, despite the fact that African Americans start smoking later in life and smoke fewer cigarettes, they have a greater likelihood of becoming sick and getting lung cancer. This is in part because African Americans have a preference for mentholated brands, which are high in tar and nicotine (Ellis, 2005). Eighty percent of African American smokers smoke mentholated cigarettes, but only 25% of white smokers smoke mentholated cigarettes. The use of menthol is associated with increased health risks and has resulted in significantly poorer health status for African Americans (Ellis, 2005).

A family tradition of soul food may be problematic for some African Americans. Soul foods traditionally have a high fat, sugar, and sodium content (Andrews, 2007). Many American-born African Americans enjoy consuming pork products with high salt content, fried foods, and heavy gravy. "Because African Americans on average have high-fat, lower-fiber diets than whites, they should be encouraged to adopt alternative diets that maintain cultural traditions where possible" (Welch, 2003).

Studies have shown that African American diets stress the consumption of meat and eggs, which results in a high-cholesterol and saturated-fat diet. African American foods also tend to be lower in complex carbohydrates and dietary fiber. This may contribute to their high incidence of being overweight. Sixty percent of African American men and 78% of African American women are considered to be overweight, and 28.8% of African American men and 50.8% of African American women are considered to be obese (Andrews, 2007). A food guide pyramid has been developed to reflect the cultural foods that African Americans eat and to help them improve their nutrition status (see Figure 9.2).

The African American pyramid of foods has a foundation of biscuits, corn (corn breads, grits, and hominy), pasta, and rice. In urban communities, store-bought

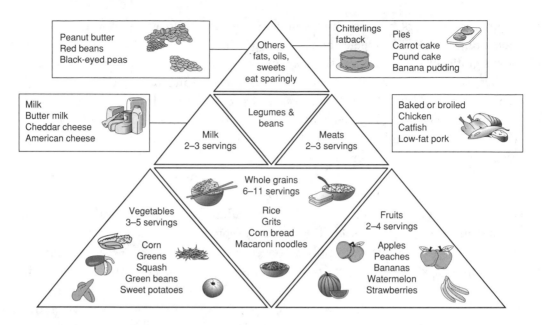

FIGURE 9.2   African American food pyramid.
Source: Adapted from sedma.org and Oldways Preservation and Exchange Trust.

breads have replaced biscuits. Vegetables (green leafy vegetables—chard, collard, kale, mustard greens—corn, okra, sweet potatoes, and yams) and fruits (apples, bananas, berries, peaches, and watermelon) make up the middle of the pyramid. Fruit consumption by today's African Americans is considered to be low when compared to other groups. Pork (chitterlings, intestines, ham hocks, and sausages) remains the primary protein source, and frying is still the most popular way of preparing foods. Fruit drinks and tea are the drinks of choice over milk (which is consumed in puddings and ice cream) (Welch, 2003).

There are many reasons that African Americans choose to eat a diet high in fat and sodium. African Americans in general accept larger body sizes, feel less guilt about overeating, and are less likely to practice unhealthy dieting behaviors, such as overexercising or purging (Andrews, 2007). Although African Americans have a healthy acceptance of a wider range of body sizes, their tolerance may lead to more obesity and serious obesity-related health problems. One problem with consuming a diet high in fat and sodium is the risk of high blood pressure. African Americans have higher rates of hypertension than any other race (Andrews, 2007).

As a result of these behavioral risk factors, African Americans have health problems. In 2003, the death rate for African Americans was higher than whites for heart diseases, stroke, cancer, asthma, influenza, pneumonia, diabetes, HIV–AIDS, and homicide (Office of Minority Health, 2008).

Over three million of all non-Hispanic blacks aged 20 years or older (13.3%) have diabetes (National Diabetes Information Clearinghouse, 2005), and many of them are not aware that they have the disease. After adjusting for population age differences, non-Hispanic blacks are 1.8 times as likely to have diabetes as non-Hispanic whites of similar age (National Diabetes Information Clearinghouse, 2005). Diabetes is particularly common among African American middle-aged and older adults and among women (Welch, 2003). Compared to whites, African Americans with diabetes are more likely to develop complications (end-stage renal disease, retinopathy, and limb amputations) and to experience greater disability as a result. The diabetes mortality rate is 27% higher among blacks than whites (Welch, 2003). Type II diabetes is the most common among African Americans, and their primary risk factors include obesity, higher levels of fasting insulin (hyperinsulinemia), gestational diabetes, and lack of physical activity (Welch, 2003). Among these risks, obesity is the most significant, and there is a disproportionate number of African Americans with both diabetes and obesity (Welch, 2003). Obesity is also believed to contribute to Type I diabetes (non-insulin-dependent diabetes) in 50% to 90% of cases (Welch, 2003).

In 2004, African Americans had 2.4 times the infant mortality rate as non-Hispanic whites. African American infants were almost four times as likely to die from causes related to low birth weight, compared to non-Hispanic white infants. They also had 2.1 times the sudden infant death syndrome mortality rate as non-Hispanic whites. African American mothers were 2.6 times more likely than non-Hispanic white mothers to begin prenatal care in the third trimester or not receive prenatal care at all (Office of Minority Health, 2008).

Heart disease is the leading cause of death for black women in the United States (CDC, 2008). As a whole, African American men and women are more likely than people of other races to have heart failure and to suffer from more severe forms of it. Also, they are more likely to have symptoms at a younger age for heart disease, have those symptoms get worse faster, have more hospital visits due to heart failure, and die from heart failure (National Heart Lung and Blood Institute, 2008).

The HIV epidemic is most prominent among African Americans. In 2005, blacks accounted for 18,121 of the estimated 37,331 new HIV/AIDS diagnoses (49%) in the United States (CDC, 2008). For African American men, the primary transmission category was sexual contact with other men, followed by injection drug use and high-risk heterosexual contact, whereas for African American women, the primary transmission category was high-risk heterosexual contact followed by injection drug use (CDC, 2008).

In addition to being at risk from sharing needles, casual and chronic substance users are more likely to engage in high-risk behaviors, such as unprotected sex (CDC, 2008). The Centers for Disease Control ranks African Americans with the highest rates of sexually transmitted diseases; furthermore, African Americans are about 18 times more likely than whites to have gonorrhea and about five times as likely to have syphilis (CDC, 2008). Linked to unprotected sex is the number of teenage pregnancies. Although the number of teenage pregnancies has declined over the years, teen pregnancy rates vary widely by race and ethnicity. In 2002, the pregnancy rate for non-Hispanic white teens was 49 per 1,000 women aged 15 to 19 years; the rate for Hispanic teens was 135.2; and for African American teens it was 138.9 (Ventura, Abma, Mosher, & Henshaw, 2006).

In 2001, the Centers for Disease Control (CDC) reported that homicide is the leading cause of death for African Americans aged 15 to 24 years and that the rate of homicide among African Americans is one of the primary reasons for the differences in life expectancy between blacks and whites (Roberts, n.d.). In an analysis of mortality data from 1998, the CDC concluded that although it is only the thirteenth leading cause of death in the United States, homicide was the third-ranking cause of death in contributing to the difference in life expectancy between blacks and whites (Roberts, n.d.). Despite making up only about 12% of the nation's population, blacks constituted 38% of all arrests for violent crime in 2002 (Roberts, n.d.). Blacks made up a disproportionate amount of arrests for aggravated assault (34.2%) and forcible rape (34%) and half of all arrests for murder and nonnegligent manslaughter (Roberts, n.d.). For individuals younger than age 18 years, blacks made up an even greater percentage of arrests for violent crimes (42%). Although arrest rates do not completely represent rates of violent acts because many acts go unreported and arrests do not always mean guilt, the tremendous disparity in the rates of arrests for violent crimes among blacks does likely indicate a higher rate of violence (Roberts, n.d.). In addition, overall, African Americans were victimized by intimate partners at significantly higher rates than persons of any other race between 1993 and 1998 (Rennison & Welchans, 2000). Black females experienced intimate partner violence at a rate 35% higher than that of white females and about 22 times the rate of women of other races (Rennison & Welchans, 2000). Black males experienced intimate partner violence at a rate about 62% higher than that of white males and about 22 times the rate of men of other races (Rennison & Welchans, 2000).

QUICK FACTS

Cancer

- In 2003, African American men were 1.4 times as likely to have new cases of lung and prostate cancer, compared to non-Hispanic white men.
- African American men were twice as likely to have new cases of stomach cancer as non-Hispanic white men.
- African American men had lower five-year cancer survival rates for lung and pancreatic cancer, compared to non-Hispanic white men.
- In 2004, African American men were 2.4 times as likely to die from prostate cancer as non-Hispanic white men.
- In 2003, African American women were 10% less likely to have been diagnosed with breast cancer than non-Hispanic white women; however, they were 36% more likely to die from breast cancer, compared to non-Hispanic white women.
- In 2003, African American women were 2.3 times as likely to have been diagnosed with stomach cancer, and they were 2.2 times as likely to die from stomach cancer, compared to non-Hispanic white women.

Diabetes

- African American adults were 1.8 times more likely than non-Hispanic white adults to have been diagnosed with diabetes by a physician.
- In 2002, African American men were 2.1 times as likely to start treatment for end-stage renal disease related to diabetes, compared to non-Hispanic white men.
- In 2003, diabetic African Americans were 1.8 times as likely as diabetic whites to be hospitalized.
- In 2004, African Americans were 2.2 times as likely as non-Hispanic whites to die from diabetes.

Heart Disease

- In 2004, African American men were 30% more likely to die from heart disease, compared to non-Hispanic white men.
- African Americans were 1.5 times as likely as non-Hispanic whites to have high blood pressure.
- African American women were 1.7 times as likely as non-Hispanic white women to be obese.

HIV–AIDS

- African Americans accounted for 47% of HIV–AIDS cases in 2005.
- African American males had more than eight times the AIDS rate of non-Hispanic white males.
- African American females had more than 23 times the AIDS rate of non-Hispanic white females.
- African American men were more than nine times as likely to die from HIV–AIDS as non-Hispanic white men.
- African American women were more than 21 times as likely to die from HIV–AIDS as non-Hispanic white women.

(Continues)

Immunization
- In 2005, African Americans aged 65 years and older were 40% less likely to have received a influenza (flu) shot in the past 12 months, compared to non-Hispanic whites of the same age group.
- In 2005, African American adults aged 65 years and older were 30% less likely to have ever received a pneumonia shot, compared to non-Hispanic white adults of the same age group.
- Although African American children aged 19 to 35 months had comparable rates of immunization for hepatitis, influenza, MMR, and polio, they were slightly less likely to be fully immunized, compared to non-Hispanic white children.

Infant Mortality
- In 2004, African Americans had 2.4 times the infant mortality rate of non-Hispanic whites.
- African American infants were almost four times as likely to die from causes related to low birth weight, compared to non-Hispanic white infants.
- African Americans had 2.1 times the sudden infant death syndrome mortality rate as non-Hispanic whites.
- African American mothers were 2.6 times as likely as non-Hispanic white mothers to begin prenatal care in the third trimester or not receive prenatal care at all.

Stroke
- African American adults were 50% more likely than their white adult counterparts to have a stroke.
- African American males were 60% more likely to die from a stroke than their white adult counterparts.
- Analysis from a CDC health interview survey reveals that African American stroke survivors were more likely to become disabled and have difficulty with activities of daily living than their non-Hispanic white counterparts.

Source: Office of Minority Health. (2008).

CONSIDERATIONS FOR HEALTH PROMOTION AND PROGRAM PLANNING

The following are some concepts to consider when planning and implementing a health promotion program for this target audience.

- Be aware and sensitive to the distrust of the medical community and the government that may exist among African American community members.
- Consider utilizing churches to disseminate information or as a place to conduct health screenings and educational interventions.
- Be aware that peer educators have not been shown to be effective in developing health programs to African American audiences.

- Develop interventions that focus on positive health changes instead of attempting to instill change through fear or negative messages.
- Until invited otherwise, greet African Americans with formal titles.
- Take special care to have congruent verbal and nonverbal communication patterns.
- Be aware of different terminology because there are various regional terms used to describe medical conditions. Among immigrants from Haiti, Jamaica, and the Bahamas, and among many Southern blacks, for example, blood may be characterized as *low* or *high*, referring to anemia as opposed to hypertension. *Spells*, also called *falling outs*, are perceived to be a result of *low blood*; elderly blacks especially may refer to *having had a spell*. *Shock* is a common term for a stroke. Other common terms include *having sugar*, *sweet blood*, or *thin blood*, referring to diabetes (Welch, 2003).
- Understand that occasional outbursts of laugher may appear to be inappropriate for the situation because African Americans find solace in laughter and playfulness.

CHAPTER SUMMARY

African Americans initially came to the United States primarily through the slave trade. Some of their beliefs about causes of illness and treatment approaches are related to their religious practices and ancestral roots, which is why some African Americans choose to use faith or spiritual healers rather than a biomedical doctor. The main behavioral risks associated with African Americans are smoking, alcohol consumption, weight management, and lack of physical activity. African Americans also experience high levels of poverty, discrimination, and violence.

In this chapter we discussed the unique aspects of the history of African Americans and how their history has had a negative impact on their trust in the medical system. We learned that religion plays a central role in this community and how that is integrated into their health belief system and practices. General tips for working with these populations were provided, but as usual we caution that there is a vast amount of diversity within this community, so it is important not to generalize.

REVIEW

1. Explain the history of African Americans in the United States.
2. Provide an overview of African Americans' socioeconomic situation.
3. Why is there is general mistrust by African Americans in the medical system?
4. What are some of the behavior risk factors and common diseases that African Americans experience?

CASE STUDY

The number of infants who die before their first birthday is much higher in the United States than in other countries, and for African Americans the rate is nearly twice as high as for white Americans. Even well-educated black women have birth outcomes worse than white women who haven't finished high school. Why?

We meet Andrea Jackson, a successful lawyer, executive, and mother. When Andrea was pregnant with her first child, she, like so many others, did her best to ensure a healthy baby; she ate right, exercised, abstained from alcohol and smoking, and received good prenatal care. Yet two and a half months before her due date, she went into labor unexpectedly. Her newborn weighed less than three pounds. Andrea and her husband were devastated. How could this have happened?

We know that, in general, health follows wealth; on average, the higher on the socioeconomic ladder you are, the lower your risk of cancer, heart disease, diabetes, infant death, and preterm deliveries. For highly-educated African American women like Andrea, the advantages of income and status do make a difference for her health, but there's still something else at play: racism.

There are several issues to consider about this case:

- How may have Andrea's race and culture played a role in her having a low-birth-weight baby?
- Are there any culture-specific protective factors that may have helped Andrea cope with the racism she has faced?

MODEL PROGRAM

SISTERS

The goal of the SISTERS program is to provide much-needed peer-oriented outreach, support, and case management to ensure the coordination of drug treatment, prenatal care, postpartum care, pediatric services, and family support services for pregnant and postpartum women. The program particularly targets African American or Hispanic women who are on public assistance, are mandated to treatment, report having experienced more than four violent traumas (e.g., sexual assault, death of a loved one), and have smoked crack cocaine during their last pregnancy. Program strategies include coordinated services, such as relapse prevention counseling, acupuncture detoxification, prenatal care, housing, transportation, child care, nutrition, assistance with child welfare, Medicaid, and sponsorship for attendance at Narcotics Anonymous meetings.

Program counselors, or "SISTERS," are women in recovery who have experienced many years of addiction, abusive relationships, life on the streets, birth of infants with positive toxicology, and removal of their child by protective services. These women have turned their lives around by getting help through available social service agencies. The SISTERS cultivate a trusting relationship with clients while serving as peer counselors. Those SISTERS who have received licensure as New York State Certified Acupuncturists administer acupuncture detoxification treatments to their clients. Additional tasks for the SISTERS include providing assistance to their clients concerning infant health services, housing, food, transportation, helping read and understand medical forms, promoting positive attitudes about the use of health and social services, and abstaining from alcohol and substance abuse.

SISTERS must qualify appropriately in five criteria: (1) professional experience or education, (2) race, ethnicity, and culture, (3) experience, age, and maturity, (4) gender, and (5) interpersonal and helping skills. Additional requirements include (1) a desire for the position, (2) having given birth to a baby with positive drug toxicology, (3) successful completion of treatment, (4) maintenance of sobriety for at least one year, and (5) the unqualified endorsement of supervisory staff in the clinic.

Evaluation

The evaluation was designed to demonstrate the effectiveness of peer counseling through (1) availability and use of services, (2) substance abuse abstinence and psychosocial functioning, and (3) birth outcomes and parenting attitudes. A repeated-measures (intake, two months, six months) evaluation design with a comparison group of non-SISTERS clients from the clinic was used. Data collection involved focus groups, individual client satisfaction surveys, and in-person interviews conducted by a social worker for which clients received stipends. Urine toxicology data from the clinic's information system was used to assess sobriety outcomes.

Outcome

Major program outcomes include the following:

- Urine samples of SISTERS clients became significantly cleaner over a one-year period, compared to the control group.
- Change scores for SISTERS clients significantly improved for measures of depression and self-efficacy in contrast to the non-SISTERS group.
- SISTERS clients, when compared to non-SISTERS clients, experienced a significant decrease in parental stress and rigidity of parenting style.

- SISTERS clients used more services than non-SISTERS clients.
- SISTERS clients were more likely to use warm expressions of empathy to describe their counselors.
- Seventy-eight percent of SISTERS clients gave birth to babies weighing at least 2,500 grams. More active clients had significantly heavier babies than less active clients.
- Eighty percent of infants born to SISTERS clients were toxicologically clean at birth.
- SISTERS clients continually regained custody of their children; at intake 60% had no children living at home, but at the end of the project this decreased to 18%. All SISTERS clients who obtained custody of their babies kept them for the duration of the program.

Source: Helping America's Youth. (n.d.).

GLOSSARY TERMS

Tuskegee study   Candomblé
voodoo

REFERENCES

Andrews, L. C. (2007). NetWellness. *African Americans and diet*. Retrieved February 10, 2008, from http://www.netwellness.org/healthtopics/aahealth/healthybody.cfm

Ansorge, R. (1999). Herbs and roots are in African-American folk medicine. *Colorado Springs Gazette*. Retrieved February 8, 2008, from http://www.texnews.com/1998/1999/ads/ads/health2/roots.html

Campinha-Bacote, J. (1998). African-Americans. In L. D. Purnell & B. J. Paulanka (Eds.), *Transcultural health care: A culturally competent approach* (pp. 53–73). Philadelphia: F. A. Davis.

Centers for Disease Control and Prevention. (2008). *Fact sheet on African Americans*. Retrieved February 11, 2008, from http://www.cdc.gov/hiv/topics/aa/resources/factsheets/aa.htm

Christopher, G. C. (2006). Strengthening black families. *Chicago Defender*, p. 13 (Document ID: 1106558821). Retrieved February 9, 2008, from Ethnic NewsWatch.

Clarke-Tasker, V. (1993). Cancer prevention and detection in African-Americans. In M. Frank-Stromburg & S. J. Olsen (Eds.), *Cancer prevention in minority populations: Cultural implications for health care professionals*. St. Louis, MO: Mosby.

Dakwar, E. (2004). Creighton University Medical Center. Complementary and Alternative Medicine. *Voodoo therapy*. Retrieved March 24, 2008, from http://altmed.creighton.edu/voodoo/

Ellis, G. (2005). Cigarette companies target African-Americans. *Philadelphia Tribune*, p. 5B (Document ID: 791096531). Retrieved February 9, 2008, from http://www.highbeam.com/doc/1P1-105266359.html

Fields, S. D. (2001). Health belief system of African-Americans: Essential information for today's practicing nurses. *The Journal of Multicultural Nursing & Health*. Retrieved from http://findarticles .com/p/articles/mi_qa3919/is_200101/ai_n8931688?tag=content;col1

Helping America's Youth.' (n.d.). *SISTERS*. Retrieved October 31, 2008, from http://guide. helpingamericasyouth.gov/programdetail.cfm?id=423

Hill, P. J. (2007). Legacy of addiction, incarceration feeds itself. *Call & Post*, pp. 9–11 (Document ID: 1369714311). Retrieved February 9, 2008, from Ethnic NewsWatch.

Jennings, K. (1996). Getting black women to screen for cancer: Incorporating health beliefs into practice. *Journal of the American Academy of Nurse Practitioners*, 8(2), 53–59.

Ladner, J., & Gourdine, R. (1992). Adolescent pregnancy in the African-American community. In R. Braithwaite & S. Taylor (Eds.), *Health issues in the black community* (pp. 206–221). San Francisco: Jossey-Bass.

Leininger, M. (1995). *Transcultural nursing: Concepts, theories, research and practice* (2nd ed.). New York: McGraw-Hill.

Moore, J. (2007). Hawaii Community College. *Traditional health beliefs*. Retrieved June 18, 2008, from http://www.hawcc.hawaii.edu/nursing/transcultural.html

National Diabetes Information Clearinghouse. (2005). *National diabetes statistics*. Retrieved June 18, 2008, from http://diabetes.niddk.nih.gov/dm/pubs/statistics/index.htm

National Heart Lung and Blood Institute. (2008). *African American health*. Retrieved February 10, 2008, from http://www.nhlbi.nih.gov/health/index.htm

Nobles, W. W., & Goddard, L. L. (1990). The Institute for the Advanced Study of Black Family Life and Culture. *An African-centered model of prevention for African-American youth at high risk*. Retrieved March 1, 2009, from http://www.iasbflc.org/Articles/AfricanModel/africanmodel01.htm

Office of Minority Health. (2008). *African-American profile*. Retrieved February 13, 2004, from http://www.omhrc.gov/

Perry, J. A. (1998). African roots of African-American culture. *Black Collegian Online*. Retrieved June 18, 2008, from http://www.black-collegian.com/issues/1998-12/africanroots12.shtml

Rennison, C. M., & Welchans, S. (2000). US Department of Justice. *Intimate partner violence* (NCJ 178247). Retrieved November 8, 2008, from http://www.ojp.usdoj.gov/bjs/pub/ascii/ipv.txt

Roberson, M. (1985). The influence of religious beliefs on health choices of Afro-Americans. *Topics in Clinical Nursing*, 7(3), 57–63.

Roberts, S. (n.d.). Black Youth Project. *Black youth, health, and society*. Retrieved November 8, 2008, from http://blackyouthproject.uchicago.edu/primers/reviews/health.pdf

Sadler, C., & Huff, M. (2007). *African-American women: Health beliefs, lifestyle, and osteoporosis*. Retrieved February 10, 2008, from http://www.nursingcenter.com/prodev/ce_article.asp?tid=710316

Savitt, T. L. (2002). *Medicine and slavery: The diseases and healthcare of blacks*. Champaign, IL: University of Illinois Press.

Spector, R. E. (2004). *Cultural diversity in health and illness* (6th ed.). Upper Saddle River, NJ: Pearson Education.

The New York Public Library. (2007). *In Motion: The African-American migration experience*. Retrieved February 11, 2008, from http://www.inmotionaame.org/home.cfm

University of Washington Medical Center. (2007). *African American culture clues: Communicating with your African American patient*. Retrieved February 9, 2008, from http://www.depts.washington .edu/pfes/pdf/AfricanAmericanCultureClue4_07.pdf

US Census Bureau. (2006). *Facts for features: African-American history month*. Retrieved February 11, 2008, from http://www.census.gov/Press-Release/www/2000/ff00-01.html

US Census Bureau. (2008). *Population density of the United States, and selected maps of race and Hispanic origin: 2000*. Retrieved November 9, 2008, from http://www.census.gov/population/www/censusdata/2000maps.html

US Department of Health and Human Services. (n.d.). *Changing demographics and the implications for physicians, nurses, and other health workers*. Washington, DC: Author. Retrieved April 19, 2009, from http://bhpr.hrsa.gov/healthworkforce/reports/changedemo/composition.htm

US Department of Health and Human Services. (2000). *Healthy People 2010: National health promotion and disease prevention objectives*. Washington, DC: Author.

Ventura, S. J., Abma, J. C., Mosher, W. D., & Henshaw, S. K. (2006, December 13). *Recent trends in teenage pregnancy in the United States, 1990–2002. Health E-stats*. Hyattsville, MD: National Center for Health Statistics.

Walker, A. (1996). Health and illness in African (black) American communities. In R. E. Spector (Ed.), *Cultural diversity in health and illness* (4th ed., pp. 191–214). New York: Appleton-Century-Crofts.

Warner, J. (2005). Folk remedies part of African American tradition. *Fox News*. Retrieved February 9, 2008, from http://www.foxnews.com/story/0,2933,149791,00.html

Welch, M. (2003). *Care of blacks and African Americans*. Retrieved June 17, 2008, from http://www.acponline.org/fcgi/search?q=welch+care+of+blacks&site=ACP_Online&num=10

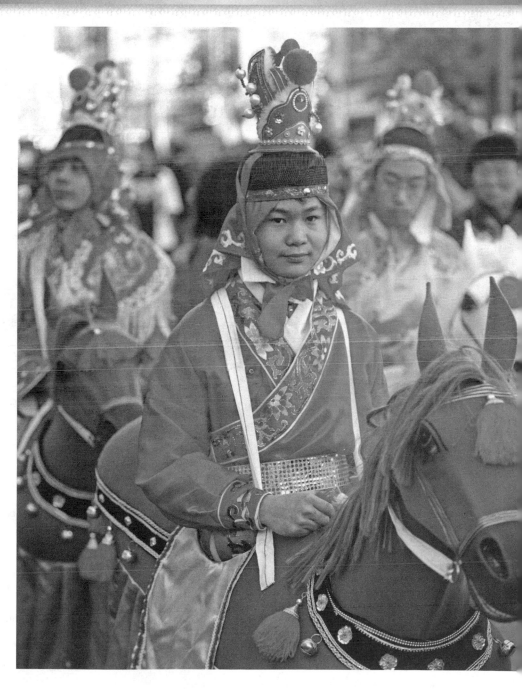

CHAPTER 10

Asian American and Pacific Islander Populations

Keeping your body healthy is an expression of gratitude to the whole cosmos—the trees, the clouds, everything.

—Thich Nhat Hanh

Always aim at complete harmony of thought and word and deed. Always aim at purifying your thoughts and everything will be well.

—Mahatma Gandhi

Sickness is a thing of the spirit.

—Japanese proverb

KEY CONCEPTS

- Hmong
- aAma and aDuonga
- Kior chi force
- Timbang
- Kava

- Betel nut
- Mana
- Lokahi
- Kahunas

CHAPTER OBJECTIVES

1. Discuss the social and economic circumstances of the various Asian Americans and Pacific Islanders in the United States.
2. Describe the beliefs about the cause of illness for Asian American and Pacific Islander cultures.
3. Discuss risk factors and illnesses that Asian Americans and Pacific Islanders are prone to.
4. Describe beliefs about healing practices for Asian Americans and Pacific Islanders.

HISTORY OF ASIAN AMERICANS AND PACIFIC ISLANDERS IN THE UNITED STATES

The experience of Asian Americans and Pacific Islanders differs depending on their country of origin, culture, and when they arrived in this country. The historical background for many of these groups is discussed below.

Chinese Americans

The background of Chinese Americans is difficult to track because no immigration records exist prior to 1820. However, stories claim that Chinese persons were brought to America as slaves by the Spanish conquistadors in the seventeenth century. There are documents that show Chinese names on the East Coast in the late eighteenth century.

Although agreement on when the first Chinese people arrived in North America cannot be reached, there is little disagreement about when their immigration exploded. When gold was discovered in California in 1849, word spread to China and immigrants flooded the West Coast. When the gold rush diminished, Chinese immigrants began working on the transcontinental railroad. They settled in great numbers in California and worked as farm laborers, in various businesses, and in factories.

Due to anti-Chinese discrimination, Chinese Americans tended to live in racially segregated areas and established enduring social structures that continue to the present. Immigration decreased for a long period as a result of the Chinese Exclusion Act of 1882, which suspended immigration and naturalization for Chinese people. This discriminatory practice was continued until the McCarran-Walter Act of 1952 made naturalization available to all races. After the reforms of the Immigration and Naturalization Act of 1965, immigration of Chinese people increased dramatically and created the basis for the strong Chinese American presence today.

Vietnamese Americans

The Vietnamese presence in the United States occurred in waves related to the American involvement in the Vietnam war. It was the continuing conflicts in Southeast Asia that led to the immigration of Laotians and Cambodians to the United States as well.

Vietnamese people who worked with the United States during that conflict fled to the United States when the Thieu government lost power in 1975. It is thought that 130,000 Vietnamese people came to the United States in 1975 alone. Most of those immigrants were young, well-educated, English-speaking city dwellers.

The second wave of immigrants was spawned by the invasion of Laos and Cambodia by Vietnamese troops. Between 1979 and 1983, 455,000 Vietnamese, Laotian, and Cambodian refugees came to the United States. These refugees tended to be made up of different ethnic groups and were more rural, less educated, and not as familiar with Western ideas as the first wave of immigrants (LaBorde, 1996).

The third group of refugees from Southeast Asia arrived from 1985 to 1991. This group tended to include both Vietnamese and Chinese people who were admitted to the country in family reunification programs (LaBorde, 1996).

Korean Americans and Asian Indians

Korean immigration to the United States began in the early twentieth century when Koreans immigrated to Hawaii to work on the plantations. Thereafter, a significant wave of immigration was related to the Korean War in the 1950s. That immigration brought many more Koreans to the U.S. mainland where most settled in the western states (Beller, Pinker, Snapka, & Van Dusan, n.d.).

Asian Indians do not have the same immigration patterns as many other Asian immigrants. Their immigration was not necessarily related to a war. Instead, they have been immigrating to the United States in greater numbers during the latter part of the twentieth century as the population in India has increased. Most came to the United States looking for greater educational and employment opportunities, and to escape the poverty of their native country.

Japanese Americans

Many Japanese people began immigrating to the United States in the nineteenth century. At first they moved to Hawaii and the Western United States to work on plantations, farms, and in the fishing and canning industry. During World War II, in one of the more shameful events in American history, Japanese Americans were interned in concentration camps because of their race and concerns that they would collaborate with the Imperial Japanese government. Even in the face of this discrimination, many Japanese Americans enlisted to assist the country in the war effort. In fact, the U.S. Army's 442nd Regimental Combat Team was composed of Japanese Americans who fought in Europe and was the most decorated unit in U.S. military history. Since the end of World War II, Japanese Americans have grown in their influence on American culture, and currently the U.S. government is engaged in a program of reparation for the suffering endured by Japanese Americans in the camps during World War II.

Native Hawaiians and Pacific Islanders

These varied islands sit in the vastness of the Pacific Ocean and were some of the last areas on Earth to be inhabited by humans. For the majority of the time during which the islands were inhabited, the people were content to remain there. It was not until recently that migration from these islands to the United States has occurred. The largest immigrations occurred after World War II and in the 1980s, with economic opportunity being the prime motivation.

The relationship of Native Hawaiians and the United States is much more controversial, because Native Hawaiians had a very distinct and proud history prior to becoming part of the union. The Hawaiian Islands were ruled by hereditary monarchs, the most famous being Kamehamcha the Great, who unified the islands prior to the arrival of Captain James Cook in 1778.

After the islands were discovered by Cook, American and European traders and planters began arriving, and the traditional way of life in the islands changed. For most of the nineteenth century, the islands were ruled by a series of monarchs descended from Kamehameha. In the latter part of the nineteenth century, the last of these monarchs, Queen Liliuokalani, was overthrown by a group of mostly Americans backed by U.S. troops. In 1898, Hawaii was annexed to the United States, and the territory of Hawaii was established. Thereafter, Hawaii became infamous for the attack on Pearl Harbor in 1942 that ushered the United States into World War II and its strategic role during that conflict.

Hawaii became the fiftieth state of the union in 1959. However, the events that led to annexation and statehood remain controversial among Native Hawaiians. A Hawaiian sovereignty movement continues to be strong and active in the islands today and pride in the Hawaiian language and traditions, such as hula, is resurging.

ASIAN AMERICANS AND PACIFIC ISLANDERS IN THE UNITED STATES

Asian Americans and Pacific Islanders (AAPI) comprise the most diverse ethnic group in the United States. According to U.S. Census Bureau data, Asians are people with origins in a number of areas of the world: the Far East, Southeast Asia, and South Asia, also known as the Indian Subcontinent. Native Hawaiians and Pacific Islanders trace their origins to Hawaii and various Pacific Islands (see Table 10.1). According to the 2004 U.S. Census Bureau data, Hawaiian and Pacific Islanders collectively comprise 5% of the population of the United States, and Asians comprise 4.2% of that number. This represents an increase of 63% from the 1990 census. These groups speak more than 100 different languages. They are the fastest growing racial/ethnic group in the United States, and it is estimated that they will comprise 1 in 10 Americans by 2050 (Office of Minority Health, 2008a).

TABLE 10.1   Asian American and Pacific Islander Origins
Far East. China, Japan, Korea, Mongolia, Okinawa, Taiwan
Southeast Asia. Borneo, Brunei, Burma, Cambodia, Celebes, Philippines, Java, Indonesia, Laos, Malaysia, Singapore, Thailand, Vietnam
South Asia (Indian Subcontinent). Afghanistan, Bangladesh, Bhutan, India, Maldives, Nepal, Pakistan, Sri Lanka, Tibet
Pacific Islands. The Flag Territories: American Samoa, Territory of Guam, Commonwealth of the Northern Mariana Islands; The Freely Associated States: Federated States of Micronesia, the Republic of Palau, the Republic of the Marshall Islands
Source: U.S. Census Bureau. (n.d.).

Notwithstanding their growing presence in the U.S. population, these groups have historically been overlooked when health research has been undertaken. Often this was due to the "myth of the model minority," a belief that Asians were quiet and did not complain and, therefore, did not have health care needs. Although these people are grouped together, they have varied cultures, traditions, religions, ancestry, languages, and health beliefs and needs. We will discuss some of what these varied peoples have in common and the specifics for many of the individual ethnic groups by exploring their history, traditional beliefs related to health and illness, risk factors, and health care needs.

QUICK FACTS

Asian Americans

Overview (demographics). Asian Americans are defined as people who have origins in any of the original peoples of the Far East, Southeast Asia, or the Indian Subcontinent. According to the 2007 U.S. Census Bureau population estimate, there are 15.2 million Asian Americans living in the United States. Asian Americans account for 5% of the nation's population. This number represents an increase of 63% from the 1990 census, thus making Asian Americans the fastest growing of all major racial/ethnic groups. In 2007, the following states had the largest Asian American populations: California, New York, Hawaii, Texas, New Jersey, and Illinois.

Language fluency. The percentage of persons aged 5 years or older who do not speak English at home varies among Asian American groups: 62% of Vietnamese, 50% of Chinese, 24% of Filipinos, and 23% of Asian Indians are not fluent in English.

Educational attainment. According to 2006 U.S. Census Bureau data, roughly 83% of all Asian Americans and all people in the United States aged 25 years and older had at least a high school diploma. However, 42% of Asian Americans, compared to 27% of the total U.S. population, had earned at least a bachelor's degree. Among Asian American subgroups, Asian Indians had the highest percentage of bachelor's degree attainment at 64%. In regards to employment, about 45% of Asian Americans were employed in management, professional, and related occupations, compared to 34% of the total population. In addition, the proportions of Asian Americans employed in highly-skilled and managerial sectors varied from 13% for Laotians to 60% for Asian Indians.

Economics. According to 2007 U.S. Census Bureau data, the median family income of Asian American families is $15,600 higher than the national median income for all households. Ten percent of Asian Americans, compared to 8.2% of non-Hispanic whites, live at the poverty level, and 2.2% of Asian Americans, compared to 1.3% of Caucasians, live on public assistance.

Source: Office of Minority Health. (2008a).

QUICK FACTS

Native Hawaiians and Pacific Islanders

Overview (demographics). Native Hawaiians and Pacific Islanders (NHPI) refers to people who have origins in any of the original peoples of Hawaii, Guam, Samoa, or other Pacific Islands. According to a 2007 U.S. Census Bureau estimate, there are roughly 1,118,000 NHPIs who reside within the United States. This group represents about 0.1% of the U.S. population. Of that number, 269,306 NHPIs reside in Hawaii. Some other states that have significant NHPI populations are California, Washington, Texas, New York, Florida, and Utah. It is also significant to note that 30% of this group is younger than 18 years of age.

Language fluency. Forty-two percent of NHPIs speak a language other than English at home.

Educational attainment. Fighty-four percent of NHPIs have high school diplomas; 10% of NHPIs have a bachelor's degree, compared to 27% of Caucasians; and 4% of NHPIs have obtained graduate degrees, compared to 11% of Caucasian Americans.

Economics. The average size of an NHPI family is four people. The median household income for this group is $50,992.

Source: Office of Minority Health. (2008b).

Geographic Distribution

As a group, Asian Americans and Pacific Islanders tend to live in the Western United States, although data indicates an increase in their populations in the East and South.

Asian Americans

Although 75% of Asian Americans resided in the 10 states shown in Table 10.2, approximately half (51%) resided in California, New York, and Hawaii. By region, 49% of Asian Americans lived in the West, 20% in the Northeast, 19% in the South, and 12% in the Midwest, as shown in Figure 10.1 (Office of Minority Health, 2008a).

Interestingly, the highest growth states for Asian Americans are not the highest population states, pointing to the emergence of new settlement and migratory patterns. The states that have exhibited some of the highest Asian American growth rates since 1990 are Nevada (219%), North Carolina (173%), Georgia (171%), Arizona (130%), and Nebraska (124%) (Office of Minority Health, 2008a).

Most Asian Americans are second and third generation in the United States. The groups with the highest percentage of foreign-born nationals living in the United States are Japanese, Pakistani, and Asian Indian (Bennett & Reeves, 2004). The largest Asian American subgroups are Filipino, Chinese, and Asian Indian (see Figure 10.2).

Native Hawaiians and Pacific Islanders

By region, approximately 73% of NHPIs lived in the West, 14% in the South, 7% in the Northeast, and 6% in the Midwest. A majority of NHPIs (58%) lived in Hawaii

TABLE 10.2 Top 10 States with Highest Number of Asian Americans	
State	**Population (Inclusive)**
California	4,155,685
New York	1,169,200
Hawaii	703,232
Texas	644,193
New Jersey	524,356
Illinois	473,649
Washington	395,741
Florida	333,013
Virginia	304,559
Massachusetts	264,814

Source: Office of Minority Health. (2008a).

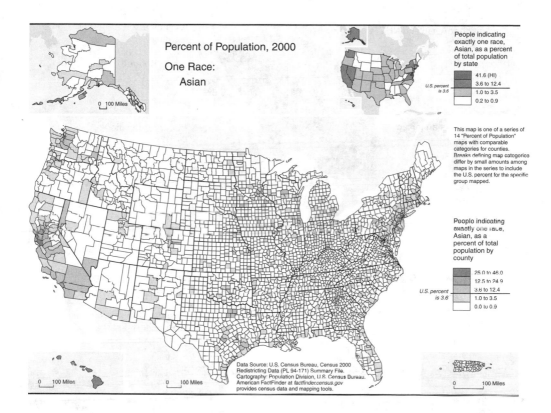

FIGURE 10.1 Percentage of population: Asian, 2000.

Source: U.S. Census Bureau, Population Division (2008). http://www.census.gov/main/www/citation.html

and California. Hawaii was home to 282,667 NHPIs (23% of the state's population), and California was home to 221,458 NHPIs (0.7% of the state's population) (see Table 10.3 and Figure 10.3).

The states with the highest growth rates for NHPIs includes both the traditionally high population states as well as some newer emerging areas. California, with the second largest NHPI population in the nation, showed one of the lowest rates of growth for NHPIs, but Nevada showed astounding growth. The NHPI population in Nevada increased 461%, and the state's total population grew 66% (U.S. Census Bureau, 2008).

Language Data

According to the 2000 census, there were over four million Asian Americans and Pacific Islanders in the United States who have limited English proficiency (LEP), which is defined as individuals who do not speak English very well.

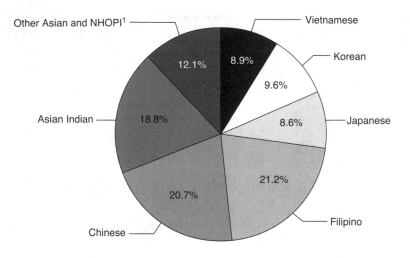

FIGURE 10.2   Percentage distribution of Asian subgroups for non-Hispanic Asian adults aged 18 years and older: United States, 2004–2006.

[1]NHOPI is Native Hawaiian or Other Pacific Islander. Estimates are age adjusted using the projected 2000 U.S. population as the standard population. Estimates are based on household interviews of a sample of the civilian noninstitutionalized population.

Source: Centers for Disease Control and Prevention. (2008).

TABLE 10.3 Top 10 States with Highest Number of NHPIs	
State	**Population (Inclusive)**
Hawaii	282,667
California	221,458
Washington	42,761
Texas	29,094
New York	28,612
Florida	23,998
Utah	21,367
Nevada	16,234
Oregon	16,019
Arizona	13,415

Source: Office of Minority Health. (2008b).

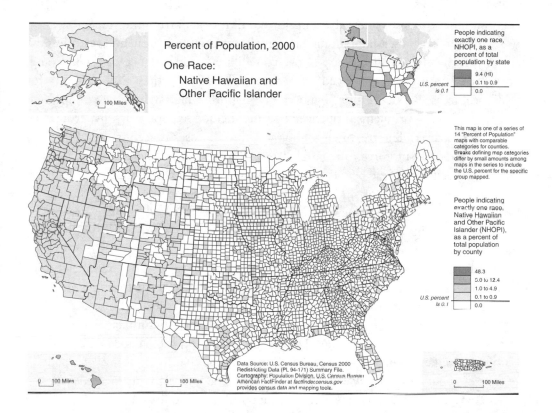

FIGURE 10.3 Percentage of population: Native Hawaiian and other Pacific Islander, 2000. *Source:* U.S. Census Bureau. (2008). http://www.census.gov/main/www/citation.html

The 2000 census also revealed that 73% of Asian Americans speak a language other than English in their homes. This represents a rate that is four times higher than the national average (18%) and more than 12 times the rate for whites (6%). When Asian Americans were disaggregated by subgroup, the results showed that many subgroups have significantly higher rates; in seven subgroups, over 90% speak a non-English language at home (Carrasco & Weiss, 2005).

BELIEFS ABOUT CAUSES OF HEALTH AND ILLNESS

Asian beliefs regarding health and illness vary from country to country and often among districts within a country. However, a common thread through many Asian health practices is the belief that the body must remain balanced to remain healthy. Many Asian cultures are incorporating Western medical systems with traditional practices.

Traditional Chinese beliefs about health and illness stem from the vital energy that flows through the body. Maintaining harmony is essential to health, and restoring the harmony of the energy is necessary to overcome illness. The balance of yin and yang, hot and cold, are often employed in traditional health practices. Yin accounts for "cold" problems like depression, hypoactivity, hypothermia, abdominal cramps, and indigestion. Health problems influenced by yang include hyperactivity, hyperthermia, stroke, and seizures. The treatment of hot and cold illnesses is accomplished through the use of the opposite force to regain balance (Beller, Pinker, Snapka, & Van Dusan, n.d.). The specifics of these beliefs are discussed at length in Chapter 3.

Vietnamese theories of illness and health vary greatly by ethnic groups. The **Hmong** mountain-dwelling people believe in the interrelatedness of medicine and religion. They believe sickness is due to being cursed or the wrath of the gods. A traditional healer is a priest who exorcises bad spirits or intercedes with the gods to remove disease. Amulets are also employed for good health. For example, babies often wear bua, an amulet of cloth containing a Buddhist verse that is worn on a string around the wrist or neck.

Urban Vietnamese people utilize a health system very similar to traditional Chinese medicine. These beliefs are based on maintaining the balance of **aAma and aDuonga**, similar to yin and yang theory. They believe that living things are made of the four elements: fire, air, water, and earth. The characteristics associated with the elements are hot, cold, wet, and dry. Treating an illness requires employment of the opposite characteristic to the one that is causing the sickness. Like Chinese medicine herbal remedies, massage, thermal treatments, and acupuncture are utilized to treat illness (LaBorde, 1996).

For traditional Koreans, illness is often seen as one's fate, and hospitalization may be seen as a sign of impending death. Illness is often attributed to yin and yang, just as in Chinese medicine. Also, the **Kior chi force**, the life force similar to chi in traditional Chinese medicine, is important in maintaining health, and efforts are made to balance this force and to not engage in activities that could diminish it. Herbal remedies are utilized for illness.

Filipino health practices incorporate a number of ideas, such as **timbang**, which is described as follows by McBride (n.d.):

> This is a key indigenous health concept that includes a complex set of fundamental principles. A range of "hot" and "cold" beliefs regarding humoral balances in the body, food, and dietary balances includes the following:
>
> - Rapid shifts from "hot" to "cold" lead to illness.
> - "Warm" environment is essential to maintain optimal health.

- Cold drinks or cooling foods should be avoided in the morning.
- An overheated body (as in childbirth or fever) is vulnerable; and heated body or muscles can get "shocked" when cooled suddenly.
- A layer of fat ("being stout") is preferred to maintain "warmth" and protect vital energy.
- Heat and cooling relate to quality and balance of air (hangin, "winds") in the body.
- Sudden changes in weather patterns, cool breezes or exposure in evening hours to low temperature, presence of hot sun immediately after a lengthy rain, or vapors rising from the soil, all may upset the body balance by simply blowing on the body surface (McBride, (n.d.), p. 3).

In the article, "Health and Illness in Filipino Immigrants", in a special issue of the *Western Journal of Medicine*, James Anderson (1983) explains that physical and mental illnesses are considered to be caused by different factors:

1. **Mystical** causes are often associated with experiences or behaviors such as retribution from ancestors for unfulfilled obligations. Some believe in soul loss and that sleep related to the wandering of the soul out of body, known as bangungot or nightmares after a heavy meal may result in death.
2. **Personalistic** causes may be attributed to social punishment or retribution by supernatural beings such as an evil spirit, witch, or mankukulam (sorcerer). A stronger spirit such as a healer or priest may counteract this force. For protection, using holy oils, wearing religious objects or an anting anting (amulet or talisman) may be recommended.
3. **Naturalistic** causes include a range of factors from nature events (thunder, lightning, drafts, etc.), excessive stress, incompatible food and drugs, infection, or familial susceptibility.

For Filipinos it is important to prevent illness by avoiding inappropriate behaviors and restoring health through the balance of the life force and the causes of illness.

Asian Indians often practice ayurvedic medicine. This ancient practice is based on the theory that the five great elements, ether, air, fire, water, and earth, are the basis for all living systems. The five elements are in constant interaction and are constantly changing. Ayurvedic medicine is discussed in detail in Chapter 3. Asian Indians also employ Western medicine.

HEALING TRADITIONS

Healing traditions among Pacific Islanders revolve around the use of naturally occurring substances, such as plant extracts and herbs. Many Pacific Islanders use **kava** root and **betel nut** for various cultural, medicinal, and ceremonial purposes. These substances are thought to overcome social barriers, ease social interactions, and cure afflictions, and they accompany ceremonial rituals. Kava is usually brewed into a tea and has been used for healing since ancient times. Betel nut is chewed and has a narcotic-like effect.

Although many Native Hawaiians utilize Western medicine for their health care needs, traditional practices continue to influence many. Like other aspects of their culture, Hawaiian health beliefs are closely related to nature. They consider the mind, body, and spirit to be one, and the body cannot maintain health without a healthy spirit. Native Hawaiians have a great regard for nature and believe the environment impacts their health through **mana**, the healing energy of the island. Thus, the concept of **lokahi**—harmony between people, nature, and the gods—is critical to maintaining health and preventing illness.

Native Hawaiian healing is practiced by **kahunas,** "keepers of the secret." Various treatments are employed, including massage and herbalism. Different types of kahunas treat different problems, not unlike specialization within Western medicine.

Many Asian Americans and Pacific Islanders use techniques discussed in Chapter 3, such as traditional Chinese medicine and ayurvedic medicine. Cambodians use coining, cupping, and pinching to treat many problems associated with "wind illness," forms of respiratory illness. Coining is rubbing or scratching the skin of the back, neck, upper chest, and arms with a coin. Cupping and pinching function in the same manner, to bring blood to an area of the body. Before or during rubbing, they apply Tiger Balm, herbal liquid medicine, skin lotion, or water on the skin. The technique helps to smooth the skin and is believed to improve the coining outcome.

BEHAVIORAL RISK FACTORS AND COMMON HEALTH PROBLEMS

Data regarding significant risks and health disparities for Asian Americans, Native Hawaiian, and Pacific Islanders include the following (Centers for Disease Control and Prevention [CDC], Office of Minority Health and Disparities, 2006):

- In 2006, the five-year relative survival rate for all cancers for Native Hawaiians was 47%, compared to 57% for whites and 55% for all races.
- In 2003, Asian American women older than age 18 years were less likely to have a Pap smear than other ethnic groups.
- In 2002, Native Hawaiians and Japanese and Filipino residents of Hawaii older than age 20 years were two times more likely to be diagnosed with diabetes as white residents of Hawaii.
- In 2002, the infant mortality rate for Native Hawaiians was 9.6 per 1,000 live births, higher than that of all other populations.
- In 2003, new AIDS cases reported among Asian Americans and Pacific Islanders was up 34.7% over the 1999 level.

- In 2001, Asian Americans and Pacific Islanders older than age 40 years were 2.5 times more likely to have hepatitis B than non-Hispanic whites.
- In 2004, Asian Americans were 5.6 times more likely to have tuberculosis than the general American population, and Native Hawaiians and Pacific Islanders were 3.3 times more likely to have the disease.

Asian Americans

Barnes, Adams, and Powell-Griner (2008) researched the utilization of health resources among Asian Americans. They found that Korean Americans were the most likely among the Asian populations to be without a regular source of health care. Vietnamese Americans were more likely than other groups to consider a clinic as their primary place for health care. Asian American adults were more likely to have never seen a dentist, compared to white or black adults, and a large percentage of Korean Americans had not been to a dentist in the last year.

Interestingly, the rate of Asian Americans who did not seek health care because of cost was relatively low. However, of this population, Korean Americas had the highest rate of not seeking care because of financial concerns (Barnes, Adams, Powell-Griner, 2008).

Data from the census and recent research has provided a much better picture of the health behaviors of Asian Americans and the common health problems they encounter. The data indicates that Asian American populations have differing personal practices and susceptibilities to disease.

Most Asian American adults have never smoked; however, for those who do, the highest rate of smoking was among Korean American and Japanese American adults. Japanese American adults also were more likely to be current moderate or heavy drinkers. Vietnamese American adults had the highest incidence of alcohol abstinence over a lifetime, and Asian Indian Americans were a close second. Most Asian American adults were in an appropriate weight range, but Filipino American adults were more likely to be obese, compared to other Asian American adults. Finally, few Asian Americans reported doing regular physical activity, and Vietnamese Americans were most likely to be inactive during their leisure time (Barnes, Adams, Powell-Griner, 2008).

Sixty percent of Asian Americans reported being in excellent or very good health (Barnes, Adams, Powell-Griner). No difference between males or females was reported for most Asian American groups. Vietnamese Americans had the highest rate of poor health, and Vietnamese American women were twice as likely to be in poor health than Vietnamese American men (see Figure 10.4).

Asian American adults are less likely to report being diagnosed with hypertension and high blood pressure than black, white, or Hispanic adults. Among Asian American

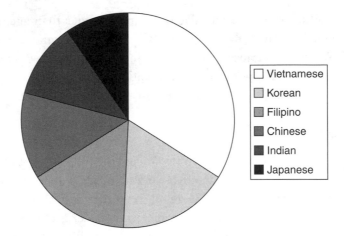

FIGURE 10.4   Asian American adults reporting fair to poor health for 2004–2006.
Source: Barnes, Adams, and Powell-Griner. (2008).

populations, Filipino Americans and Japanese Americans are more likely to be diagnosed with hypertension than Chinese Americans, Korean Americans, or Asian Indian Americans. Asian Americans were also less likely to have diabetes than black or Hispanic Americans. However, within the Asian American population, Asian Indian Americans had a significantly greater incidence of diabetes than Chinese or Japanese Americans. Compared to white, black, and Hispanic Americans, Asian Americans are less likely to suffer from migraines. Among the Asian American population, Vietnamese Americans and Filipino Americans have the highest incidence of migraines.

Immunization rates for Asian American populations are lower than the other groups overall. Asian Americans were less likely to have received a pneumonia vaccine. They received the hepatitis B vaccine at the same rate as white and black adults, but they were less likely to obtain HIV testing. Asian Americans report psychological distress less frequently than white, black, or Hispanic adults (Barnes, Adams, Powell-Griner, 2008).

Asian Americans are most at risk for a number of health problems, including cancer, heart disease, stroke, diabetes, and unintentional injuries. They also have a high incidence of chronic obstructive pulmonary disease, hepatitis B, HIV–AIDS, smoking, tuberculosis, and liver disease (CDC, 2006).

Although heart disease occurs less frequently among Asian Americans than any other minority group, it is still a leading cause of death among Asian Americans (see Table 10.4). Asian Americans are at risk for silent heart attacks, a painless form of the disease that can lead to a fatal outcome as a result of the lack of warning of a problem.

TABLE 10.4	Ten Leading Causes of Death in Asian American and Pacific Islander Populations	
1. Cancer		6. Influenza and pneumonia
2. Heart disease		7. Chronic lower respiratory disease
3. Stroke		8. Suicide
4. Unintentional injuries		9. Kidney disease
5. Diabetes		10. Alzheimer disease

Source: Centers for Disease Control and Prevention, Office of Minority Health and Disparities. (2007).

Stroke within the Asian American population is higher than within the white American population.

In addition to the various pathologies that Asian Americans are susceptible to, there are other factors that negatively impact their health. They tend to avoid visits to medical practitioners because of language and cultural barriers, fear of deportation, and lack of insurance (Office of Minority Health, 2008a). Figure 10.5 depicts

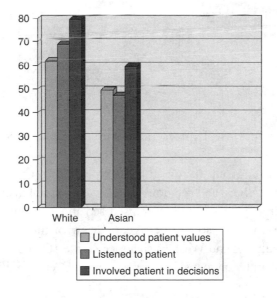

FIGURE 10.5 Asian Americans' and white Americans' perceptions of relationship with physicians.
Source: Ngo-Metzger, Legedza, and Phillips. (2004).

TABLE 10.5 Comparison of Eastern and Western Values		
Values	**Eastern/Traditional**	**Western/Modern**
Societal orientation	Family	Individual
Family makeup	Extended	Nuclear
Primary relationship	Parent–child	Marital
Family values	Well defined	Flexible
Relationship emphasis	Interpersonal and harmony	Self-fulfillment and development
Gender roles	Male dominant	Opportunity for females
Control	Authoritative	Democratic
Emotional expression	Suppressive	Expressive
Beliefs	Fatalism/karma	Personal control
	Harmony with nature	Control of nature
	Cooperation	Competition
	Spiritualism	Materialism

Source: Carrasco and Weiss. (2005).

Asian Americans' perceptions of interactions with physicians, compared to white Americans' perceptions.

Asian Americans as a group have similar perspectives on mental health issues. Many traditional Asian cultural and religious beliefs view mental health problems to be shameful and disgraceful. They often are not discussed and, consequently, seeking help is often avoided. These views also instruct Asians' view of the world and the differences between Asian cultures and Western societies. Table 10.5 compares the differing approaches to society, family, and behavioral issues between Asian and Western societies.

Native Hawaiians and Pacific Islanders

Native Hawaiians and Pacific Islanders (NHPI) have poorer health than the American population as a whole. The most common health disorders for Pacific Islanders include cancer, diabetes, heart disease, and obesity. Some of the leading causes of death are cancer, heart disease, stroke, and unintentional injuries, and premature death is caused by obesity, cardiovascular disease, cancer, and diabetes (CDC, 2006) (see Table 10.4). Some other health conditions and risk factors that are prevalent among NHPIs are hepatitis B, HIV–AIDS, and tuberculosis.

It is significant to note that in comparison to other ethnic groups, NHPIs have higher rates of smoking, alcohol consumption, and obesity. This group also has little access to cancer prevention and control programs (Office of Minority Health, 2008b).

The infant mortality rate (deaths per 1,000 live births) for Native Hawaiians in 2002 was 9.6, higher than the rate for all Asian American and Pacific Islander groups combined (4.8 deaths per 1,000 live births) and for the general population (7.0 deaths per 1,000 live births). The tuberculosis rate (cases per 100,000 patients) for NHPIs in 2007 was 21 times higher than the white population; the NHPI rate was 23.0 cases per 100,000, compared to 1.1 cases per 100,000 for the white population (Office of Minority Health, 2008b).

QUICK FACTS

Cancer
- In 2004, NHPI men were 40% less likely to have prostate cancer than non-Hispanic white men.
- In 2004, NHPI women were 30% less likely to have breast cancer than non-Hispanic white women.
- NHPI men and women have higher incidence and mortality rates for stomach and liver cancer.

Diabetes
- In Hawaii, Native Hawaiians have more than twice the rate of diabetes as whites.
- NHPIs are 20% less likely than non-Hispanic whites to die from diabetes.
- In Hawaii, Native Hawaiians are more than 5.7 times as likely as whites to die from diabetes.
- In Hawaii, Filipino Americans have more than three times the death rate of whites.

Heart Disease
- Overall, NHPI adults are less likely than white adults to have heart disease, and they are less likely to die from heart disease.
- NHPIs are 40% more likely to be diagnosed with heart disease, compared to non-Hispanic whites.

(Continues)

HIV–AIDS
- NHPIs have lower AIDS rates than their non-Hispanic white counterparts, and they are less likely to die of HIV–AIDS.
- One NHPI child was diagnosed with AIDS in 2006.

Immunization
- In 2005, NHPI adults aged 65 years and older were 40% less likely to have ever received a pneumonia shot, compared to non-Hispanic white adults of the same age group.
- In 2005, NHPI children aged 19 to 35 months reached the *Healthy People 2010* goal for Hib-Imune, hepatitis B, MMR, polio, and chicken pox vaccines.

Infant Mortality
- Among NHPIs, sudden infant death syndrome (SIDS) is the fourth leading cause of infant mortality.
- The infant mortality rate for NHPIs was 40% greater for mothers younger than age 20 years, compared to mothers aged 25–29 years.

Stroke
- In general, NHPI adults are less likely to die from a stroke.
- In general, NHPI adults have lower rates of being overweight or obese, lower rates of hypertension, and they are less likely to be current cigarette smokers, compared to white adults.

Source: Reprinted from Office of Minority Health. (2008b).

Diet

As a group, Asian Americans are not as concerned with nutrition as people from Western cultures. The texture, flavor, color, and aroma of food is much more important in Chinese cooking. The balance of yin and yang, hot and cold, is much more important than food groups.

Because many Asian Americans are lactose intolerant, dairy products are not a large part of their diet. Soy milk and tofu are the staples that provide protein and calcium. The primary food groups for Asian Americans are grains, vegetables, fruit, and meat or fish, and rice and noodles are daily staples (see Figure 10.6).

The Asian Indian diet and cooking involves the use of aromatic spices. Asian Indian dietary practices have religious influences from the Hindu and Muslim traditions. Hindus are vegetarians and believe that food was created by a Supreme Being for the benefit of man. Muslims have several dietary restrictions (Bhungalia, Kelly, VanDeKeift, & Young, n.d.).

Pacific Islanders have been experiencing poor nutrition related to dietary changes that incorporate more Western practices like fast food and highly processed foods. Coupled with more sedentary lifestyles, these dietary changes have placed more Pacific Islanders at risk for obesity and diabetes.

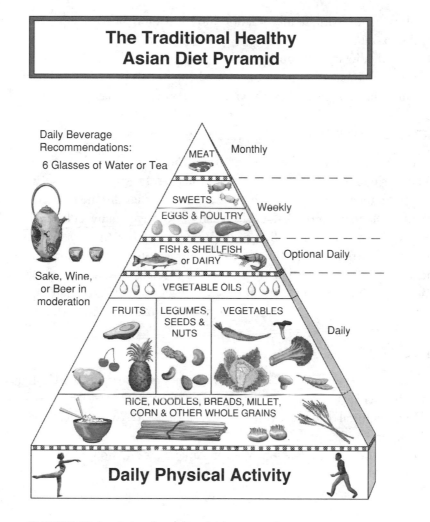

FIGURE 10.6 Asian food pyramid.
Source: © 2000 Oldways Preservation & Exchange Trust.
www.oldwayspt.org. Reproduced with permission.

CONSIDERATIONS FOR HEALTH PROMOTION AND PROGRAM PLANNING

Health promotion for Asian Americans and Pacific Islanders creates a unique challenge given the varied cultures and traditions involved. Points to consider for Asian American and Pacific Islander programs should include:

- Ensure good communication by thorough explanation and language translation where necessary.

- Show respect for family relationships and their needs, and include family in discussions.
- Provide dietary-appropriate meals.
- Inquire about other treatments used for health problems and obtain specific information regarding herbs and other substances that are being used.

CHAPTER SUMMARY

The term "Asian American" is a generality for many people who trace their heritage to numerous countries, cultures, and traditions across Asia. They continue the traditions of their ancestors and experience health care issues unique to their heritage.

Pacific Islanders and Native Hawaiians also have many cultural backgrounds. Many people in the United States are unaware of the history of Hawaii and its controversial entry into the United States. This chapter has provided an introduction to the varied cultures and health practices that comprise Asian Americans, Pacific Islanders, and Native Hawaiians through a discussion of their heritage, history in America, traditional health practices, and common health risks.

REVIEW

1. Discuss Asian Americans' and Pacific Islanders' history in the United States and the influence it has had on their health.
2. What cultural influences impact the health of Asian Americans and Pacific Islanders?
3. Discuss the health behaviors of Asian Americans and how those behaviors impact their health.
4. Discuss the health behaviors of Pacific Islanders and how those behaviors impact their health.

CASE STUDIES

Case #1. An elderly Japanese American woman lived alone in her apartment. Recently it was noted that she was not keeping her apartment and garden up as she did in the past, she has locked herself out of her apartment four times this year, she has forgotten to pay the rent, and last week she left the stove on and burned a pot.

Her friends and family made an appointment for her with a geriatric consultant through her health care provider. She was evaluated by a social worker, and a Caucasian caregiver was hired to assist her with activities of daily living. Since the caregiver has been cooking, the woman has been experiencing diarrhea, cramping, and abdominal pain. She has been using over-the-counter medications for the problem and is being evaluated at the hospital for her symptoms.

Among the things to be considered by the doctors is the possibility that the woman is lactose intolerant, which is prevalent among Japanese people. Because a non-Japanese caregiver now cooks her meals, she may be eating food she is not used to that possibly contains lactose, and she may not be able to discuss this with the caregiver due to communication problems.

Consider the following:

- What can be done to assist this woman in a manner more appropriate to her traditions?

Case #2. A healthy Japanese American man was declared brain dead after a motor vehicle accident. His children consented to donate his organs. The decedent's siblings arrived from Japan and were very upset that his organs had been donated. They believed the decedent would not have wanted that, and they could not understand how he had died because his heart was still beating. They made overtures that the children had improperly let him die, and a terrible split occurred within the family.

Organ donation among traditional Japanese is not well received. Education and counseling is needed to assist the family during the loss of a loved one.

Consider the following:

- How could the health care providers have helped to reduce the likelihood of the family rift?
- How might health care providers deal with family members who don't understand the decisions that were made?

Source: Tanabe. (n.d.).

MODEL PROGRAMS

Families In Good Health

The Families in Good Health Program was designed in Long Beach, California to improve cardiac health by decreasing the sedentary lifestyle among Southeast Asians. The program focused on families and spent considerable effort in identifying the needs of the various communities. Since the main place for socialization was the temples and churches attended by the various groups, fitness activities were developed and offered at those sites.

Activities offered included health education, traditional dances, youth classes, walking groups, water aerobics for elders, and an exercise cassette with traditional music and nutritional information for those who could not read English. Community groups donated exercise equipment, and the YMCA worked with the program to lower costs for program participants.

Source: National Institutes of Health, Office of Prevention, Education, and Control. (2000).

Strengthening Hawaii Families

The Strengthening Hawaii Families program is a culturally relevant, family-focused program designed to prevent substance abuse and other problems through improving parenting skills, family relations, and reducing childhood behavioral problems.

Evaluation

The program consists of 14 weeks of training in parenting, child skills, and family skills. Topics covered include family values, culture and generational continuity, goal setting, communication problem solving, anger management, and wellness, among others.

Outcomes

At the end of the program, follow-up found that the program had the following positive outcomes:

- Significant reduction in family conflict
- Significant improvement in family cohesion and organization
- Significant improvement in family communication

Source: SAMHSA's National Registry of Evidence-based Programs and Practices. (2009).

GLOSSARY TERMS _____

Hmong

aAma and aDuonga

Kior chi force

timbang

kava

betel nut

mana

lokahi

kahunas

REFERENCES

Anderson, J. (1983). Health and illness in Filipino immigrants. In Cross-Cultural Medicine [Special issue]. *Western Journal of Medicine, 139*(6), 811–819.

Barnes, P., Adams, P., & Powell-Griner, E. (2008). *Health characteristics of the Asian Adult population: United States, 2004–2006.* Advance data from vital and health statistics, no. 394. Hyattsville, MD: National Center for Health Statistics. Retrieved May 22, 2008, from http://www.meps.ahrq.gov/mepsweb/data_files/publications/st224/stat224.pdf

Beller, T., Pinker, M., Snapka, S., & Van Dusan, D. (n.d.). *Korean-American health care beliefs and practices.* Retrieved April 25, 2008 from http://bearspace.baylor.edu/Charles_Kemp/www/korean_health.htm

Bennett, C., & Reeves, T. (2004, December). *We the people: Asians in the United States. Census 2000 special reports.* Retrieved May 16, 2008 from http://www.census.gov/prod/2004pubs/censr-17.pdf

Bhungalia, S., Kelly, T., VanDeKeift, S., & Young, M. (n.d.). *Indian health care beliefs and practices.* Retrieved April 25, 2008, from http://bearspace.baylor.edu/Charles_Kemp/www/korean_health.htm

Carrasco, M., & Weiss, J. (2005). NAMI. *Asian American and Pacific Islander outreach resource manual.* Retrieved April 25, 2008, from http://www.NAMI.org/Content/ContentGroups/Multicultural_Support1/AAPIManual.pdf

Centers for Disease Control and Prevention. (2008). *CDC advance data from vital and health statistics, number 394. Health characteristics of the Asian adult population: United States, 2004–2006.* Retrieved May 22, 2008, from http://www.cdc.gov/nchs/data/ad/ad394.pdf

Centers for Disease Control and Prevention, Office of Minority Health and Disparities. (2006, May). *Highlights in minority health & health disparities May 2006; Asian American Pacific Islander heritage month* 2006. Retrieved April 25, 2008, from http://www.cdc.gov/omhd/Highlights/2006/HMay06AAPI.htm

Centers for Disease Control and Prevention, Office of Minority Health and Disparities. (2007). *Asian American populations.* Retrieved April 25, 2008, from http://www.cdc.gov/omhd/Populations/AsianAm/AsianAm.htm

Hilgenkamp, K., & Pescaia, C. (2003). Traditional Hawaiian healing and western influence [Special issue: Hawaii]. *California Journal of Health Promotion, 1,* 34–39. Retrieved May 30, 2008, from http://www.hawaii.edu/hivandaids/Traditional_Hawaiian_Healing_and_Western_Influence.pdf

LaBorde, P. (1996, July). *Vietnamese cultural profile.* Retrieved April 25, 2008, from http://www.ethnomed.org/ethnomed/cultures/vietnamese/vietnamese_cp.html

McBride, M. (n.d.). *Health and health care of Filipino American elders.* Retrieved May 23, 2008, from http://www.stanford.edu/group/ethnoger/filipino.html

National Institutes of Health, Office of Prevention, Education, and Control. (2000). *Addressing cardiovascular health in Asian Americans and Pacific Islanders* (NIH Publication No. 00-3647).

Ngo-Metzger, Q., Legedza, A., & Phillips, R. (2004). Asian Americans reports of their health care experiences. *The Commonwealth Fund.* Retrieved May 16, 2008, from http://www.commonwealthfund.org/Content/Publications/In-the-Literature/2004/Feb/Asian-Americans-Reports-of-Their-Health-Care-Experiences.aspx

Office of Minority Health. (2008a). *Asian American/Pacific Islander profile.* Retrieved April 25, 2008, from http://www.omhrc.gov/templates/browse.aspx?lvl=2&lvlid=53

Office of Minority Health. (2008b). *Native Hawaiians/other Pacific Islanders profile*. Retrieved November 21, 2008, from www.omhrc.gov/templates/browse.aspx?lvl=2&lvlID=71

Oldways Preservation & Exchange Trust. (2008). *Asian diet pyramid*. Retrieved July 23, 2008, from http://www.oldwayspt.org/asian_pyramid.html

SAMHSA's National Registry of Evidence-based Programs and Practices. (2009). *Strengthening Hawaii families*. Retrieved January 26, 2009, from http://nrepp.samhsa.gov/legacy_fulldetails. asp?LEGACY_ID=1038

Tanabe, M. (n.d.). *Health and health care of Japanese-American elders*. Retrieved May 23, 2008, from http://www.stanford.edu/group/ethnoger/japanese.html

US Census Bureau. (n.d.). *Race and Hispanic origin in 2005*. Retrieved May 27, 2008, from http://www.Census.gov/population/pop-profile/dynamic/RACEHO.pdf

US Census Bureau. (2008). *Population density of the United States, and selected maps of race and Hispanic origin: 2000*. Retrieved November 9, 2008, from http://www.census.gov/population/www/censusdata/2000maps.html

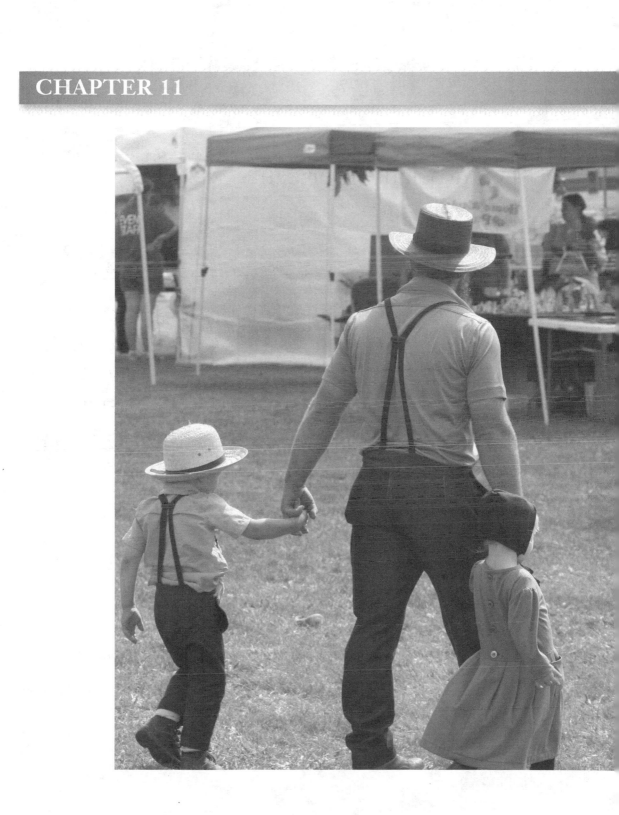

CHAPTER 11

Caucasian American Populations

Sometimes God calms the storm, but sometimes God lets the storm rage
and calms his child.

—Amish proverb

May God give you luck and health.

—Roma (Gypsy) blessing

It is well to give when asked, but it is better to give unasked,
through understanding.

—Kahlil Gibran

KEY CONCEPTS

- Rumspringa
- Brauche
- Ellis-van Creveld syndrome
- Romany
- Gadje
- Wuzho
- Marime
- Drabarni

CHAPTER OBJECTIVES

1. Describe the cultural impact on health for the Amish, Roma, and Arab Americans.
2. Discuss the common health risks for these groups.
3. Describe the behavioral health challenges for these groups.

The U.S. Census Bureau's term "white" applies to a person having origins among any of the original peoples of Europe, the Middle East, or North Africa. That is a very broad area that encompasses numerous ethnic and cultural groups. Much has been written about the dominant European groups that inhabit the United States. Figure 11.1 illustrates the distribution of non-Hispanic whites in the United States. In this chapter we will discuss some of the cultural and health care issues that impact cultures and ethnic groups that are less well known.

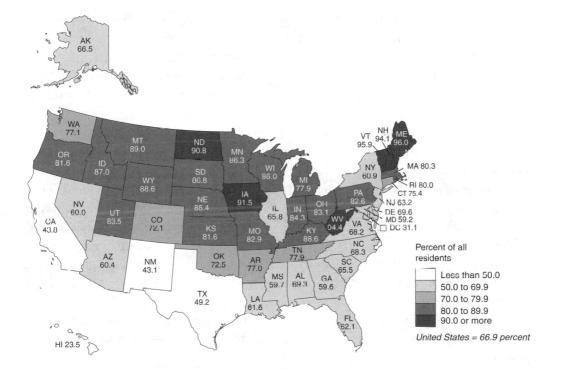

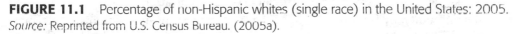

FIGURE 11.1   Percentage of non-Hispanic whites (single race) in the United States: 2005. *Source:* Reprinted from U.S. Census Bureau. (2005a).

HISTORY OF AMISH AMERICANS IN THE UNITED STATES

Jakob Amman, a Swiss Anabaptist leader, is the namesake of the Amish. Their religion can be traced back to sixteenth century Europe during Martin Luther's Protestant Reformation. Questions about whether the government or the Bible should be the supreme authority arose, and further divisions occurred, resulting in a new religious sect, the Anabaptists. The Anabaptists would experience further subdivision, resulting in groups we know today as the Amish, Mennonites, Church of the Brethren, Hutterites, and many more. The Amish have five religious orders: Old Order, New Order, Andy Weaver, Beachy, and Swartzentruber, with Old Order being the most traditional.

AMISH AMERICANS IN THE UNITED STATES

Religious persecution forced the Amish and Mennonites to find a safe haven in the New World. In the 1730s, a group of Amish immigrants joined Mennonite colonists who had already established a community in Lancaster, Pennsylvania. Lancaster houses the oldest Amish community in North America. "More than 90 percent of Lancaster's Amish are affiliated with the Old Order Amish" (Kraybill, 2001, p. 12).

Amish families live in common geographic areas. In the present day, they have established 1,300 congregations and have grown to a population of about 180,000 throughout 24 states, as well as Ontario, Canada. Although the oldest settlement is found in Pennsylvania, the most heavily populated area is Ohio, where over 150 congregations exist, and 70% of the Amish are found in Indiana, Ohio, and Pennsylvania. (Kraybill, 2001). They speak a specific Pennsylvania German dialect commonly called Pennsylvania Dutch.

The Amish strive for homogeneity. They have deep agricultural roots and believe that farming is the glue that holds their communities together. Traditionally, farming has also leveled the occupational profiles of the Amish. Although increases in land values and new business ventures have challenged the level of equality in Amish communities, the society is still a relatively egalitarian one; thus, great monetary wealth and relative poverty are nearly nonexistent. Consequently, the Amish frown upon the use of government assistance in times of need. Their society is structured such that any assistance required is provided by the community itself. This isolation from mainstream society makes it difficult to track Amish poverty levels in terms of federal poverty guidelines.

Unlike typical Western societies, social class and education are not revered in the Amish community; preserving religion and way of life is of primary importance. Traditionally, Amish children attended one-room public schools where the curriculum reflected Amish values. The Amish believe that education in evolution, science, and sex education is contradictory to their value system and consider higher education to be vain. For the most part, the Amish have successfully resisted governmental and societal movements to change their educational practices. Today, most Amish students in Lancaster, Pennsylvania still attend one-room private schools taught by Amish teachers. In 1972, the Supreme Court ruled in favor of allowing Amish families to remove their children from school at the conclusion of eight years of education.

The Amish social environment, including the family structure, child-rearing practices, religion, communication, and pregnancy beliefs, greatly influences the health of this population. The Amish live a simple lifestyle that abstains from material luxuries and resembles the lifestyle of sixteenth century European peasants. For example, they still utilize horses and buggies for transportation, and their lifestyle is agriculturally based. Their unique heritage is ingrained in a belief system that seeks to retain their traditional values while avoiding the influences of the dominant culture. The two most valued aspects of their lives include their family and their church district.

The Amish generally have large families, mostly because they do not routinely practice birth control. Children are believed to be economic blessings, because they help with maintaining the farm and household. It is not unusual for generations of family members to live in the same house and operate as one unit. Single people and single-parent homes are rare: "Only five percent of Amish households are single-person units, compared to twenty percent for the county" (Kraybill, 2001, p. 100). The average number of people in a household is 12, which may include extended family.

The gender roles within the family are traditional; the males are the dominant figures within the household, directing the farming operations and overseeing their children's work in the fields. Many husbands will assist in child care, lawn care, and gardening, but they usually do not assist in other household work. Wives are responsible for washing, cooking, canning, sewing, mending, and cleaning. Church leaders teach that wives must submit to the authority of their husbands according to religious doctrine. Women are not usually employed outside of the home. Their main duties revolve around raising the children, gardening, and assisting with barn chores. They find opportunities to host quilting parties and attend special events like weddings to maintain some form of socialization. The women who have their own businesses like their male counterparts, which include nearly 15% of the business owners in the Amish community, are believed to be acting in direct violation of God's created order (Kraybill, 2001). They are believed to be more susceptible to divorce, having unruly children, and disrupting the family order. The Amish are such strong believers in a patriarchal society that if divorce occurs because a woman does not subject herself to her defined gender role, she can be excommunicated from the community. Likewise, a man that chooses to divorce his wife must also be excommunicated. His wife can remain in the church, but she cannot remarry until her former husband dies.

The Amish religion is deeply integrated with their family structure. The Amish believe that the Bible is a guide for parents to teach their children the values of their religion while training them to conform to the Amish ways. Cultural beliefs are passed down through the generations in such a way that young Amish children are not exposed to cultural diversities that modern youth outside of the Amish community are exposed.

The church district is the other primary location of activity besides the home. The Amish practice a religion that has its roots in Christianity but has no specific identification. Some Amish would consider themselves to be conservative Protestant, but the majority would consider themselves to be Anabaptist. The ordained leaders of the church are always men and are usually elderly. Old age is respected among the Amish community as a symbol of wisdom and knowledge. Congregations meet to worship and attend baptisms, weddings, excommunications, and funerals. Sinful members must confess their major sins before other members of the congregation. One bishop, two or three ministers, and a deacon usually lead two congregations in two separate districts. The power that bishops have is the ability to recommend an excommunication and the ability to reinstate a penitent member upon approval of the congregation through a majority vote. Bishops are also responsible for making their own interpretations of religious doctrine for a district. Some bishops are more lenient than others. For example, some bishops will permit power lawn mowers, but others do not. The role of the ministers is to preach to the congregation and provide spiritual direction. These ministers do not need to have credentials or special training to become a minister; they are selected by the congregation to serve the people without monetary compensation. Ministers earn their livelihood by farming, carpentry, or other related occupations, including business (Kraybill, 2001).

Technology and electricity are believed to be products of modernity and are addressed and integrated into the Amish community under meticulous law. Amish people may use technology to communicate with one another or with non-Amish acquaintances, but the technology must be kept at a distance yet be easily accessible to all individuals within the Amish community. For example, a telephone may be located at the end of a lane and used by all families within that vicinity (Armer & Radina, 2006). Certain electric appliances are used more often by men who work in the barns than women who work in the kitchen or house. Electric mixers, blenders, dishwashers, microwave ovens, and clothes dryers are usually banned from the kitchen. Washing machines, sewing machines, mixers, beaters, and blenders are operated by air pressure.

A unique part of the Amish culture is **Rumspringa**, which means "running around." This practice is the focus of a documentary directed by Lucy Walker entitled *Devil's Playground*. Walker describes Rumspringa as a time when adolescents are free to explore the world outside of the Amish culture. Rumspringa is practiced by young males and females between the ages of 16 and 21 years. During this period, individuals may partake in activities of their choosing, which may include drinking alcohol, using illicit drugs, and experimenting with sexual activities. Rumspringa ends when the young person makes the decision to either live in the outside world or become baptized within the Amish community (Cantor & Walker, 2002).

BELIEFS ABOUT CAUSES OF HEALTH
AND ILLNESS AMONG AMISH AMERICANS

The Amish believe that sin is the cause of illness; therefore, their approach to health care in the United States is unique compared to other white Americans (Palmer, 1992). The way in which the Amish make decisions about health is affected by their separation from the world and modern technology.

Health care practitioners should be sensitive to the unique perspective of their Amish patients. For example, considering that the Amish have little contact with medical professionals and technology, health care practitioners should convey descriptions of treatment procedures accordingly, avoiding complex medical language (Lee, 2005). Moreover, health care professionals should expect to talk to spouses and family members who are likely to gather in support of the patient. Finally, as much treatment as possible should take place in one visit due to transportation difficulties. These issues should be considered to provide Amish patients with the best possible health care outcomes (Lee, 2005).

HEALING TRADITIONS AMONG AMISH AMERICANS

The Amish tend to approach health care as organically as possible with the use of holistic, natural, herbal, and folk medicine, which are readily accessible in Amish communities (Palmer, 1992). Basic natural and herbal remedies may include iron pills, vitamins E and C, herbal tea, and sage tea. Other natural remedies include corn silk tea for an enlarged prostate, aloe vera gel for minor trauma, and poho oil (peppermint oil in a petrolatum base) for respiratory problems (Kriebel, 2000). Additionally, the Amish have been known to utilize reflexology, which is the practice of applying pressure to specific parts of the feet and hands to affect the nervous system (Julia, 1996). The Amish utilize chiropractic procedures and **brauche** practices in which the brauche healer lays his hands over a patient's head or stomach while quietly reciting verses to "pull out" the ailment (Wenger, 1995).

Amish women try to limit their use of technology, even during pregnancy and while giving birth. For example, amniocentesis and other invasive prenatal diagnostic tests are not acceptable. Amish women prefer to use nurse midwives and lay midwives, and to have home deliveries, because it limits the use of technology as well as reduces the number of visits to the doctor, which may be costly (Lemon, 2006).

Women practice certain folk traditions during pregnancy to prepare themselves for giving birth. These practices include not walking under a clothesline because that is believed to cause a stillbirth. Another practice includes not climbing through a window or under a table because both can cause the umbilical cord to wrap around the baby's neck (Lemon, 2006). Women use a medley of herbs, called 5-W, five weeks before their pregnancy ends. These herbs include a mixture of red raspberry leaves, black cohosh root, butcher's broom root, dong quai root, and squaw vine root. The formula is believed to ease the labor by quieting the nerves and relaxing the uterus (Lemon, 2006).

BEHAVIORAL RISK FACTORS AND COMMON HEALTH PROBLEMS AMONG AMISH AMERICANS

The Amish have few behavioral risk factors due to various health-promoting behaviors, which, among the adult population, include low rates of tobacco use and alcohol consumption, high levels of physical activity, and low levels of obesity. However, the Amish are cautious and conservative and may refuse health care services (Armer & Radina, 2006). Furthermore, Amish youth are prone to alcohol abuse, which inspired the Drug Abuse Resistance Education (D.A.R.E.) program to conduct outreach in Amish communities (Ohio Department of Alcohol and Drug Services, 2005).

Amish children and adolescents live in nontechnological farming communities, which results in a population that is physically active and that has a low rate of obesity (Basset, Schneider, & Huntington, 2004). Amish adults also showed very high levels of physical activity, which includes consistently walking at moderate to vigorous levels and farming daily. This type of lifestyle, one that promotes physical activity, results in the low prevalence of obesity and positive health outcomes in general for the Amish community (Basset, et al., 2007).

The Amish do not completely prohibit the use of modern medical technology, but they tend to be extremely cautious and may refuse intervention if it is not approved by community leaders. For example, Amish families vary in receptivity to the practice of immunizations for communicable diseases, leading to increased vulnerability to those illnesses. Although the Amish account for less than 0.5% of the national population, they were responsible for nearly all cases of rubella reported in the United States in 1991 (Armer & Radina, 2006). Moreover, the lack of immunizations puts the Amish at risk when they travel outside of their communities, because they may not be protected against diseases to which they become exposed.

According to the *Encyclopedia of Medical Anthropology*, certain Amish communities live by laws and precepts that have been passed down for generations. Such customs include marrying within their own community and allowing first cousins to marry. Consequently, a growing number of distinctive genetic recessive disorders among the

Amish have arisen (Ember & Ember, 2004). Individuals who have a genetic recessive disorder, such as **Ellis-van Creveld syndrome** (EVC), receive a defective recessive gene from each parent. EVC, a form of dwarfism, is an autosomal recessive disorder in which individuals exhibit postaxial polydactyly of the hands; this is indicated by an extra digit located next to the fifth digit. In addition, EVC is characterized by individuals having short forearms and legs as well as congenital heart failure (Leach, 2007).

Cartilage-hair hypoplasia, another form of dwarfism, is a genetic disorder that is rarely seen outside of Amish communities (ClinicalTrials.gov, 2007). This rare disorder was not recognized until the mid-1960s when Amish children began to present with features similar to, but more pronounced than, EVC. These signs include fine and underdeveloped hair (hypoplasia of the hair) and underdeveloped cartilage (hypoplasia of the cartilage), resulting in skeletal abnormalities and an inability to fully extend the upper limbs (McKusick, 2000). Researchers are currently attempting to verify the causes of such health problems to find solutions to these disorders. As the homogenous Amish population continues to grow, further research is necessary to understand their propensity toward genetic recessive disorders (ClinicalTrials.gov, 2007).

Another rising health concern, particularly among young Amish community members, is the use of drugs and alcohol. It has been noted that the use of drugs and alcohol was not initially taken seriously because of the Amish adolescent participation in the Rumspringa ritual (Donnermeyer & Lora, 2002).

For some individuals, the use of drugs and alcohol during the period of Rumspringa has been linked with depression (Donnermeyer & Lora, 2002). Drug- and alcohol-related depression may exist in part because of the pressure to either join the church or become shunned and leave the community (Cantor & Walker, 2002). This issue has become so severe in Holmes County, Ohio, that Amish church elders set up a private mental health center for their community. Because the center is not directed by the outside medical community, the elders are responsible for counseling members who suffer from depression or other mental illnesses (Donnermeyer & Lora, 2002). Although teen depression has risen within Amish communities, depression among adults has not been an issue. Studies have revealed that Amish adults tend to live relatively stress-free lives (Cantor & Walker, 2002).

Humility and simplicity are characteristics that form the underpinning of Amish society in the United States. The Amish practice a conservative form of Christian idealism, which was founded on early Anabaptist practices (Kraybill, 2001). The Amish interpret the Bible literally and strive to retain their traditional values while avoiding the influences of outside norms. The Amish limit their contact with the dominant culture and generally reject the use of modern technology (Armer & Radina, 2006).

The Amish tend to prefer natural home remedies; however, they may seek health care services from medical doctors and complementary health providers, such as reflexologists and chiropractors (Julia, 1996). Due to a relatively stress-free and active lifestyle, positive health outcomes among the population include low rates of obesity, smoking, and cancer (Ferketich, et al., 2008). As a result of the lack of vaccinations among the Amish, they are more susceptible to communicable diseases (Armer & Radina, 2006). Finally, common health problems found among the Amish are birth defects as a result of recessive genetic disorders due to intermarriage practices (Leach, 2007).

CONSIDERATIONS FOR HEALTH PROMOTION AND PROGRAM PLANNING FOR AMISH AMERICANS

When working with members of the Amish community, the following recommendations should be considered to improve cultural understanding:

- Be cognizant of the cultural differences this group has with society as a whole.
- Recognize the importance of privacy.
- Recognize that Amish people might not understand things you consider to be everyday occurrences.
- Be cognizant of the formality of family relationships.
- Explain all procedures and instructions to ensure understanding.

HISTORY OF ROMA AMERICANS IN THE UNITED STATES

A cultural group that is very misunderstood and often overlooked is the Roma. Commonly known as Gypsies, that term is considered a pejorative by these people, and the proper term for this group is the Roma or the Romani. They are an isolated group that maintains a strong social and cultural bond separate and apart from everyday American society.

The Roma are originally from northern India and migrated throughout middle and eastern Europe beginning around 1000 AD. They immigrated to the United States mainly in two stages: in the eighteenth century as a result of being deported from various European countries and at the end of the nineteenth century primarily from Eastern Europe.

They speak primarily **Romany**, a language derived from Sanskrit, and English as a second language. Interestingly, until recently Romany was a wholly spoken language.

Most older Roma are not literate, and some younger members have some education. Written forms of the Romany language have been occurring with the education of the younger generations.

ROMA AMERICANS IN THE UNITED STATES

It is difficult to determine the exact number of Roma in the United States, because they do not believe in recording births and deaths, and no census data exists. However, it is estimated that there are between 200,000 and 500,000 members of various Roma groups in the United States (Sutherland, 1992). Roma populations are concentrated in urban areas such as San Francisco, New York, Los Angeles, Chicago, Boston, Atlanta, Seattle, and Houston.

Roma Americans have a very complicated social structure to their culture. In general they have four loyalties to their nation, clan, family, and vista. They are first divided into nations; the most common nations are the Machwaya, Kalderasham, Churara, and Lowara. The nations are further divided into clans. A clan is a group of families united by ancestry, profession, and historic ties. Each clan has a leader, but there is no such thing as "Gypsy kings" as characterized in popular lore. Some clans are further divided into tribes, but most are composed of families. It is the family that is the most important social group for the Roma. A vista is extended family (Ryczak, Zebreski, May, Traver, & Kemp, n.d.).

Roma Americans purposely isolate themselves from the larger community and tend to be ethnocentric. They maintain separation from people and things that are **gadje**, non-Roma, who are considered to be unclean. The strict code that they live by limits acculturation.

BELIEFS ABOUT CAUSES OF HEALTH AND ILLNESS AMONG ROMA AMERICANS

Roma Americans' beliefs regarding health and illness stem from two concepts: impurity and fortune. The first concept is related to the ideas of **wuzho** (pure) and **marime** (impure). Roma Americans have very strict traditions about what is polluted and how things are to be kept clean. Secretions from the upper half of the body are not polluted, but secretions from the lower half of the body are. Therefore, separate soap and towels are used for the upper and lower halves of the body. Failing to keep the two secretions separate can result in serious illness. Also, because gadje (non-Romas) do not practice body separation, they are considered to be impure and diseased.

Fortune also plays a role in health. Good fortune and good health are thought to be related. Illness can be caused by actions that are considered to be contaminating and, therefore, create bad fortune.

Roma Americans distinguish between illnesses that are of a gadje cause and those that are part of their beliefs. Gadje illnesses can be cured by gadje doctors. Hospitals are avoided by Roma Americans because they are unclean and are separate from Roma society. Illness is a problem to be dealt with by the entire clan. Therefore, if a clan member is hospitalized, family and clan members are expected to stay with them and provide curing rituals and protect them. An exception to the aversion to hospitals is childbirth. Women are considered to be unclean during pregnancy and for a number of weeks after delivery. Childbirth should not happen in the family home because it can cause impurity in the home. Therefore, delivery in hospitals is accepted in the culture.

Finally, older members of a family are very important in health care decision making. They are considered to be the authority in the family and carry great weight in all decisions.

HEALING TRADITIONS AMONG ROMA AMERICANS

As previously discussed, illnesses can be characterized as those of the Roma or those that are gadje. Roma health treatment is the prerogative of the older women of the clan who are known as **drabarni**, women who have knowledge of medicines. Roma diseases are not connected to gadje diseases and can only be cured by Roma treatments. Some diseases are caused by spirits or the devil. One spirit, called Mamioro, spreads disease among dirty houses, so keeping a clean home is imperative. The devil has been known to cause nervous diseases. Herbs and rituals are utilized to address these problems.

BEHAVIORAL RISK FACTORS AND COMMON HEALTH PROBLEMS AMONG ROMA AMERICANS

There are reports that the life expectancy of Roma Americans is reduced from the general population. A European study found they have a life expectancy of less than 50 years (Ryczak, et al., n.d.). It has been reported that the life expectancy of a Roma person in the United States is between age 48 and 55 years (Sutherland, 1992). In Romani culture, the larger a person is, the luckier he or she is considered to be. A fat person is considered to be healthy and fortunate, and a thin person is considered to be ill and to have poor luck. This belief and other cultural beliefs are sources of health concerns for this group.

As a group, Roma Americans are resistant to immunization because it does not comport with their beliefs regarding purification. Thus, they are at risk for many communicable diseases.

The Roma American diet is high in fat and salt. A great percentage of Roma Americans smoke and are obese. These practices put them at risk for cardiovascular disease, hypertension, and diabetes. The closeness of living conditions leads to an increased risk of infectious diseases such as hepatitis. Romani children are more likely to be born prematurely or with low birth weight, and the increased incidence of consanguineous marriages has led to an increased risk of birth defects (Ryczak, Zebreski, May, Traver, Kemp, n.d.).

CONSIDERATIONS FOR HEALTH PROMOTION AND PROGRAM PLANNING FOR ROMA AMERICANS

In working with Roma Americans, the following issues should be considered:

- Understand that illness is an issue for the entire society, and the entire clan will be involved in visiting the sick person in the hospital.
- Recognize the primacy of the elders in the family and the clan in making decisions.
- Always remember the importance of what is considered to be clean and unclean and provide separate soap, washcloths, and towels for the upper and lower body parts.
- Understand that this population is mistrustful of non-Roma people and things.
- Understand that Roma Americans are an ethnocentric culture and believe that they must be provided with the best doctors and treatment even if such treatment is not indicated.

HISTORY OF ARAB AND MIDDLE EASTERN AMERICANS IN THE UNITED STATES

Being Arab is not based on race. Arabs are usually associated with the geographic area extending from the Atlantic coast of Northern Africa to the Arabian Gulf. The people who descend from this area are classified as Arabs based largely on a common language (Arabic) and a shared sense of geographic, historic, and cultural identity. Arabs include peoples with widely-varied physical features, countries, or origin and religions.

There are 10 Arab countries in Africa (Algeria, Djibouti, Egypt, Eritrea, Libya, Mauritania, Morocco, Somalia, Sudan, and Tunisia) and 11 countries in Asia (Bahrain, Iraq, Jordan, Kuwait, Lebanon, Oman, Qatar, Saudi Arabia, Syria, United Arab Emirates, and Yemen), including the Palestinian people who live either in Israeli territory or under semiautonomous conditions in the West Bank and Gaza (Ahmad, 2004).

Although it is believed that between 2–3 million Arabs live in the United States, the 2000 U.S. census found that only 850,000 people in the country voluntarily reported Arab ancestry, which is 0.3% of the total population, an increase from 0.2% in 1990 (see Figure 11.2). More than half of the respondents were American born, and 46% of foreign-born respondents arrived in the United States between 1990 and 2000 (see Figure 11.3).

Middle Easterners who trace their ancestry to Iran are not considered to be Arab. They are of Persian descent, and their primary language is Farsi. However, Arab and

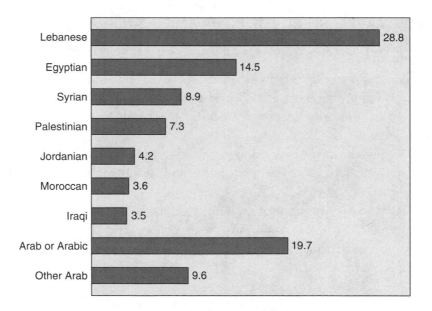

FIGURE 11.2   Arab population by ancestry: 2000.

Percent distribution. Data based on sample. For information on confidentiality protection, sampling error, nonsampling error, and definitions, see www.census.gov/prod/cen2000/doc/sf4.pdf.

Other Arab (9.6%) includes Yemeni, Kurdish, Algerian, Saudi, Tunisian, Kuwaiti, Libyan, Berber, Emirati (United Arab Emirates), Omani, Qatari, Bahraini, Alhuceman, Bedouin, Rio de Oro, and the general terms Middle Eastern and North African.

Source: Reprinted from U.S. Census Bureau. (2005b).

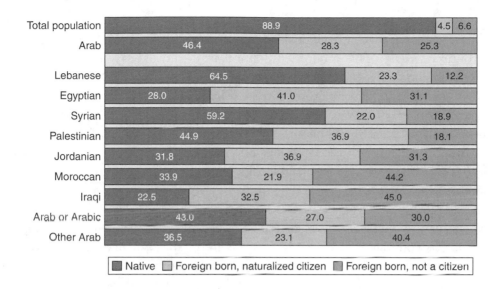

FIGURE 11.3   Nativity and citizenship status: 2000.
Percent distribution. Data based on sample. For information on confidentiality protection, sampling error, nonsampling error, and definitions, see www.census.gov/prod/cen2000/doc/sf4.pdf.
Source: Reprinted from U.S. Census Bureau. (2005b).

Persian Middle Easterners have a significant factor in common: The great majority of them are Muslim. Although some Arabs are Christian and Jewish, the great majority of Arabs in the world (92%) are Muslim (Ahmad, 2004).

ARAB AND MIDDLE EASTERN AMERICANS IN THE UNITED STATES

Persons of Arab and Middle Eastern descent are a growing demographic in American society and, not unlike the Amish and Romani, are not well understood by the larger society. This cultural group has also experienced increased discrimination and suspicion since 9/11 events.

Arabs immigrated to the United States in three waves. The first occurred between the late 1800s and World War I from the area of Palestine for economic reasons. Many of these immigrants were Christians, and their descendants have become firmly acculturated. The second wave began after 1948 and the establishment of the State of Israel. This group included many professionals and Muslims. This wave tended to settle in the Midwest and accounts for the large concentration of Arab descendants in the Detroit and Chicago areas. The third wave began with the 1967 Arab–Israeli War and continues today. This group fled political instability. Today the area with the largest Arab population is the Dearborn, Michigan area (Ahmad, 2004).

Because the vast majority of Arabs are Muslim, the tenets of the Islamic religion are very influential in Arab Americans' lives. Arab American culture is centered around family relationships. The simplest relationship is the nuclear family, but each Arab American belongs to a large, extended family and often to an even more extended clan that is related by blood kinship (Hammad, Kysia, Rabah, Hassoun, & Connelly, 1999).

The Arab American family is the center of Arab American culture. It is a paternalistic structure, but women are respected, especially mothers. Marriage is highly valued and is considered to be the basic structure of society. Divorce is highly discouraged. Having children is very important in the Arab American culture, and a marriage with many children is considered to be highly blessed. Sickness, birth, and death are events that involve participation by the community.

Cleanliness is a basic tenet of Islam. The Quran, the Islamic holy book, proscribes eating certain foods, including pork or pork products, meat of dead animals, blood, and all intoxicants. Fasting from dawn to dusk every day during the month of Ramadan is required by the religious tenets (Athar, n.d.).

BELIEFS ABOUT CAUSES OF HEALTH AND ILLNESS AMONG ARAB AND MIDDLE EASTERN AMERICANS

Middle Eastern health beliefs arise from the long-standing traditions of the great Islamic healers of the seventh and eighth centuries. Western theories from Hippocrates and Galen came to Arab medicine through trading routes and were incorporated into the Arabs' knowledge base. They advanced human knowledge of anatomy, physiology, and medical treatments. Thus, the tenets of allopathic medicine form the basis of most Arab beliefs about health and illness.

However, traditional religious-based beliefs still exist. There is a tradition that bad thoughts toward someone can cause illness and that the evil eye can cause adverse consequences. Amulets and verses from holy works are utilized to offset the effect. Such beliefs are not uncommon in the Middle East and may be found among those who live in the United States (Hammad, et al., 1999).

Muslims consider an illness to be atonement for their sins, and they receive illness and death with patience and prayers. Death is part of their journey to meet Allah (God) (Athar, n.d.).

HEALING TRADITIONS AMONG ARAB AND MIDDLE EASTERN AMERICANS

The great majority of Arab and Middle Eastern Americans utilize the Western allopathic medical care, much of which derived from the great Arab healers of the past, but there are a few traditional practices still in evidence. Traditional practitioners are in existence in the Arab world, although not frequently within the United States. The most utilized traditional practitioners are bonesetters, who are considered to be superior in skill to Western providers. Midwives are used for childbirth, although birth in hospitals is considered to be more prestigious (Hammad, et al., 1999).

Almost all Middle Eastern people believe in maintaining good health through hygiene and a healthy diet. Women and men are modest and may refuse treatment by practitioners of the opposite gender.

Iraqis have a significant history of traditional healing practices. Some common practices include the following (Iraqi Refugees, 2002):

- Cumin, in conjunction with various other ingredients, is used to treat fever, abdominal pain, and tooth pain.
- Respiratory complaints are treated with honey and lemon.
- Infertility can be treated by a placenta being placed over the doorway of the infertile couple's home.
- Henna is believed to have magic healing properties and will be painted on the body to protect against the evil eye and spirits.

Middle Eastern diets have the following characteristics (Nolan, 1995):

- *Dairy products*. The most common dairy products are yogurt and cheese; feta cheese is preferred. Milk is usually only used in desserts and puddings.
- *Protein*. Pork is eaten only by Christians and is forbidden by religion for Muslims and Jews. Lamb is the most frequently used meat. Many Middle Easterners will not combine dairy products or shellfish with the meal. Legumes, such as black beans, chickpeas (garbanzo beans), lentils, navy beans, and red beans, are commonly used in all dishes.
- *Breads and cereals*. Some form of wheat or rice accompanies each meal.
- *Fruits*. Fruits tend to be eaten as dessert or as snacks. Fresh, raw fruit is preferred. Lemons are used for flavoring. Green and black olives are present in many dishes, and olive oil is most frequently used in food preparation.
- *Vegetables*. Vegetables are preferred raw.

The Mediterranean diet pyramid is shown in Figure 11.4.

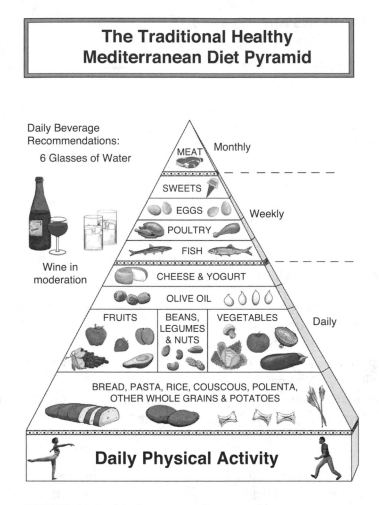

FIGURE 11.4   Mediterranean diet pyramid.
Source: © 2000 Oldways Preservation & Exchange Trust.
www.oldwayspt.org. Reproduced with permission.

BEHAVIORAL RISK FACTORS AND COMMON HEALTH PROBLEMS AMONG ARAB AND MIDDLE EASTERN AMERICANS

As a group, Arab and Middle Eastern Americans face the same health concerns as the majority of Caucasian American citizens. Recent immigrants may be at greater risk for certain inborn genetic disorders as a result of interfamily marriages. Otherwise, their health risks mirror the majority of the population, with heart disease and cancer among the major morbidity factors.

CONSIDERATIONS FOR HEALTH PROMOTION AND PROGRAM PLANNING FOR ARAB AND MIDDLE EASTERN AMERICANS _____

A number of points that should be considered when dealing with Arab and Middle Eastern Americans in health care include the following:

- Arab and Middle Eastern Americans prefer treatment by a medical provider of the same gender, especially for women.
- Arab and Middle Eastern Americans consider nurses to be helpers, not health care professionals, and their suggestions and advice are not taken seriously.
- Arab and Middle Eastern Americans prefer treatment that involves prescribing pills or giving injections rather than simple medical counseling.
- For orthodox Muslims, follow a halal (Muslim diet), which prohibits some types of meat, like pork, and medications and foods that contain alcohol. Meat needs to be prepared according to Islamic requirements. Also, provide for religious requirements for prayer as often as five times a day, starting before sunrise and ending at night, and provide fasting during the holy month of Ramadan between sunrise and sunset. Although those who are ill are exempted from this practice, devout Muslims may desire to fast anyway.
- Allow for receipt of food into the right hand for Muslim patients. The left hand is considered to be unclean because it is used for cleaning during toileting.
- Respect modesty and privacy.
- Allow for visits and input by the imam, a prayer leader.

CHAPTER SUMMARY _____

People who are characterized as white or Caucasian are not composed of just those of northern European descent. They contain people of very divergent backgrounds, such as the Amish, Roma, and those of Arab and Middle Eastern descent. It is important to remember that culture and ethnicity have a significant impact on people's health activities and perspectives on health, and merely characterizing a person as white does not describe those beliefs.

REVIEW _____

1. Describe the health and illness beliefs of the Amish and Roma Americans.
2. Prepare three recommendations to provide culturally competent care for a clinic that deals with Amish or Roma American clients.
3. Describe how Arab American clients might view American health practices differently than other patients.

CASE STUDIES

Case #1. After his wife gave birth, an Arab man would not allow a male lab technician to enter his wife's room to draw blood. The nurses explained to the man the need for the blood test, and the man eventually agreed to allow the technician into the room. He made sure his wife was completely covered in the bed and exposed only her arm for the lab technician to draw the blood. This protected his wife's modesty and the family honor.

Male providers should be aware of these sensitivities when dealing with Arab American families. In this situation the family's concerns were addressed and respected.

Case #2. A nurse found an Iranian patient on the floor when she entered her room. The nurse was concerned that the patient had fallen, and the patient became upset when the nurse tried to help her out. Because the patient did not speak English, she could not explain to the nurse what she was doing. The nurse later learned that the patient was praying.

Muslims pray to Mecca five times per day. The patient was merely practicing her religious tenets. It is important to be aware of such practices when treating ethnic patients.

Source: Fernandez and Fernandez. (2005).

MODEL PROGRAM

Dental Services for Amish Families

In the late 1990s a team from Indiana University organized a program to provide dental services to families of the local Amish communities. They obtained a grant from the Robert Wood Johnson Foundation to undertake dental screening, care, education, and ongoing access. The primary goal of the program was to address serious deficiencies in oral health among the Amish community related to cultural isolation, economics, and transportation problems. The Amish bishop was enlisted to assist in spreading the word about the services and to encourage participation.

The program focused on four areas:

- A series of dental clinics that provided direct dental care
- Testing area water wells for fluoride levels
- Dental education
- Creating a fluoride rinse program in 25 schools

The plan further called for the Amish community to create a plan to provide for their dental needs after the end of the grant. That resulted in the Amish community building and equipping a dental clinic to provide ongoing services to the community.

Source: Robert Wood Johnson Foundation. (2005).

GLOSSARY TERMS

Rumspringa	gadje
brauche	wuzho
Ellis-van Creveld syndrome	marime
Romany	drabarni

REFERENCES

Ahmad, N. (2004). *Arab-American culture and health care.* Retrieved June 16, 2008, from http://www.case.edu/med/epidbio/mphp439/Arab Americans.htm

Armer, J. M., & Radina, M. E. (2006). Definition of health and health promotion behaviors among Midwestern old order Amish families. *The Journal of Multicultural Nursing & Health, 12*(3), 44–53.

Athar, S. (n.d.). *Information for health care providers when dealing with a Muslim patient.* Retrieved June 12, 2008, from http://www.islam-usa.com

Basset, D., Jr., Schneider, P. L., & Huntington, G. E. (2004, January). Physical activity in an old order Amish community. *Medicine & Science in Sports & Exercise, 36*(1), 79–85.

Basset, D. R., Jr., Tremblay, M. S., Esliger, D. W., Copeland, J. L., Barnes, D., & Huntington, G. E. (2007, March). Physical activity and body mass index of children in an older Amish community. *Medicine & Science in Sports & Exercise, 39*(3), 410–415.

Cantor, S. (Producer), & Walker, L. (Director). (2002). *Devil's playground* [Documentary]. United States: Stick Figure Productions.

ClinicalTrials.gov. (2007, September). *Genetic studies in the Amish and Mennonites.* Retrieved May 23, 2008, from http://clinicaltrials.gov

Donnermeyer, J. F., & Lora, F. (2002). Amish society: An overview reconsidered. *Journal of Multicultural Nursing & Health.* Retrieved May 24, 2008, from http://findarticles.com/p/articles/mi_qa3919/is_200610/ai_n17194972

Ember, C. R., & Ember, M. (2004). *Encyclopedia of medical anthropology: Health and illness in the world's culture* (Vol. 2). New York: Kluwer/Plenum.

Ferketich, A. K., Katz, M. L., Paskett, E. D., Lemeshow, S., Westman, J. A., Clinton, S. K., et al. (2008, Winter). Tobacco use among the Amish in Holmes County, Ohio. *Journal of Rural Health, 24*(1), 84–90.

Fernandez, V. M., & Fernandez, K. M. (2005). *Transcultural nursing: The Middle Eastern community.* Retrieved June 16, 2008, from http://www.culturediversity.org/mide.htm

Hammad, A., Kysia, R., Rabah, R., Hassoun, R., & Connelly, M. (1999). Arab Community Center for Social and Economic Services. *Guide to Arab culture: Health care delivery to the Arab American community.* Retrieved June 16, 2008, from http://www.accesscommunity.org/site/DocServer/health_and_research_cente_21.pdf?docID=381

Iraqi Refugees. (2002). Retrieved June 19, 2008, from http://www3.baylor.edu:80~Charles_Kemp/Iraqi_refugees.htm

Julia, M. C. (1996). *Multicultural awareness in the health care professions.* Needham Heights, MA: Simon and Schuster.

Kraybill, D. B. (2001). *The riddle of Amish culture.* Baltimore: Johns Hopkins University Press.

Kriebel, D. W. (2000). *Belief, power, and identity in Pennsylvania Dutch brauche, or powwowing.* Ann Arbor, MI: UMI

Leach, B. (2007, February 1). Scienceline. *The road to genetic cures.* Retrieved May 23, 2008, from http://www.scienceline.org/2007/02/01/biology-hapmaps-leach/

Lee, D. (2005). *Our Amish neighbors: Providing culturally competent care* (Multicultural Health Series) [Videotape and handout]. UMHS, PMCH, Cultural Competency Division.

Lemon, B. C. (2006, Fall). Amish health and belief systems in obstetrical settings. *The Journal of Multicultural Nursing & Health*, 1–7.

McKusick, V. A. (2000). Ellis-van Creveld syndrome and the Amish. *Nature Genetics.* Retrieved May 24, 2008, from http://www.nature.com/ng/journal/v24/n3/full/ng0300_203.html

Nolan, J. (1995). *Cultural diversity: Eating in America. Middle Eastern.* Retrieved June 12, 2008, from http://ohioline.osu.edu/hyg-Fact/5000/5256.html

Ohio Department of Alcohol and Drug Services. (2005, Spring/Summer). Amish D.A.R.E. program shining example of SDFSC funds, innovation at work. *Perspectives, 3*(1), 5–6.

Oldways Preservation and Exchange Trust. (2000). Retrieved February 4, 2009, from www.oldwayspt.org.

Palmer, C. V. (1992). The health beliefs and practices of an old order Amish family. *Journal of the American Academy of Nurse Practitioners, 4*, 117–122.

Robert Wood Johnson Foundation. (2005). *Providing modern dentistry for folk who cling to old ways.* Retrieved January 23, 2009, from http://www.rwjf.org/reports/grr/035938.htm

Ryczak, K., Zebreski, L., May, M., Traver, S. & Kemp, C. (n.d.). *Gypsy (Roma) culture health refugees immigrants.* Retrieved June 16, 2008, from http://bearspace.baylor.edu/Charles_Kemp/www/gypsy_health.htm

Sutherland, A. (1992). Cross-cultural medicine: A decade later. Gypsies and healthcare. *The Western Journal of Medicine, 157*, 3. Retrieved June 16, 2008, from http://www.pubmedcentral.nih.gov/picrender.fcgi?artid=1011276&blobtype=pdf

US Census Bureau. (2005a). *Race and Hispanic origin in 2005.* Retrieved June 10, 2008, from http://www.census.gov/population/www/pop-profile/files/dynamic/RACEHO.pdf

US Census Bureau. (2005b). *We the people of Arab ancestry in the United States. Census 2000 special reports.* Retrieved June 16, 2008, from http://www.census.gov/prod/2005pubs/censr-21.pdf

Wenger, A. F. Z. (1995). Cultural context, health and health care decision making. *Journal of Transcultural Nursing, 7*(1), 3–14.

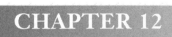

CHAPTER 12

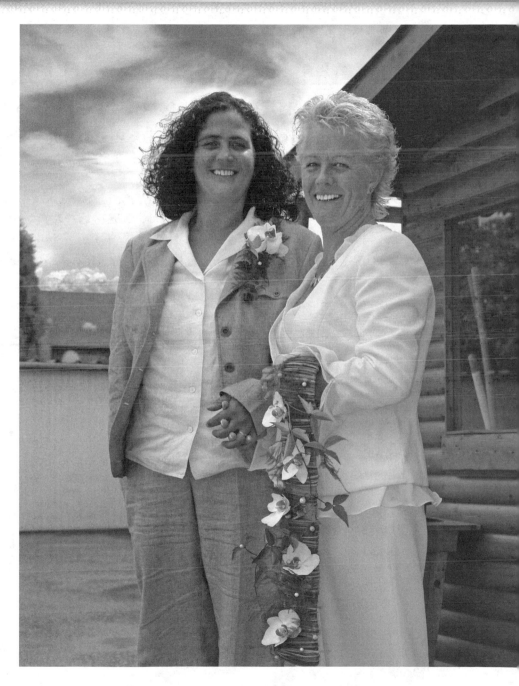

Nonethnic Populations: Lesbian, Gay, Bisexual, and Transgender (LGBT) Individuals; Migrant Farmworkers

Gay and lesbian people fall in love. We settle down. We commit our lives to one another. We raise our children. We protect them. We try to be good citizens.

—Senator Sheila Kuehl

If God had wanted me otherwise, He would have created me otherwise.

—Johann Wolfgang von Goethe

We draw our strength from the very despair in which we have been forced to live. We shall endure.

—Cesar Chavez

KEY CONCEPTS

- Sexual identity
- Gender identity
- Homosexual
- Transgender

- Bisexual
- Gay
- Lesbian

CHAPTER OBJECTIVES

1. Describe the differences among lesbian, gay, bisexual, and transgender (LGBT) persons.
2. Discuss the health risks encountered by LGBT persons.
3. Describe the problems often encountered by LGBT persons in accessing health care services.
4. Discuss steps that can be taken to improve cultural competence within the medical community in caring for LGBT patients and their families.
5. Describe the challenges migrant farm workers encounter in obtaining health care.
6. Discuss ways to decrease migrant farm workers' health risks.

Although culture can be easily identified in ethnic and racial groups, it also exists in other human relationships. Culture is not restricted to race, ethnicity, or heritage; it includes customs, beliefs, values, and knowledge that influence our behavior and impact our health. Therefore, understanding the health influences on nonethnic cultural groups is necessary to complete a discussion of cultures and health.

This concept of culture becomes clear when we examine the lesbian, gay, bisexual, and transgender communities, as well as migrant farmworkers, and how these cultural relationships impact health.

INTRODUCTION TO LESBIAN, GAY, BISEXUAL, AND TRANSGENDER (LGBT) INDIVIDUALS

Lesbian, gay, bisexual, and transgender (LGBT) individuals exist in all cultures, communities, and subgroups of American society. Therefore, LGBT persons tend to be as different as the varied cultures from which they arise. LGBT culture has its own values, beliefs, traditions, and behaviors. Unlike other cultures, however, LGBT culture is often concealed within society as a result of homophobia, heterosexism, prejudice, and discrimination.

It is difficult to identify members of this culture without their self-identification or resorting to stereotypical prejudices. LGBT culture, to a great extent, remains hidden from the larger society and is not taught or transmitted through usual cultural vehicles, such as family and society. Historically, the secrecy of the culture has been an effort at self-preservation. Today, the LGBT culture is emerging and demanding a place in society.

Perhaps we should begin our discussion of this unique and varied cultural group by defining some terms. **Sexual identity** is usually defined as a person's physical, romantic, emotional, and/or spiritual attraction to another person. **Gender identity** references a person's internal, personal sense of being male or female, boy or girl, man or woman. Gender identity and sexual identity are not the same thing. **Homosexual** individuals' gender identity is consistent with their physical sexual characteristics, but their sexual identity is to persons of the same sex. For transgender people, their physical, birth-assigned gender does not match their internal sense of their gender. **Transgender** is usually defined as individuals who live full- or part-time in the gender role opposite to the one in which they were physically born. They may be heterosexual or homosexual. **Bisexual** refers to those whose sexual identity is to both men and women. Finally, the term **gay** refers to homosexuals in general, and it is usually used to refer to male homosexuals more specifically. **Lesbian** refers to homosexual women specifically.

HISTORY OF LGBT AMERICANS IN THE UNITED STATES

History has references to homosexuality throughout the ages. It was not until the twentieth century in the United States that homosexuals began to emerge as a culture and demand their rights. For the greatest part of American history, homosexual activity has been outlawed through state sodomy laws. The members of the LGBT community lived underground to avoid legal entanglements.

LGBT AMERICANS IN THE UNITED STATES

In the post–World War II, anticommunist era of the 1950s, small groups of gay men and lesbian women began to form to end discrimination. Most notably were the Daughters of Bilitis, which is credited as the first lesbian rights group, and the Mattachine Society, the first group to advocate on behalf of gay men.

Societal changes in the 1960s heralded a new wave of gay activism. As civil rights were being obtained by black Americans, gay Americans were beginning to object to the restraints placed by the law on their lives. Years of resentment came to a head in the Stonewall riots in 1969. Prior to this event, it was common for police to raid gay and lesbian bars and arrest the patrons. In a New York bar named the Stonewall Inn, the patrons protested and a riot broke out. Over the next few days, gays and lesbians continued to riot, demanding their right to assembly. This event sparked gay and lesbian activism across the country, resulting in the birth of the gay rights movement, which overturned many laws and other restrictions on personal activity.

LGBT persons have made significant strides in obtaining equal status in the United States; however, discriminatory practices still exist. In 1973 the American Psychiatric Association declassified homosexuality as a mental disorder. The diagnosis of "ego-dystonic homosexuality" was removed from the *Diagnostic and Statistical Manual of Mental Disorders (DSM)*, and for the first time homosexual Americans were no longer considered to be mentally ill. Legal advances, though slow, have been made as well. Many states have overturned their sodomy laws and now offer domestic partner benefits to same-sex couples. As this book is being written, the California Supreme court has followed the lead of the Massachusetts Supreme Court in ruling that depriving same-sex couples the right to marry is a denial of equal protection under the state constitution. In response, a proposition was placed on the California ballot for the November 2008 election to limit marriage to a man and a woman. That initiative passed and its constitutionality is being reviewed by the California Supreme Court as this book is being printed. Despite these legislative changes, homosexuality is still criminalized by sodomy laws in 16 states. Thus, the struggle for equality within the LGBT community continues, and discrimination based on homophobia and heterosexism continues in basic civil rights, employment, and housing.

HEALING TRADITIONS AMONG LGBT AMERICANS

A major hurdle to understanding the interaction of the LGBT community and health care is that little research is available to guide the discussion. In fact, there is not even good data on the number of LGBT persons in the United States. The classic assumption about the size of the LGBT population comes from the 1949 Kinsey Report. There it was postulated that 10% of the male population and 5% to 6% of the female population of the United States was homosexual. The 1990 U.S. census allowed respondents to classify themselves as unmarried partners. Of those over the age of 15 years, 1.63% reported themselves as the unmarried partner of the householder (Gay & Lesbian Medical Association, 2001). There is no data on the number of transgender individuals in the United States, but 25,000 have undergone sexual reassignment surgery, and another 60,000 consider themselves to be candidates for the surgery (Gay & Lesbian Medical Association, 2001).

Due to their minority status and history of discrimination, clinical and public health studies regarding the needs of LGBT persons are infrequent. Therefore, researchers have to depend on small studies that are often uninformative in describing the needs of this community.

It is widely reported that LGBT persons experience discrimination in health care. It has been reported that they encounter substandard care and often do not report important health issues because of fear of stigmatization. One study reported that 40% of responding physicians were uncomfortable providing care to LGBT patients. In a survey of LGBT physicians, 67% of the respondents reported their belief that they had seen gay and/or lesbian patients receive substandard care or be mishandled as a result of their sexual orientation (Dean, et al., 2000).

Access to care is often a major problem for this group. Although as a group LGBT persons have higher education levels than average, they experience a lower socioeconomic status than heterosexuals. Those in committed relationships experience difficulty with insurance companies recognizing them, and they are often denied the privileges that are extended to married partners (O'Hanlan, Cabaj, Schatz, Lock, & Nemrow, 1997). Discrimination in insurance and public entitlement programs creates roadblocks to public programs, and they often do not cover needed services. Even if an LGBT couple can obtain insurance coverage through employment, they are often reluctant to utilize it for fear that it would expose their sexual orientation and submit them to job discrimination.

TABLE 12.1	Factors That Impact Health in LGBT Persons			
Sexuality	**Cultural**	**Disclosure of Sexual Orientation**	**Prejudice/ Discrimination**	**Concealed Sexual Identity**
HIV–AIDS	Socialization Parenting	Family conflicts	Health care provider bias	Reluctance to seek care
Hepatitis	Nulliparity in women	Psychological problems	Harassment	Delayed treatment
Human papillomavirus		Depression Anxiety Suicide	Limited access	Suppression of medical information
Sexually transmitted disease			Violence Pathologizing of behavior	
Anal cancer				

Source: Dean, et al. (2000).

Stigmatization, lack of sensitivity, and reluctance to address sexual issues has been reported as interfering with mental health care. LGBT persons report discriminatory care in nursing homes and senior centers (Dean, et al., 2000). Table 12.1 describes many social and behavioral factors that are of significant concern to this community.

LGBT couples encounter difficulty obtaining the rights granted to married couples in health care settings, such as hospitals. Unless they have a signed durable power of attorney for health care or an advance directive, authorization for medical treatment will be made by the closest relative, not the homosexual partner. Further, those same family members could override the decision of the partner, even in circumstances where the partner is in a much better position to know what the sick individual would want.

LGBT persons report difficulty in communication with health care providers. LGBT persons find it difficult to discuss their sexual history and related health needs with their health care providers. A 1990 survey of Michigan lesbians found that 61% of the respondents felt they could not disclose their sexual identity to their provider (Dean, et al., 2000). Medical education has not informed providers about the health needs of this population. Removing the barriers to communication and educating practitioners about the unique health needs of the LGBT community is imperative.

More specifically, misconceptions and assumptions about lesbians' health and their health care needs have been identified. Lesbians' care can be compromised as a result of their sexual orientation. Lesbians are less likely to receive Pap smears for cervical cancer due to a false assumption that because they are not currently sexually active with men, they are not at risk for developing the disease. They remain at risk for sexually transmitted diseases, specifically human papillomavirus, which has been associated with cervical cancer. Therefore, they should be treated for all risks (U.S. Department of Health and Human Services, Office on Women's Health [HHS OWH], 2000).

The Office on Women's Health of the U.S. Department of Health and Human Services has identified the need for research to improve the health care of lesbians and to identify health conditions for which they are at risk. It was noted that improved cultural competency, with physicians being better informed about lesbian health issues and more understanding of lesbians' reluctance to seek care due to homophobia, was needed (HHS OWH, 2000).

To investigate U.S. hospitals' policies and procedures related to LGBT concerns, the Human Rights Campaign Foundation and the Gay and Lesbian Medical Association devised the Healthcare Equality Index to evaluate how the health care community responds to the needs of the LGBT community. The focus of the inquiry was on five criteria: patient nondiscrimination, hospital visitation, decision making, cultural competency training, and employment policies.

The project began in 2007, and all participants were given anonymity for their responses. Requests for participation were sent to 1,000 hospitals. Responses from 78 hospitals in 20 states were obtained. The results showed that 50 hospitals had policies providing the same access to same-sex partners as is provided to married spouses, 56 allowed the designation of a domestic partner or someone else as medical surrogate, only 45 had a policy allowing same-sex parents the same access to medical decision making for their minor children as married spouses, and 57 provided staff training on specific issues impacting the LGBT patients and their families (HRC, GLMA, 2007).

The 2008 results were provided by 88 hospitals in 21 states. Forty-five of the responding hospitals responded affirmatively to the 10 survey questions. The question with the most positive results involved having a patient bill of rights with a nondiscrimination policy, including sexual orientation. The question with the least affirmative responses involved having equal employment opportunity policies that include gender identity and/or expression (HRC, GLMA, 2007).

BEHAVIORAL RISK FACTORS AND COMMON HEALTH PROBLEMS AMONG LGBT AMERICANS

The LGBT community is at risk for unique health problems. These risks can be exacerbated by misunderstanding and stigmatization.

HIV–AIDS

The onset of acquired immunodeficiency syndrome (AIDS) in the 1980s brought devastation to the lives of gay men. Since the early 1980s, it is estimated that 702,000 Americans have been diagnosed with the disease, and 54% of that number are men who have had sexual interactions with other men. African and Latino men have constituted the majority of cases reported since 1998 (Dean, et al., 2000). Although discrimination and a belief that these men deserved their fate was the initial response to the epidemic, with time, a better understanding of the disease and its risk factors have enlightened the discussion. The importance of distinguishing between sexual identity and sexual behavior has been emphasized in dealing with this disease.

Recent research has found that men who have sex with men are most at risk. Those men characterize themselves as gay, bisexual, and heterosexual. Therefore, focus must be placed on behaviors and not labels. Studies have shown that bisexual behavior in men was associated with a reduced use of condoms and a weaker perception of safe sexual practices. Also, bisexual men were often unlikely to disclose their bisexuality to their female partners (Dean, et al., 2000).

Impacting behavior remains the primary way of reducing the spread of this disease. Education about safe sex practices has been strongly supported within the gay community, and research has shown that most gay men report having protected sex most of the time.

There is little research on AIDS in the lesbian community. The few studies that have occurred indicate a small incidence and no evidence for female-to-female transmission. It is presumed that lesbians who contract the disease have either used intravenous drugs or had intercourse with a man. However, research to determine the true risk factors within this population is needed.

Like the lesbian population, little information is available regarding the incidence of AIDS within the transgender community. It is suspected that the rate of AIDS within the population is high based on the few studies available. In a self-reporting study, 25% of respondents indicated they were HIV positive, and a study of those seeking hormone therapy reported that 15% of respondents were HIV positive (Dean, et al., 2000).

Cancer

Although definitive studies are lacking, the information to date indicates that gay men and lesbians are at higher risk for certain cancers. Gay men are at higher risk for Kaposi sarcoma, which is associated with HIV infection, and AIDS-related non-Hodgkin lymphoma. Bisexual and gay men are at increased risk for anal cancer and Hodgkin disease, according to recent research. It has also been noted that survival time for gay men with cancer is less than the population at large. It is speculated that this is due to HIV–AIDS comorbidity and delay in detection and treatment (Dean, et al., 2000).

Lesbians have been found to be at higher risk for breast cancer than heterosexual women due to increased risk factors, including alcohol consumption, obesity, and nulliparity. Lesbians have been found to receive less frequent gynecologic care and breast cancer screening.

Substance Use

Studies of substance use in the LGBT population are varied at best. Some have shown no greater use of alcohol in this population than in the general population. Others have found higher rates of both heavy drinking and abstention in both gay men and lesbians.

Limited data also indicates that lesbians report greater use of cocaine, inhalants, and marijuana than women in the general population. The data for gay men is similar. However, no good study has been undertaken for this population.

Mental Health

As previously noted, declassification of homosexuality as a mental illness occurred in 1973. However, the LGBT population is at increased risk for certain mental health issues as a result of stressors related to antigay societal attitudes and internalization of negative social attitudes. Significant among the problems encountered by this group are mental disorders and distress, substance use, and suicide.

As with other health issues faced by this population, few scientifically significant studies are available in this area. Studies have found higher rates of depression, generalized anxiety disorder, and conduct disorders in the LGBT population. Various studies have identified increased rates of bipolar disorder and affective disorders in the gay male population.

The studies that address suicide in this population are controversial. Studies have indicated an increased rate of suicidal ideation and attempts in gay and bisexual men and lesbians. However, others have found no increased rates of completed suicides in that population.

The American Psychiatric Association's *Diagnostic and Statistical Manual of Mental Disorders (DSM)* contains four diagnoses that may be applicable to transgender individuals. The most common is gender identity disorder. According to the *DSM*, for the diagnosis to apply, other symptoms evidencing distress and functional impairment are necessary. Therefore, being transgender does not itself mean the person has a mental disorder (Dean, et al., 2000).

However, the transgender population is at risk for mental health problems comparable to others who undergo major life changes, minority status, discrimination, and chronic medical conditions. Studies indicate increased rates of depression, substance use, and anxiety disorders. Unfortunately, suicide attempts and completed suicides are more common in the transgender population, and genital mutilation is also reported at significant rates (Dean, et al., 2000).

Aging

Not surprisingly, there is little information about the needs of LGBT elders. Although they are at risk for the health problems that are common to all, it is believed that they encounter specific problems not usually faced by the general population.

Recent surveys have shown that LGBT elders are more likely to live alone than elders in the population at large (Gay & Lesbian Medical Association, 2001). Furthermore, few agencies exist to meet the social service needs of this group, and the availability of long-term care facilities to meet the needs of this group is virtually nonexistent. Finally, due to their age, LGBT elders are less able to deal with the discrimination in the health care system than younger members of the LGBT community.

CONSIDERATIONS FOR HEALTH PROMOTION AND PROGRAM PLANNING FOR LGBT AMERICANS

To provide appropriate care to any patient population necessitates reliable information on which the practitioner can base care decisions. The lack of reliable information regarding the health needs of the LGBT community is a significant hindrance to providing proper care to this group. Improved research is necessary to provide dependable data to guide care.

Like all cultural minorities, the LGBT community experiences barriers to accessing care. The lack of health insurance for themselves and their partners, discrimination in health care services, cultural barriers, and a poor understanding of their health care needs all impact the health of this group. For health promotion to occur, efforts need to be made to address these problems. Cultural competency must be addressed within the provider community as well. Table 12.2 and Table 12.3 provide objectives for creating LGBT cultural competence.

TABLE 12.2   LGBT Cultural Competence Strategies

Use gender-neutral language in forms and practice.

Do not make assumptions about sexuality.

Utilize nonbiased behavior and communication.

Do not use labels; focus on behavior.

Conduct a thorough sexual-risk evaluation.

Be aware of LGBT health risks.

Be knowledgeable about the health needs of the LGBT community.

Source: Gay & Lesbian Medical Association. (2001).

TABLE 12.3   Recommended Community Standards for Gay, Lesbian, and Transgender Persons

1. Create and promote open communication and a safe and nondiscriminatory workplace.

2. Create comprehensive policies to ensure that services are provided to LGBT clients and their families in a nondiscriminatory manner.

3. Have procedures available for clients to resolve complaints concerning violation of policies.

4. Prepare and implement assessment tools to meet the needs of LGBT clients and their families.

5. Maintain a basic understanding of LGBT issues within the organization.

6. All personnel who provide direct care to LGBT clients shall be competent to identify and address the health issues encountered by LGBT clients and their families and be able to provide appropriate treatment or referrals.

7. The organization shall ensure the confidentiality of client information.

8. Community outreach shall include the LGBT community.

9. The board of directors of the organization should have an LGBT representative.

10. The organization shall provide appropriate and safe care and treatment to all LGBT clients and their families.

Source: Gay & Lesbian Medical Association. (2001).

TABLE 12.4   Four Steps for Culturally Competent Care
1. Maintain a nonhomophobic attitude.
2. Distinguish sexual behavior from sexual identity.
3. Communicate clearly and sensitively using gender-neutral terms.
4. Be aware of how your attitudes affect your clinical judgment.

Source: Gay & Lesbian Medical Association. (2001).

Health care providers should provide a nonjudgmental environment for LGBT patients and their families so that avoidance of care can be overcome. Harrison and Silenzio suggested four steps for improving cultural sensitivity and increasing equality of treatment and access (Gay & Lesbian Medical Association, 2001) (see Table 12.4).

INTRODUCTION TO MIGRANT FARMWORKERS

Migrant farmworkers in the United States are the backbone of the farming community. It has been postulated that their work constitutes a new form of slavery to support the United States (Moore, 2004).

HISTORY OF MIGRANT FARMWORKERS IN THE UNITED STATES

Migrant farmworkers are referred to as the "invisible population" (Gonzalez, 2008). Statistics regarding the actual size of this population vary from 3 to 5 million individuals (National Center for Farmworker Health Inc. [NCFH], 2002; Fisher, Marcoux, Miller, Sanchez, & Ramirez Cunningham, 2004; U.S. Department of Homeland Security, 2002). A National Agricultural Workers Survey (NAWS) is conducted every year by the U.S. Department of Labor, and the Current Population Survey (CPS) is updated by the U.S. Bureau of Labor Statistics monthly, yet it is difficult to track trends in this population. Even with these surveys it is difficult to find accurate statistics due to the fact that "52 out of every 100 of all farm workers do not have authorization or any legal status in the U.S." (Gonzalez, 2008). Because many workers and their families are unauthorized, they are reluctant to provide any demographic information about themselves or their community because of the risk of deportation.

MIGRANT FARMWORKERS IN THE UNITED STATES _____

Today, Mexican workers are the largest population of migrant farmworkers in American agriculture. Migrant farmworkers are also from other countries, including Guatemala, Honduras, Puerto Rico, Dominican Republic, Southeast Asia, Philippines, Jamaica, Haiti, and other Caribbean islands. Farmworkers are predominantly Hispanic, and 7 out of 10 farmworkers are foreign born. Of the foreign-born workers, 94% are from Mexico (U.S. Department of Labor, Employment and Training Administration, 2009). Prior to the Mexican workers' emergence, Chinese workers filled the labor pool. Nearly 200,000 Chinese were legally contracted to cultivate California fields until the Chinese Exclusion Act. Thereafter, Japanese workers replaced the Chinese field hands (PBS, 1999).

Mexican immigration began during the 1850s to geographic land regions that were still considered to be part of Mexico (i.e., California). In the 1920s, the Mexican government addressed complaints of abuse with the United States by securing contracts with the United States to try to trace immigration and provide some type of labor protection to their citizens who traveled to the United States for work. The first was the de facto Bracero Program, which allowed workers to bring their families. During World War II, the United States signed another Bracero treaty to legalize immigration for Mexican workers to fill the labor gaps left by soldiers who were participating in the war. Under this program, approximately 4 million Mexican farmworkers came to support the agriculture industry between 1942 and 1964 (PBS, 1999).

Besides the Bracero Program, the United States has entered into more recent trade agreements that directly affect migrant laborers, like the General Agreement on Tariffs and Trade (GATT) and North American Free Trade Agreement (NAFTA). More recently, the Immigration Reform and Control Act has played a role in the legalization and fluctuation of migrant workers and their services.

According to the National Center for Farmworker Health Inc. and the Atlas of Migrant and Seasonal Farmworkers, migrant workers can be found in almost every state. The states with the most concentrated populations heavily rely on agriculture as a part of their state's economy. California leads with the highest population (approximately 1.3 million), with Texas, Florida, Washington, and North Carolina rounding out the top five (NCFH, 2002).

Recent data indicates that almost 75% of farmworkers earned less than $10,000 per year, and three out of five farmworker families lived in poverty. Few farmworkers had assets of any import, and about one-third owned, or were buying, a house or trailer in the United States (U.S. Department of Labor, Employment and Training Administration, 2009).

Given their meager incomes, many households qualify for social services and housing assistance. However, many migrant workers do not apply for those services for fear of deportation.

According to the National Agricultural Workers Survey (NAWS), migrant farmworkers are poorly educated. More than one-third are school dropouts, and of those who attend school, 17% are at a grade level lower than their same-age peers (U.S. Department of Labor, Employment and Training Administration, 2009). The most recent data shows that the approximate median level of education for the population is at the sixth-grade level, and there is only a 50.7% high school graduation rate among migrant teenagers (U.S. Department of Labor, Employment and Training Administration, 2009). High illiteracy rates are a contributing factor to poor education: 20% of the population are completely illiterate; 38% are functionally illiterate; and 27% are marginally illiterate. Poor English proficiency also contributes to poor education levels.

BELIEFS ABOUT CAUSES OF HEALTH AND ILLNESS AMONG MIGRANT FARMWORKERS

Migrant farmworkers, mostly Hispanic, believe that an imbalance between a person and the environment causes physical and mental illness. Emotional, spiritual, social, and physical ailments are often expressed as having too much "hot" or "cold." In general, cold diseases and conditions are characterized by vasoconstriction and low metabolic rate (such as menstrual cramps, pneumonia, and colic). Hot diseases and conditions are characterized by vasodilatation and high metabolic rate (such as pregnancy, hypertension, diabetes, and acid indigestion).

Mal de ojo is known as the "evil eye." It is also thought to cause illness more in women and infants than in men. Evil eye is caused by a person with a "strong eye" (especially green or blue) who looks with admiration or jealousy at another person. Susto is "soul loss" caused by fright. Susto may be acute or chronic and includes a variety of vague complaints. Folk or ethnomedical illnesses are health problems associated with members of a particular group for which the culture provides etiology, diagnosis, prevention, and a regimen of healing. These illnesses also have psychological and/or religious overtones (Leybas-Amedia, Nuno, & Garcia, 2005).

Fatalism or inevitable predetermination is an attitude possessed by many migrant farmworkers. It is a broad concept that encompasses a religious commitment to acceptance of the conditions in one's life. Hispanic migrant farmworkers reject the concept of germ theory. They believe that the cause of disease or illness is spirit and not germs, making them less likely to seek preventive care and treatment (Kelz, 1999).

HEALING TRADITIONS AMONG MIGRANT FARMWORKERS

Migrant farmworkers are prone to skin diseases, and they usually treat the diseases themselves. "Latino migrant and seasonal farm workers experience high rates of skin disease that result from their working and living conditions" (Arcury, Vallejos, Feldman, & Quandt, 2006). Working conditions expose them to many toxins that cause various types of skin diseases and irritations. Causes of occupational skin disease among agricultural workers are diverse and include exposure to wind and sun, pesticides, fertilizer, petroleum products, plants, and infectious agents (Arcury, et al., 2006). Ultraviolet rays, allergic reactions, and the use of untested healing methods may contribute to damaged and sensitive skin.

Farmworkers tend to use home remedies, such as household products and herbs, to cure skin symptoms (Arcury, et al., 2006). Plant products are used as remedies to heal certain types of wounds and sores.

BEHAVIORAL RISK FACTORS AND COMMON HEALTH PROBLEMS AMONG MIGRANT FARMWORKERS

Many factors impact migrant farmworkers' health. They tend to be geographically isolated and constantly move from place to place, which makes access to care difficult. In addition, a lack of health education contributes to poor knowledge of good health practices.

Health standards for migrant farmworkers are similar to that of third-world countries, even though they work in the United States. Unsanitary working and housing conditions place farmworkers at risk for many health problems. Most farmworkers cannot afford to take time off from work and also risk losing their jobs to attend doctor appointments (NCFH, 2002).

Farmworkers are exposed to many different types of diseases and injuries, many of which are related to the chemicals and machinery they use, including musculoskeletal injuries, respiratory illness, tuberculosis, HIV, and others.

Musculoskeletal injuries are very common in farmworkers. The labor done by farmworkers consists of heavy lifting and constant, quick movements of certain body parts, such as the wrists. Workers are also encouraged to work at a quicker pace to finish early (NCFH, 2002).

Respiratory illnesses, including asthma, occur due to exposure to pesticides, dust, pollen, and molds. Exposure to these pollutants for long periods of time can have long-term effects on the workers (NCFH, 2002).

Tuberculosis is common among migrant farmworkers due to the prevalence of tuberculosis in their home countries. The disease is transmitted to workers in the United States and spreads amongst the population (NCFH, 2002).

AIDS is prevalent in migrant populations and is associated with increased rates of sexually-transmitted diseases and prostitution in labor camps. Wives of the men who travel to the United States for work are at risk for infection transmitted by their husbands (NCFH, 2002).

CONSIDERATIONS FOR HEALTH PROMOTION AND PROGRAM PLANNING FOR MIGRANT FARMWORKERS

Guidelines for dealing with migrant farmworkers include the following:

- Recognize the concern migrant farmworkers have regarding immigration issues and the possibility of deportation.
- Ensure that appropriate translations services are available.
- Remember to include family members in decision making.
- Determine a person's living situation before planning.
- Understand that fear and mistrust exist.

CHAPTER SUMMARY

Lesbians, gay men, bisexuals, and transgender people have faced significant discrimination as a result of their sexual orientation, and discrimination continues today. The LGBT culture tends to hide from society at large as a survival technique.

In this chapter we have discussed the barriers to care and challenges encountered by these people in their interactions with health care services. We found that they are less likely to seek care because of fear of discrimination, and they tend to have higher incidences of certain diseases as a result. Unfortunately, there are few studies to guide our understanding of the health problems this group encounters outside of HIV–AIDS, which has been closely studied. Therefore, for many health issues there is little reliable information to guide practitioners. Finally, we learned that steps need to be taken to improve the cultural competence of health care providers and facilities to ensure equal care for the LGBT community.

Migrant farmworkers account for approximately 3 to 5 million people in the United States. They are mostly Hispanic people who work in almost every state. Poverty, unsettlement, legal issues, low education level, and harsh working conditions are their main challenges. They are at major risk to skin diseases and exposure to the sun and pesticides. AIDS is common among migrant farmworkers due to lack of education, an increase in sexually-transmitted diseases, and prostitution.

REVIEW

1. Describe three roadblocks to accessing health care that are encountered by the LGBT community and migrant farmworkers.
2. Prepare three cultural competence recommendations for a clinic that provides services to migrant farmworkers.
3. Outline what areas should be covered in a staff training session to address the needs of LGBT clients.
4. Describe how discrimination toward migrant farmworkers and LGBT people impacts their health and health care.

CASE STUDY

In 2008, the Human Rights Campaign Foundation Family Project, in conjunction with the Gay and Lesbian Medical Association, conducted a survey of hospitals to determine the health care industry's practices related to LGBT issues. The 23 questions focused on baseline institutional information and LGBT-specific policies.

Some of the findings were as follows (HRC, GLMA, 2007):

- 98% of the respondents reported including sexual orientation in their patient's bill of rights or nondiscrimination policies. Only 66% included gender identity or gender expression in those policies.
- 69% had a written visitation policy to provide LGBT partners the same access as spouses or next of kin.
- 68% had a visitation policy that allowed same-sex parents the same access to their minor children as opposite-sex parents.
- 88% of the respondents had policies that provided for the LGBT partner to be named as the decision maker in a patient's advance directive.
- 64% provided same-sex parents the same decision-making authority for their minor children as that afforded opposite-sex parents.
- 69% had cultural competency training that addressed LGBT patients and their families.
- 84% had policies barring employment discrimination based on sexual orientation, but only 58% included gender identity or expression.

There are several issues to consider about this case:

- Why do you think only 88 out of 1,000 hospitals responded to the survey?
- What does the survey tell us about the health care provided to LGBT patients and their families?
- What is the relationship between the findings regarding employment and the findings about health care?

MODEL PROGRAM

The Mpowerment Project

The Mpowerment Project is a program in San Francisco conducted by the University of California, San Francisco in conjunction with the Diffusion of Effective Behavioral Interventions (DEBI) project. The program was designed to reduce the rate of AIDS transmission among young gay and bisexual men. It is a community-based prevention program that has the goal of reducing risky behavior in men aged 18–29 years.

The guiding principles of the program are as follows:

- Personal and community empowerment
- Diffusion of new behavior through social networks
- Peer influence
- Placing HIV prevention in context with other issues in young men's lives
- Building community
- Utilizing gay-positive approaches to prevention

The program utilizes a group of young men along with a group of volunteers for outreach to the community. They attend popular events and embark on publicity campaigns to promote safe sex practices. A hallmark of the program is meetings where discussions related to safe sex practices are conducted. The goal of the program is to improve health and prevent disease through a peer group within the community.

Source: Mpowerment Project. (2009).

GLOSSARY TERMS

sexual identity
gender identity
homosexual
transgender

bisexual
gay
lesbian

REFERENCES

Arcury, T. A., Vallejos, Q. M., Feldman, S. R., & Quandt, S. A. (2006). Treating skin disease: Self-management behaviors of Latino farmworkers. *Journal of Agromedicine, 11*(2). Retrieved May 17, 2008, from http://cha.wa.gov/english/documents/TreatmentofSkinDiseaseamongLatino-Farmworkers.pdf

Cason, K. L., & Snyder, A. (2004, November). *The health and nutrition of Hispanic migrant and seasonal farm workers.* Retrieved May 18, 2008, from http://www.ruralpa.org/migrant_farm_workers.pdf

Centers for Disease Control and Prevention. (2004). Health disparities experienced by Hispanics—United States. *Morbidity and Mortality Weekly Report, 53*(40), 935–937.

Dean, L., Meyer, I. H., Robinson, K., Sell, R. L., Sember, R., Silenzio, V. M. B., et al. (2000). Lesbian, gay, bisexual and transgender health: Findings and concerns. *Journal of the Gay and Lesbian Medical Association, 4*(3). Retrieved May 28, 2008, from http://glma.org/document/docWindow.cfm?fuseaction=document.viewDocument&documentid=17&documentFormatID=26

Fisher, K. E., Marcoux, E., Miller, L. S., Sanchez, A., & Ramirez Cunningham, E. (2004). Information behaviour of migrant Hispanic farm workers and their families in the Pacific Northwest. *Information Research, 10*(1) paper 199. Retrieved May 20, 2008, from http://informationr.net/ir/10-1/paper199.html

Franzini, L., Ribble, J. C., & Keddie, A. M. (2001, Autumn). Understanding the Hispanic paradox. *Ethnicity and Disease, 11*(3), 496–518.

Gay & Lesbian Medical Association. (2001). *Healthy People 2010 companion document for lesbian, gay, bisexual and transgender (LGBT) health.* Retrieved May 28, 2008, from http://www.glma.org/_data/n.0001/resourceslive/HealthyCompanionDoc3

Gonzalez, E., Jr. (2008, May 27). *Migrant farm workers: Our nation's invisible population.* Retrieved May 23, 2008, from http://www.extension.org/pages/Migrant_Farm_Workers:_Our_Nation's_Invisible_Population

HRC, GLMA release inaugural healthcare equality index. (2007, October 7). *The Advocate.* Retrieved May 20, 2008 from http://www.advocate.com/news_detail_ektid49485.asp

Huang, G. G. (n.d.). *What federal statistics reveal about migrant farm workers: A summary for education. ERIC Digest.* Retrieved May 23, 2008, from www.ericdigests.org/2003-4/migrant-farmworkers.html

Hunt, L. M., Arar, N. H., & Akana, L. L. (2000). Herbs, prayer, and insulin: Use of medical and alternative treatments by a group of Mexican-American diabetes patients. *Journal of Family Practice, 49*(3), 216–223.

Kelz, R. K. (1999). *Conversational Spanish for health professionals: Essential expressions, questions, and directions for medical personnel to facilitate conversation with Spanish-speaking patients and coworkers.* Albany, NY: Delmar.

Kemp, C. (2005, March). *Mexican & Mexican-Americans: Health beliefs & practices.* Retrieved May 20, 2008, from http://bearspace.baylor.edu/Charles_Kemp/www/hispanic_health.htm

Leybas-Amedia, V., Nuno, T., & Garcia, F. (2005). Effect of acculturation and income on Hispanic women's health. *Journal of Health Care for the Poor and Underserved, 16*(4)(Suppl. A). Retrieved May 23, 2008, from http://muse.jhu.edu/journals/journal_of_health_care_for_the_poor_and_underserved/v016/16.4Aleybas-amedia.html

Moore, M. (2004, March 31). *Migrant farmworkers: America's new plantation workers.* Retrieved May 25, 2008, from http://www.foodfirst.org/node/45

Mpowerment Project. (2009). Retrieved January 23, 2009, from http://www.mpowerment.org/

National Center for Farmworker Health Inc. (2002). *Factsheets About Farmworkers*. Retrieved May 23, 2008, from http://www.ncfh.org/?pid=5

O'Hanlan, K., Cabaj, R. B., Schatz, B., Lock, J., & Nemrow, P. (1997). A review of the medical consequences of homophobia with suggestions for resolution. *Journal of the Gay and Lesbian Medical Association, 1*(1), 25–40.

Palerm, J. V. (2006). *Immigrant and migrant farm workers in the Santa Maria Valley, California.* Retrieved May 23, 2008, from http://repositories.cdlib.org/cgi/viewcontent.cgi?article=1005& context=ccs_ucsb

PBS. (1999). *Mexican immigrant labor history*. Retrieved May 24, 2008, from http://www.pbs.org/ kpbs/theborder/history/timeline/17.html

Rangel, I. (2002). *Overview of America's farm workers*. Retrieved May 19, 2008, from http:// www.ncfh.org/?pid=4

US Department of Health and Human Services, Office on Women's Health. (2000). *Lesbian health fact sheet*. Retrieved June 9, 2008, from http://www.womenshealth.gov/pub/faq.cfm

US Department of Homeland Security. (2002). *Fiscal year 2002 yearbook of immigration statistics* (formerly, *Statistical yearbook of the Immigration and Naturalization Service*). Retrieved May 23, 2008, from http://www.dhs.gov/ximgtn/statistics/publications/YrBk02En.shtm

US Department of Labor, Employment and Training Administration. (2009). *The national agricultural workers survey*. Retrieved May 24, 2008, from www.doleta.gov/agworker/report/ch1.cfm

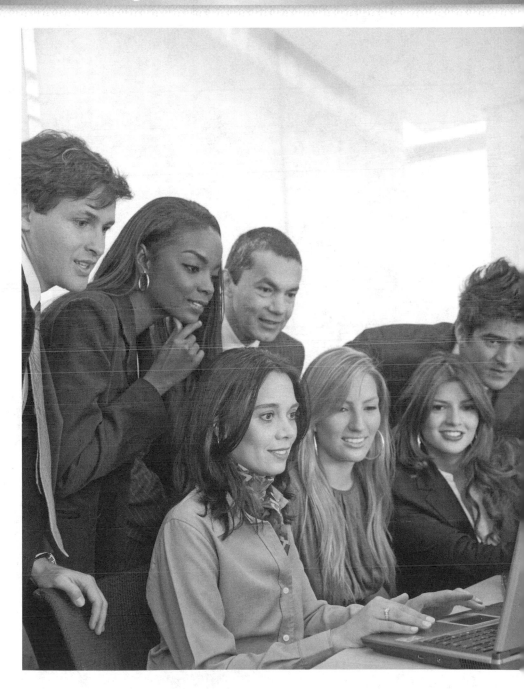

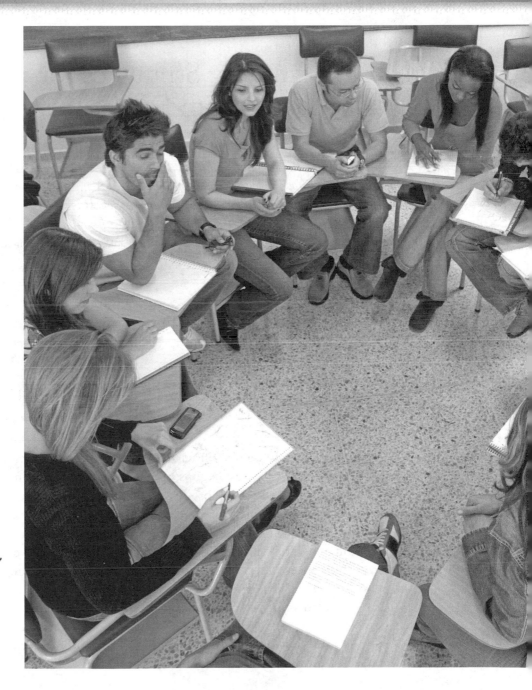

CHAPTER 13

Closing the Gap: Strategies for Eliminating Health Disparities

The future health of the nation will be determined to a large extent by how effectively we work with communities to reduce and eliminate health disparities between non-minority and minority populations experiencing disproportionate burdens of disease, disability, and premature death.

—Guiding principle for improving minority health
(Office of Minority Health & Health Disparities, 2007)

KEY CONCEPTS

- Best practices
- Telemedicine

- Cultural Competence

CHAPTER OBJECTIVES

1. List the six priority areas for eliminating health disparities.
2. Describe at least six strategies for reducing or eliminating health disparities.

Throughout this book, we have discussed the fact that the health disparities in the United States are extensive as demonstrated by the differences in the incidence and consequences of diseases and mortality rates. The causes of health disparities are complex, systemic, personal, integrated, and multifactorial, and there are no easy and immediate solutions to reduce or eliminate them. The complexity of the problem should not deter our efforts to work on reducing, and eventually eliminating, these differences in health, because these disparities have a negative impact on the people of our nation and are viewed as morally wrong by many. The problem will continue to be magnified because the changing demographics that are anticipated over the next decade will amplify the problem; hence the importance of addressing disparities in health. Groups who are currently experiencing poorer health status are expected to grow as a proportion of the total U.S. population;

therefore, the future health of America as a whole will be influenced substantially by our success in improving the health of these groups. A national focus on disparities in health status is particularly important as major changes unfold in the way in which health care is delivered and financed (Office of Minority Health & Health Disparities, 2007).

The government has highlighted the need to reduce health disparities, and this focus is reflected in the *Healthy People 2010* objectives. *Healthy People 2010* is designed to achieve two overarching goals: (1) increase quality and years of healthy life; and (2) eliminate health disparities. The second goal of *Healthy People 2010*, to eliminate health disparities, includes differences that occur by gender, race, ethnicity, education, income, disability, geographic location, or sexual orientation. Compelling evidence indicates that race and ethnicity correlate with persistent, and often increasing, health disparities among U.S. populations in all these categories and demands national attention (Office of Minority Health & Health Disparities, 2007).

The U.S. Department of Health and Human Services (HHS) has selected six focus areas in which racial and ethnic minorities experience serious disparities in health access and outcomes:

1. Infant mortality
2. Cancer screening and management
3. Cardiovascular disease
4. Diabetes
5. HIV infection and AIDS
6. Immunizations

These six health areas were selected for emphasis because they reflect areas of disparity that are known to affect multiple racial and ethnic minority groups at all life stages (Office of Minority Health & Health Disparities, 2007). Many other federal agencies and states have developed strategic plans to eliminate health disparities. These plans can be useful to organizations when they are developing their own objectives and interventions.

Eliminating health disparities will require enhanced efforts and changes in research, improving the environments of people who are affected by health disparities, increasing access to health care, improving the quality of care, and making policy and legal changes. These five areas are the spokes of the overarching goal of this chapter, which is to provide information about strategies for reducing health disparities.

STRATEGIES FOR REDUCING OR ELIMINATING HEALTH DISPARITIES

A variety of approaches are needed to reduce health disparities. This task requires a systematic, coordinated, and collaborative effort to effectively implement the strategies. The methods necessitate implementation at different ecological levels with community, local, state, and national organizations and politicians at the helm.

Research

Eliminating health disparities will require new knowledge about the determinants of disease, causes of health disparities, effective interventions for prevention and treatment, and innovative ways of working in partnership with health care systems. The advances in knowledge about topics such as genetics and best practices need to be put into action and applied to the health care industry and not just lie in the pages of professional journals.

Best practices (also known as promising practices) of disparity reduction initiatives and programs are being identified and shared. This needs to continue and be magnified. We recommend that government organizations and researchers work to document and publicize those programs and policy changes that have been proven to be effective, but it is just as important to identify programs that do not work! Most of what is published in journals and on Web sites illustrates the successes, but the unsuccessful programs and policies add to the knowledge as well. Knowing what does not work eliminates health care professionals from channeling valuable resources to interventions that have already been shown to not produce positive effects.

There also is a need for data on specific populations. A majority of the data report on broad categories of race and ethnicities, such as Asians and American Indians. In addition, much of the research combines groups, such as Asians with Pacific Islanders and American Indians with Alaska Natives. There is great diversity within these groups, so more specific data is needed to help identify the health problems within the subpopulations and successful strategies for reducing them. Researchers and government agencies are encouraged to collect and report on data for racial and ethnic subgroups instead of the current commonly used broad categories.

In the United States, socioeconomic status has traditionally been measured by education and income. Surveys also should capture information about a range of contextual variables that have been found to be explanatory in health differences, such as social support, social networks, family supports, levels of acculturation, social cohesion, community involvement, perceived financial burdens, discrimination, and differences in the health status of foreign-born versus U.S.-born individuals, which at times also are linked to socioeconomic status.

Improving the Environments of People Affected by Health Disparities

There is little doubt that neighborhood characteristics are an important association with health. Residents of socially and economically deprived communities experience worse health outcomes on average than those living in more prosperous neighborhoods. This is because neighborhoods may influence health through relatively short-term influences on behaviors, attitudes, and health care utilization, thereby affecting health conditions that are more immediate. Neighborhoods also can impact health on a long-term basis through "weathering," whereby the accumulated stress, lower environmental quality, and limited resources of poorer communities experienced over many years negatively impacts the health of residents.

Minorities are more likely to live in poor neighborhoods. These neighborhoods often have poor-performing schools, crime, substandard housing, few health care providers and pharmacies, more alcohol and tobacco advertising, and limited access to grocery stores with healthy food choices. These social determinants of health can accumulate over the course of a life and can be detrimental to physical and emotional health.

Policies have historically led to racial segregation through regulations such as legal restrictions on which racial and ethnic groups may purchase property in certain geographic regions. Policies continue to have an impact on minorities, such as decisions related to regions with a high number of minorities often being targeted for placement of waste sites, for example. Policies are needed to reduce or eliminate environmental inequalities. An example of such a policy is that, in 2004, Senator Hillary Rodham Clinton (D-NY) and Congresswoman Hilda L. Solis (D-CA) announced the introduction of the Environmental Justice Renewal Act. The legislation championed by Senator Clinton and Congresswoman Solis was designed to increase the federal government's efforts in addressing the disproportionate impact of environmental pollution upon racial and ethnic minority and low-income populations. The purpose of the act was to expand existing grant programs and create new grant opportunities to help community-based groups and states address environmental justice, require the U.S. Environmental Protection Agency (EPA) to engage in additional outreach at the community level, and create the position of Environmental Justice Ombudsman to investigate the agency's handling of environmental justice complaints. It also was designed to increase accountability by requiring routine, independent evaluation of the government's actions to reduce and eliminate the disparate impact of environmental pollution upon minority and low-income communities.

Increasing Access to Health Care

More than half of the uninsured people in the United States are racial and ethnic minorities (McDonough, et al., 2004). Our nation needs to make coverage more accessible and equitable. Accessibility is not just related to financial barriers, because there are people who can afford coverage but are denied based on their medical history. Is universal health care coverage the answer? That is a major debate that we will not wrestle with here, but some consider it to be a possible solution.

Access to care also is related to having health care providers within your geographic region. There are imbalances in how the health care workforce is distributed, and this leads to lower access to care in some geographic regions of the United States. Poor neighborhoods tend to have a lower person-to-health care provider ratio than more affluent regions. **Telemedicine**, which offers incentives and competitive salaries to providers who work with low-income regions, and training community members as peer educators and outreach workers are all possible solutions to be explored.

Improving Quality of Care

Improving quality of care is related to training of health care providers, providing equal care, reducing language barriers, and increasing diversity in the workforce. Each of these four areas is discussed in the following paragraphs.

With regard to training health care providers, fostering a culturally-competent health care system that reflects and serves the diversity of America must be a priority for health care reform. States and academic centers that train health care professionals can develop, and some already have, requirements for training in this area. This can assist with providing equal treatment.

The groundbreaking report *Unequal Treatment: Confronting Racial and Ethnic Disparities in Health Care*, released in 2002 by the National Academies' Institute of Medicine (IOM), showed that racial and ethnic minorities receive lower-quality health care than Caucasians, even when insurance status, income, age, and severity of conditions are comparable. The report's first recommendation for reducing these disparities is to increase awareness of the issue among the public, health care providers, insurance companies, and policy makers. It also recommended the standardized collection of data on health care access and utilization by patients' race, ethnicity, socioeconomic status, and, where possible, primary language.

Language barriers can lead to numerous problems, such as damage to the patient and provider relationship, miscommunication with regard to the health problem and treatment approach, medication and correct-dosage mistakes, and legal problems. Health care has a language of its own and can make communication with people with limited English proficiency (LEP) skills even more difficult. Barriers can be reduced by multilingual signage, providing interpretive services, making record of a patient's native language and communication needs, and having documents (i.e., consent forms and educational materials) available in languages that reflect the demographics of the region served.

Diversity in the workforce is another goal. The health care workforce is under-represented by people who are nonwhite, yet people of color are more likely than white physicians to practice in federally-designated underserved areas, to see patients of color, and to accept Medicaid patients. As stated in a Commonwealth Fund report (McDonough, et al., 2004), racial concordance of patient and provider leads to greater participation in care and greater adherence to treatment.

Policy Changes and Laws

Policies and laws that mandate cultural competency training for medical professionals have been shown to be effective. A few of these laws are discussed here.

In 2005, New Jersey became the first state to enact a law, Senate Bill (SB) 144, to address the issue of equity in health care and cultural competency training of physicians. The law requires medical professionals to receive cultural competency training to receive a diploma from medical schools located in the state or to get licensed or relicensed to practice in the state. Each medical school in New Jersey is required to provide this training.

California has taken several steps to ensure cultural competency across the state's health care infrastructure. In 2005, Assembly Bill 1195 required mandatory continuing medical education courses to include cultural and linguistic courses. In the previous session, SB 853 was enacted, which requires commercial health plans to ensure members' access to linguistic services and to report to state regulators steps being taken to improve the cultural competency of their services. Similarly, the state's Medicaid program, Medi-Cal, requires all health plans providing services for Medicaid patients to ensure their linguistic needs are met, including 24-hour access to interpretive services and documents in native languages.

The state of Washington enacted SB 6194 in 2006, which requires all medical education curricula in the state to include multicultural health training and awareness courses. All of these laws strive to establish cultural competence among health care professionals.

CULTURAL COMPETENCE

There is no universally-accepted definition of cultural competency in health care. In general, **cultural competence** is a set of congruent behaviors, attitudes, structures, and policies that come together to work effectively in intercultural situations (National CASA Association, 1995–1996). That set of behaviors can be adopted and practiced by a solitary professional or an entire organization. Cultural competence requires a set of skills by individuals and systems that allows an increased understanding and appreciation of cultural differences as well as the demonstrated skills necessary to work with and serve diverse individuals and groups.

According to the National CASA Association (1995–1996), the culturally competent organization:

- values diversity
- conducts cultural self-assessments
- is conscious of and manages the dynamics of difference
- institutionalizes cultural knowledge
- adapts services to fit the cultural diversity of the community served

Cultural competency entails the willingness and ability of individuals and a system to value the importance of culture in the delivery of services to all segments of the population at all levels of an organization. It includes activities such as policy development and implementation, governance, education, promoting workforce diversity, and the reduction of language barriers.

Becoming culturally competent is an ongoing process. It requires a dedication to growing with a changing society that is becoming more diverse and to serving the individuals and communities with the most culturally appropriate, and hence highest quality care possible.

Improving cultural competency levels should begin with an assessment to determine where an individual and/or organization can improve. It can assist with directing training and education for the workforce, policy development, and other systematic changes. We included an individual and an organizational cultural competency assessment tool in Chapter 2.

CHAPTER SUMMARY

To achieve quality and affordable health care for all, health care reform must include concrete steps to reduce health disparities. Ensuring access to coverage is only part of the answer. Other strategies include reducing barriers to quality health care for people of color by requiring cultural competency training of medical professionals, recruiting a diverse workforce, eliminating language barriers, coordinating public and private programs that target disparities, providing more funding to community health centers, and improving chronic disease management programs by making them more responsive to minorities. Health disparities reflect and perpetuate the inequity and injustice that permeates American society. Eliminating health disparities will help create equal opportunity for all Americans in all sectors of our society

In this chapter, we discussed a variety of methods for reducing health disparities. These include strategies such as diversifying the health care workforce, changing policies, training health care professionals in the area of cultural competency, and conducting additional research. These changes can help reduce the gap in health among Americans, and this needs to continue to be a priority for our nation, particularly in light of the changing demographics of the United States.

We hope that you have achieved a higher level of cultural competency as you complete the final chapter of this textbook. As we have mentioned, cultural competency is a process, and you still have a lot to learn. You will never learn all there is to know about the numerous cultures, but what is important is that you are aware of the major differences, challenge your assumptions, respect and embrace values and beliefs that are different from your own, and provide the same high standards of care to all humans, regardless of race, ethnicity, gender, sexual preference, or other attribute. We hope that you will go beyond this by advocating for equality and striving to improve health care systems to help close the gaps in the levels of health that exist among certain groups. We leave you with this quote:

Cultural differences should not separate us from each other, but rather cultural diversity brings a collective strength that can benefit all of humanity.
—Robert Alan

REVIEW

1. List the six priority areas for eliminating health disparities.
2. Describe strategies to reduce or eliminate health disparities.
3. Describe what cultural competency is and why it is important.

CASE STUDY

Confronting Disparities While
Reforming Health Care
A Look at Massachusetts

Health Reform in the States

As health care costs and the number of uninsured rise steadily throughout the nation, the lack of a federal solution to this growing crisis has prompted more and more states to take matters into their own hands. Innovative health reform plans have been popping up across the country, from Maine to California. These reform efforts present a unique opportunity to harness the growing political momentum to fix our health care system and to bring attention to the persistent racial and ethnic disparities that plague the system.

It is a common misconception that efforts to provide universal health care will automatically translate into equitable, quality health coverage for all. This is simply not the case: Access alone will not eliminate health disparities.[1] The issue of health disparities must be specifically addressed within health care reform efforts so that inequities can be eliminated.[2]

In 2006, Massachusetts made national headlines when it passed health reform legislation that extended coverage to nearly all Bay Staters. Health advocates from across the country have looked to Massachusetts as an example of how to successfully enact bold health policy reform. However, Massachusetts can serve as a model for more than its work to expand coverage—recent experience there can also provide guidance in how to address health disparities in the context of health reform.

Massachusetts: A Unique Health Policy History

Massachusetts has a long history of progressive health reform, which has served as a necessary foundation for its most recent expansion.[3] In 1985, the state legislature created the Uncompensated Care Pool, which reimburses hospitals and community health centers (CHCs) that provide free care to eligible low-income uninsured people. That same year, the legislature also established a special commission charged with developing a plan for achieving universal health coverage in Massachusetts. A bill based on the commission's plan was signed into law in 1988, and parts of this legislation are still in place today, including programs that provide coverage for children, pregnant women, uninsured workers, adults with disabilities, and college students.

In 1996, the state undertook a massive reform that reinvented its Medicaid program and created MassHealth, which extended Medicaid coverage to an additional 300,000 residents. That legislation also included expanded coverage for children, limits on the amount of out-of-pocket money seniors were required to pay for prescriptions, as well as assistance for low-wage workers purchasing health insurance.

In 2004, health care advocates in Massachusetts once again saw the opportunity to move forward with new health reforms. Health Care for All (HCFA), a prominent health policy organization in the state, led a diverse coalition of stakeholders in drafting legislation that would expand health coverage to virtually all state residents. The coalition was made up of consumers, patients, community and religious organizations, businesses, labor unions, doctors, hospitals, health plans, and community health centers. It came to be known as the Affordable Care Today (ACT!) Coalition.

ACT! was largely responsible for the passage of the most recent health care reform legislation, commonly known as Chapter 58. Passed in 2006, Chapter 58 was designed to expand health coverage to nearly all Massachusetts residents through several mechanisms, including the creation of the Commonwealth Health Insurance Connector (a program designed to help individuals and small employers purchase affordable insurance more easily), a modest expansion of MassHealth, and an individual mandate.

Racial and Ethnic Health Disparities in Massachusetts

As all of this work to expand health coverage was taking place, momentum was also building around the effort to eliminate health disparities. Soon after the landmark Institute of Medicine report, *Unequal Treatment: Confronting Racial and Ethnic Health Disparities in Health Care*, was released in 2002, Boston Mayor Thomas Menino called for city hospitals and community clinics to develop concrete strategies to reduce racial and ethnic health disparities. Menino later established the Mayor's Task Force to Eliminate Racial and Ethnic Disparities and charged it with developing a set of standards and recommendations to help eliminate health disparities in Boston.

In 2005, Menino declared health disparities to be the city's most pressing health care issue and, drawing on recommendations from the task force, launched The Disparities Project to combat health disparities.[4] The Boston Public Health Commission took the lead and created a "blueprint" that laid out 12 sweeping recommendations designed to eliminate disparities in Boston. Mayor Menino raised more than $1 million to fund implementation of the blueprint recommendations through contracts with local groups that were already working to eliminate racial and ethnic health disparities.[5]

The effort to eliminate disparities was not limited to Boston. At the state level, a Special Legislative Commission on Racial and Ethnic Health Disparities was investigating health disparities and developing recommendations and an action plan for addressing such disparities statewide. HCFA played a leadership role in writing this commission into state statute.

The key political support of Mayor Menino and the array of disparities reduction campaigns helped move health disparities into the public eye. Suddenly, people who had never heard of health disparities were opening *The Boston Globe* to find stories on The Disparities Project. The strong support of the health research community also helped to make health disparities a serious legislative issue. The general public and, perhaps more importantly, state legislators, were hearing about health disparities around the same time that they were hearing about broader health reform efforts. This timing created a political climate that was favorable to the inclusion of provisions that addressed racial and ethnic health disparities in the new health reform legislation.

In addition to Mayor Menino, Governor Deval Patrick, who took office in 2007, has shown a real commitment to eliminating health disparities. Not only did he speak at the state's first ever disparities advocacy event [see page 367], leading officials in his administration have also pledged to work with disparities advocates around developing the state's health disparities agenda.

Chapter 58 Legislation and Health Disparities

The Chapter 58 legislation contains four provisions that address racial and ethnic health disparities: [6]

1. **Section 160** calls for the creation of an ongoing **Health Disparities Council** that is charged with developing recommendations on several minority health issues, including workforce diversity, disparate disease rates among communities of color, and social determinants of health.
2. **Section 16 L. (a)** calls for the creation of a **Health Care Quality and Cost Council,** which will focus on health care quality issues with the goals of lowering costs, improving health care quality, and reducing disparities.
3. **Section 13B** develops standards for **Hospital Performance and Rate Increases**, with a specific stipulation regarding hospital rate increases being based on quality issues such as reducing racial and ethnic health disparities.
4. **Section 110** requires a **Community Health Worker Study** to be conducted by the Public Health Department to determine the effectiveness of community health workers in reducing racial and ethnic health disparities.

The Health Disparities Council mandated by Section 160 convened its first meeting in December 2007. The council established several broad initial goals, such as implementing the recommendations of the State Commission to End Racial and Ethnic Health Disparities, as well as ensuring that implementation of Chapter 58 included a consideration of the unique needs of communities of color. More specifically, the council discussed how to integrate the disparities agenda into larger efforts around improvements in health care quality via the Health Care Quality and Cost Council, which was also established by Chapter 58.

Including these provisions in Chapter 58 was an important and necessary step in beginning to tackle health disparities. However, disparities advocates in Massachusetts recognized that reducing disparities would require more than these provisions: Although these measures created a solid foundation, many advocates working on minority health issues felt it was necessary to build more substantive policy on this foundation.

Expanding Health Disparities Legislation

To build on the disparities provisions in Chapter 58, and to more thoroughly address the host of issues that affect health disparities, a coalition came together to file omnibus legislation whose sole focus was reducing racial and ethnic health disparities. HCFA once again took the lead in bringing the project together, and it was joined by a wide range of individuals, organizations, and institutions, ranging from the Boston Public Health Commission to the local chapter of the Service Employees International Union (SEIU). Others involved in the process included legal associations, research organizations, community health organizations, large health care providers, health policy organizations, as well as multi-issue organizations concerned with equity and justice in health policy. Together, they formed the Disparities Action Network (DAN).[7,8]

The DAN formally convened for the first time in June 2006 with the goal of drafting omnibus disparities legislation for the 2007–2008 state legislative session. Its work was based partly on recommendations put forth by the Special Legislative Commission on Racial and Ethnic Health Disparities. From there, the group determined what it thought was missing from Chapter 58, drawing upon the collective knowledge of its diverse membership to come up with real policy solutions.

The DAN wrote its legislation using a collaborative work group process, meeting several times throughout the summer and fall of 2006 to write and review the legislation before it was filed. First, the coalition held a brainstorming session to determine what should be included in the legislation, which yielded an exhaustive list of policy recommendations and ideas. The final legislation grew from one key premise, which was the need to create a Health Equity Office. The members of the DAN believed

MEMBERS OF THE DISPARITIES ACTION NETWORK (DAN)[9]

- Action for Boston Community Development
- AIDS Action Committee
- Alliance for Community Health
- American Cancer Society
- American Diabetes Association
- American Heart/American Stroke Association
- American Red Cross of Massachusetts Bay
- Association of Haitian Pastors
- Association of Haitian Women
- Berkshire Area Health Education Center
- Boston Center for Community & Justice
- Boston Medical Center Haitian Health Institute
- Boston Public Health Commission
- Boston University Center for Excellence in Women's Health
- Boston Urban Asthma Coalition
- Cambridge Health Alliance
- Caring Health Center
- Center for Community Health Education Research and Service
- Community Catalyst
- Community Change Inc.
- Conference on Boston Teaching Hospitals
- Critical MASS
- Diabetes Association Inc.
- Greater Lawrence Family Health Center
- Haitian Multi-Service Center
- Haitian Nurses Association
- Health Care for All
- International Medical Interpreters Association
- Jewish Alliance for Law and Social Action
- La Alianza Hispana
- Latin American Health Institute
- The Lawyers' Committee for Civil Rights under Law of the Boston Bar Association
- Lowell Community Health Center
- Lynn Health Task Force
- Mass CONECT, Harvard School of Public Health
- Massachusetts Asian and Pacific Islanders for Health
- Massachusetts Association of Community Health Workers
- Massachusetts Breast Cancer Coalition
- Massachusetts General Hospital, Disparities Solutions Center
- Massachusetts Hospital Association
- Massachusetts League of Community Health Centers
- Massachusetts Medical Society
- Massachusetts Public Health Association
- Medical-Legal Partnership for Children
- Multicultural AIDS Coalition
- NAACP Boston
- NARAL Pro-Choice Massachusetts
- ¿Oíste?
- Oral Health Advocacy Task Force
- Physicians for Human Rights
- Planned Parenthood League of Massachusetts
- Project RIGHT
- SEIU 1199
- Tobacco Free Massachusetts
- Vietnamese American Civic Association
- Whittier Street Health Center
- YMCA of Greater Worcester, Central Community Branch
- Youth and Family Enrichment Services

that the abundance of projects, programs, and other efforts to eliminate racial and ethnic health disparities in Massachusetts could be greatly strengthened if they were not so fragmented. A Health Equity Office could serve as a coordinating body for all of the disparities work within the state. Under the guidance of such an office, disparities could be addressed in a systematic, cohesive approach through strategic planning and coordination of efforts on multiple fronts.

These efforts include programs that address both disparities in health and disparities in health care. More specifically, these programs involve developing standards based on best practices from across the state. These standards focus on health literacy, healthy communities initiatives that address environmental and social determinants of health, and workforce diversity (through coordination of existing labor standards). Other programs include support for medical interpreter services, community health workers, wellness education, community-based participatory research, and coordination of racial and ethnic data collection projects across public and private agencies.[10]

The legislation, entitled *An Act Eliminating Racial and Ethnic Health Disparities in the Commonwealth* (H. 2234), was introduced in the Massachusetts legislature on January 9, 2007, by Representative Byron Rushing. In anticipation of the bill's hearing, the DAN formed several committees to build momentum around ending health disparities. This included a grassroots advocacy committee to help bring a community voice to the policy process and to reach out to communities to help them understand more about disparities and why passing this legislation is important. The network also formed lobbying and communications workgroups to educate members of the Joint Committee on Public Health both about the bill and about health disparities in general, as well as to gain more publicity in local media to broadly publicize information on disparities and the DAN legislation.[11]

The bill was heard on May 16, 2007, and it remains in the Public Health Committee. A panel comprised of health care and disparities experts, community members, and the legislative leads for the bill used their testimony as an opportunity to further educate legislators about the importance of addressing health disparities within health reform efforts.

Since that hearing, the DAN has submitted one redraft of the legislation, which made the following minor changes per the recommendation of the committee chair: the grant programs have been consolidated and made less prescriptive by the language; all grant programs have been clearly designated as subject to appropriation; and the Environmental Justice provision has been shortened and simplified.

The redrafted bill was submitted in late November 2007, and it remains in committee. In the meantime, in November 2007, the Patrick administration announced that it would distribute $1 million in grants to agencies throughout Massachusetts to eliminate health disparities, and it released a report that documented widespread disparities in health across the state. Many of the grant recipients were DAN member organizations.

An Act Eliminating Racial and Ethnic Health Disparities in the Commonwealth includes the following provisions:[12]

- **Office of Health Equity**
  The Office of Health Equity will be housed under the State Executive Office of Health and Human Services and will be advised by the Health Disparities Council that was created by Chapter 58. The Office of Health Equity will be responsible for coordinating all disparities elimination efforts in the state. The office will publish annual disparities impact statements, put out annual disparities report cards on regional progress, set evaluation standards, determine reimbursement rates for medical translation services, and manage programmatic provisions of the legislation.

- **Community Agency Grants Program**
  The Office of Health Equity will run a grant program to support efforts by community-based health agencies to eliminate disparities in underserved populations.

- **Data Collection Coordination**
  The Office of Health Equity may choose to publish best standards on data collection. The office will also coordinate the data collection, analysis, and dissemination activities of all parties involved in the collection of data on patient race, ethnicity, and language spoken.

- **Community Health Workers**
  The Office of Health Equity will run a competitive grant program to provide funds to hospitals, community health centers, and nonprofit community organizations to employ community health workers to better the health of the communities in which they live.

- **Community-Based Participatory Research**
  The Office of Health Equity will run a competitive grant program to provide funding for research partnerships between community-based organizations and academic researchers focusing on the elimination of health disparities.

- **Health Literacy**

  The Office of Health Equity will designate and disseminate best practice guidelines for the creation of health-related materials and literature drawing on federal and public health standards. The goal is to make materials widely accessible to patients, including those with limited educational attainment and limited English proficiency.

- **Workforce Development**

  The Office of Health Equity will establish a council to coordinate state, local, and private-sector efforts to establish health care workforce diversity and development.

- **Environmental Justice**

  A statewide community health index will be created to demonstrate which communities suffer from high rates of death and illness based on a weighted set of primary and secondary indicators of health outcomes.

- **Chronic Disease Management**

  A chronic disease management program will be established in the Department of Public Health to begin wellness education of individuals who suffer from chronic disease.

Lessons Learned

The goals and ideas put forth by the DAN are far from unique. There was already an enormous amount of work going on around the elimination of health disparities prior

---

DAN ADVOCACY ACTIVITIES

Legislative Advocacy

The DAN has advocated broadly throughout the legislature, and it has rallied black and Latino caucus members in support of the legislation. In October 2007, the DAN hosted the first ever health disparities advocacy event at the State House. The event drew more than 350 attendees from around the state, many of whom were consumers of color. What's more, representatives from 42 legislative offices came to the event. One highlight of the program was a surprise visit from Governor Patrick, who affirmed his commitment to eliminating health disparities. After the event, DAN members and consumers visited those legislative offices to further educate members of the State House about the bill and about health disparities.

(Continues)

Budget Advocacy

The DAN has begun working on another approach to accomplishing the objectives of the original legislation. Because the bill has remained in committee since early 2007, the DAN has looked to the governor's budget as a vehicle for moving specific pieces of the legislation. In November 2007, the DAN submitted a request to the governor's office to include in his budget funding for many of the programs contained in the bill, such as the creation of an Office of Health Equity that would administer grant programs for community health agencies, community health workers, and community-based participatory research. The budget is expected to be released in late January 2008, and while this approach would provide immediate funding for some much-needed programs, the DAN will also continue to pursue its legislative strategy so that these programs become codified into state law.

WHAT ABOUT THE SOCIAL AND ENVIRONMENTAL DETERMINANTS OF HEALTH?

Racial and ethnic health disparities are not simply the result of disparities in access to quality health care. Rather, they result from complex social, economic, and environmental factors. After the initial brainstorming process, the DAN work group realized that many of the provisions it had discussed were focused on the structural and social determinants of health, as opposed to reforms of the health care system itself. For example, there were several provisions that addressed access to healthy grocers, green space, healthy school lunches, and safe places for children to play within communities of color.

These provisions presented a challenge because the legislation was meant to be a "health care bill," and the group did not want to weaken the bill by spreading its focus too broadly. At the same time, the group did not want to develop a bill that focused solely on health care and ignored the larger environmental determinants of health—such a bill would send the message that policies that improve quality and access in the health care system are all that is needed to eliminate racial and ethnic health disparities.

Although the majority of the legislation was focused on reforms within the health care system, DAN advocates wanted to acknowledge the deeper roots of health disparities. They therefore included a provision that requires the Office of Health Equity to monitor social and environmental effects on health. The Office of Health Equity will be responsible for addressing these effects by engaging other state agencies, such as the housing and transportation authorities, and by generating annual disparities impact statements on the major initiatives of these agencies. The Boston Public Health Commission, a member of the DAN, also filed smaller-scale legislation on environmental equity issues (this legislation is currently on hold), while the DAN made a concerted effort to emphasize the important role of environmental and social justice in the effort to eliminate disparities.

to the convening of the DAN. Yet there is much to learn from the experiences of minority health advocates in Massachusetts as they move forward with their health disparities legislation.

- **Framing the Message and Getting Media Coverage**

  The DAN showed that by harnessing the political and media attention surrounding health care expansions and reforms, it is possible to successfully elevate a disparities policy agenda to the state level. As more and more states begin to develop their own health care expansion legislation, disparities advocates must be ready to seize any political opportunities that can move the issue of health disparities into the public eye. The DAN advocates were successful because they were able to use all of the public attention surrounding health reform in Massachusetts, as well as the media attention garnered by the mayor's Disparities Project, to successfully raise awareness about health disparities and simultaneously put forth a substantive strategy aimed at eliminating those disparities.

  At the same time, the DAN has faced some challenges in framing its message and fully addressing the disparities issue within the context of Chapter 58. For example, some stakeholders believe that the issue of health disparities is only an issue of health access, and they point to health care reform as the key to eliminating all disparities. The DAN continues to work hard to educate those audiences about factors other than access that can lead to health disparities, such as the social determinants of health and unequal treatment.

  Another challenge the DAN faces is garnering media attention that examines the nuances of disparities in health and health care. The group has found that when media outlets do report on health disparities, they tend to focus only on overt discrimination in health care settings, and they have less interest in investigating or reporting on the full breadth of disparities issues, or on possible solutions. Media outlets have also shown a bit of fatigue when it comes to reporting on health care issues, including disparities.

- **Coalition Strategy and Engagement**

  The collaboration among multiple groups coming together to write legislation focused on disparities demonstrated the political power that advocates can wield through collective action. The DAN has been a powerful driving force because it uses the knowledge, skills, resources, and political power that its diverse membership brings to the table. By drawing on these resources and developing a defined agenda, the DAN was well-positioned to raise awareness about health disparities and to move its policy agenda forward.

Advocates need to keep in mind that raising awareness around disparities is only part of the battle. Introducing disparities legislation is not easy, which is why collaboration is so crucial. Minority health advocates must look beyond their traditional partners and seek out diverse partners. For instance, advocates who are working to expand health coverage may not be the same advocates who are trying to eliminate disparities and ensure health equity. However, these issues must go hand in hand: Conversations around expanding access are a natural place to discuss efforts to ensure health care equity and reduce disparities. Each of these individual efforts can be strengthened through collaboration.

The DAN has found it challenging to diversify its membership so that it includes more community-based minority organizations. Many of these groups have prioritized other important issues (such as housing, violence, or education) over disparities, and they have not had the capacity to join the DAN table. Disparities advocates can address some of these hurdles by taking a few practical steps, such as holding meetings outside normal business hours to attract interested volunteers, helping groups make the connection between larger social issues and policy goals and their own organizational goals, as well as recognizing that not all groups can devote staff time to health disparities efforts.

- **Policy and Advocacy**
  Another important lesson to be learned from the experiences of the DAN is that policy is a tool that minority health advocates can, and should, use to help eliminate health disparities. Advocates who work on minority health issues often focus on direct service or disease-specific issues in their efforts to reduce disparities in health and health care. Although these efforts are critical, it is important to look beyond these traditional strategies and use policy as a tool to help eliminate health disparities. Health disparities are a systemic problem that calls for systemic answers, and policy can serve as a powerful tool to address inequities. While the political and historical circumstances in Massachusetts were clearly unique factors that allowed the disparities legislation to advance, minority health advocates can still look to the state as a model for legislation in their own states.

  Finally, although expansion of health coverage can be a useful vehicle from which to address disparities in health care access and quality, because disparities are rooted in many sources, advocates must not limit their work to health care access. Disparities result from a wide range of factors, including social and cultural circumstances, physical environment, and individual socioeconomic status. With so many factors contributing to health disparities, it is unrealistic to believe that disparities can be eradicated by pursuing narrow policies that focus solely on health care access and delivery systems. To combat the complex ways in which health disparities affect minorities, advocates must explore program and policy solutions that can address the environmental and social determinants of disparities as well.

Health disparities are complex. By looking at success stories like that of the DAN, minority health advocates can develop and strengthen tools that will eliminate racial and ethnic health disparities and, ultimately, lead to health equity.

Endnotes

[1]Kate Meyers, *Racial and Ethnic Health Disparities* (Oakland, CA: Kaiser Permanente Institute for Health Policy, 2007), available online at http://www.kpihp.org/publications/docs/disparities_highlights.pdf.

[2]Jack Geiger, "Race and Health Care—An American Dilemma?", *New England Journal of Medicine* 335 (September 1996): 815–816.

[3]ACT! Affordable Care Today, *Previous Health Care Reform Efforts in MA: A Brief Background* (Boston: Health Care for All, 2006), available online at http://www.hcfama.org/act/reform101.asp.

[4]Boston Public Health Commission, *The Disparities Project: Year One Report* (Boston: Boston Public Health Commission, 2007), available online at http://www.bphc.org/reports/pdfs_222.pdf.

[5]Ibid.

[6]ACT! Affordable Care Today, *Chapter 58 of the Acts of 2006: An Act Providing Access to Affordable, Quality, Accountable Health Care* (Boston: Health Care for All, 2006), available online at http://www.hcfama.org/act/mahealthreformlaw.asp.

[7]Health Care for All, *Disparities Action Network* (Boston: Health Care for All, 2006), available online at http://www.hcfama.org/index.cfm?fuseaction=page.viewPage&pageID=516.

[8]Camille Watson, "Policy and Advocacy Efforts to Eliminate Disparities in Massachusetts," presentation at Universal and Equal: Ensuring Health Equity in Health Reform meeting, March 9, 2007.

[9]Health Care for All, op cit.

[10]Camille Watson, op cit.

[11]Ibid.

[12]Health Care for All, *An Act Eliminating Racial and Ethnic Health Disparities in the Commonwealth: Summary* (Boston: Health Care for All, 2006), available online at http://www.hcfama.org/_uploads/documents/live/Dan%20Summary.pdf.

Source: Families USA. (2008). Reproduced with permission.

GLOSSARY TERMS

best practices   cultural competence
telemedicine

REFERENCES

Families USA. (2008). *Confronting disparities while reforming health care: A look at Massachusetts.* Retrieved October 27, 2008, from http://www.familiesusa.org/assets/pdfs/ma-disparities-case-study.pdf

McDonough, J. E., Gibbs, B. K., Scott-Harris, J. L., Kronebusch, K., Navarro, A. M., & Taylor, K. (2004). A state policy agenda to eliminate racial and ethnic health disparities. The Commonwealth Fund.

National CASA Association. (1995–1996, Fall/Winter). *What is cultural competence? Family Resource Coalition's report.* Retrieved April 20, 2008, from http://www.casanet.org/library/culture/competence.htm

Office of Minority Health & Health Disparities. (2007). *Eliminating racial & ethnic health disparities.* Retrieved April 6, 2008, from http://www.cdc.gov/omhd/About/disparities.htm

Smedley, B. D., Stith, A. Y., & Nelson, A. R. (Eds) (2003). *Unequal treatment: Confronting racial and ethnic disparities in health care.* Washington, DC: The National Academies Press.

GLOSSARY

aAma and aDuonga: Vietnamese belief of balance in all things, similar to yin and yang in traditional Chinese medicine.

acculturation: The process of adapting to another culture by acquiring the majority group's culture.

acupuncture: Traditional Chinese medicine treatment that involves stimulating specific points along the meridians to achieve a therapeutic purpose. The usual practice involves inserting a needle into one of the acupoints along a meridian that is associated with that organ or function.

advance directives: Pertains to treatment preferences and the designation of a surrogate decision maker in the event that a person should become unable to make medical decisions on his or her own behalf.

ahimsa: A Buddhist and Hindu doctrine that expresses belief in the sacredness of all living creatures and urges the avoidance of harm and violence.

alternative medicine: A variety of therapeutic or preventive health care practices, such as homeopathy, naturopathy, chiropractic, and herbal medicine, that do not follow generally accepted medical methods and may not have a scientific explanation for their effectiveness; used instead of Western medicine.

animal sacrifice: The ritual killing of an animal as part of a religion.

assimilation: The process of becoming absorbed into another culture, adopting its characteristics, and developing a new cultural identity.

autonomy: The ethical principle that embodies the right of self-determination.

ayurvedic medicine: India's ancient and traditional natural system of medicine that provides an integrated approach to preventing and treating illness through lifestyle interventions and natural therapies.

beneficence: The state or quality of being kind and charitable; a principle that requires doing good or removing harm.

best practices: An assertion that there is a strategy that is more effective at delivering a particular outcome than any other technique, method, or process.

betel nut: A seed used by many Pacific Islanders for cultural purposes.

bisexual: Individuals whose sexual identity is to both men and women.

brauche: Amish practice whereby a healer lays his hands over a patient's head or stomach while quietly reciting verses to "pull out" the ailment.

Candomblé: A religion developed in Brazil by enslaved Africans that involves rituals such as animal sacrifice, drumming, and dancing.

chiropractic: The diagnosis and treatment of disorders of the muscular, nervous, and skeletal systems, with special emphasis on the spine. Spinal adjustment is the predominate treatment tool.

complementary medicine: Treatments that are utilized in conjunction with conventional Western medical therapies that are prescribed by a physician.

cultural adaptation: The degree to which a person or community has adapted to the dominant culture and retained its traditional practices.

cultural competence: The ability to interact effectively with people of different cultures; a set of congruent behaviors, attitudes, structures, and policies that come together to work effectively in intercultural situations.

cultural relativism: The principle that one's beliefs and activities should be interpreted in terms of one's own culture and that no culture is superior to another.

culture: The set of learned behaviors, beliefs, attitudes, values, and ideals that are characteristic of a particular society or population.

curandero (male) or curandera (female): A traditional folk healer or shaman who is dedicated to curing physical and/or spiritual illnesses.

digital divide: The disparity in access to electronic information resources.

discrimination: The practice of treating people differently on a basis other than merit.

dominant culture: The total, generally organized way of life, including values, norms, institutions, and symbols.

doshas: In ayurvedic medicine, the three vital energies that regulate everything in nature.

drabarni: Roma women who have knowledge of medicines.

Ellis-van Creveld syndrome: Genetic disorder found among the Amish in which there is a defective recessive gene from each parent.

empacho: In the Hispanic culture, a description of stomach pains and cramps.

Espiritismo: A Latin American and Caribbean belief that good and evil spirits can affect human life, such as one's health and luck.

ethnicity: Large groups of people who are classified according to common racial, national, tribal, religious, linguistic, or cultural origin or background.

ethnocentricity: When a person believes that his or her culture is superior to that of another.

euthanasia: Act or practice of ending the life of an individual who is suffering from a terminal illness or an incurable condition by lethal injection or the suspension of extraordinary medical treatment.

evil eye: Also referred to as mal de ojo. In the Hispanic culture, an illness thought to be caused by jealousy; the Spanish translation is "bad eye." This belief is held by many migrant farmworkers.

fidelity: Ethical principle that entails keeping one's promises or commitments.

five elements: The traditional Chinese medicine theory based on the perception of the relationships among all things. These patterns are grouped and named for the five elements: wood, fire, earth, metal, and water.

fotonovela: An illustrated novel.

gadje: All things non-Roma; considered to be not clean.

gay: Term that refers to homosexuals in general and is usually used to refer to male homosexuals specifically.

gender identity: A person's internal, personal sense of being male or female, boy or girl, man or woman.

healing: Also referred to as laying on of hands. An energy and spiritual healing practice.

health disparities: Also referred to as health inequalities. Gaps in the quality of health and health care across racial, ethnic, sexual orientation, and socioeconomic groups.

Healthy People 2010: A program that provides a prevention framework for the nation. It is a statement of national health objectives designed to identify the most significant preventable threats to health and to establish national goals to reduce these threats.

heritage consistency: The degree to which people identify with their culture of origin.

Hill-Burton Act: Also referred to as the Hospital Survey and Construction Act of 1946. It provided federal assistance to state governments for the construction and modernization of hospitals and other health care facilities. The original statute required recipient hospitals to make services available "to all persons residing in the territorial area of the application, without discrimination on account of race, creed, or color."

Hmong: Mountain-dwelling people from Cambodia and Vietnam.

homeopath: A practitioner of homeopathy.

homeopathy: The premise that "like cures like," a belief in the body's ability to heal itself. A system for treating disease based on the administration of minute doses of a drug that in massive amounts produces symptoms in healthy individuals similar to those of the disease itself.

homosexual: An individual whose gender identity is consistent with his or her physical sexual characteristics but whose sexual identity is to persons of the same sex.

humour: A fluid (or semifluid) substance.

hydrotherapy: A treatment used by naturopathic practitioners based on the therapeutic effects of water. Thought to assist in ridding the body of waste and toxins, it utilizes hot and cold baths, compresses, wraps, and showers as treatment modalities.

integrative medicine: A process in which complementary and alternative medicine practices are incorporated into conventional care.

justice: The ethical principle in which people should be treated equally and fairly.

kahuna: Native Hawaiian leader known as "keeper of the secret."

karma: The total effect of a person's conduct during the successive phases of the person's existence, which is expected to determine the person's destiny.

kava: A root used by Pacific Island cultures for various cultural and healing traditions.

Kior chi force: Korean belief in a life force similar to chi in traditional Chinese medicine; it is important in maintaining health, and efforts are made to balance this force and to not engage in activities that could diminish it.

Law/Principle of Similars: The concept upon which homeopathy is based; the premise that "like cures like," a belief in the body's ability to heal itself.

lesbian: Term that refers to homosexual women specifically.

living will: A set of instructions that documents a person's wishes about medical care that is intended to sustain life.

lokahi: Native Hawaiian belief in harmony between people, nature, and the gods, which is critical to maintaining health and preventing illness.

magnet therapy: Treatments involving the use of electromagnetic energy.

mal de ojo: Also referred to as evil eye. In the Hispanic culture, an illness thought to be caused by jealousy; the Spanish translation is "bad eye."

mana: Native Hawaiian belief in the healing energy of the island.

marime: Roma concept of impurity, which is foundational to their health beliefs.

medicine bundle: A wrapped package used by American Indians for religious and healing purposes.

meditation: A group of mental techniques intended to provide relaxation and mental harmony as well as to quiet one's mind and increase awareness.

meridians: The traditional Chinese medicine concept of channels through which qi, blood, and information flow to all parts of the body.

mindfulness meditation: The concept of increasing awareness and acceptance of the present.

minority: A group that is smaller in number than another group; a part of a population that differs in characteristics, often resulting in differential treatment.

multicultural evaluation: Integrates cultural considerations into an evaluation's theory, measures, analysis, and practice.

multicultural health: The provision of health services in a sensitive, knowledgeable, and nonjudgmental manner with respect for people's health beliefs and practices when they are different from your own.

naturopath: A person who practices naturopathy.

naturopathy: Healing practice based on ancient beliefs in the healing power of nature and that natural organisms have the ability to heal themselves and maintain health. The body strives to maintain a state of equilibrium, known as homeostasis, and unhealthy environments, diets, physical or emotional stress, and lack of sleep or fresh air can disrupt that balance. Natural remedies, such as herbs and foods, are used instead of surgery or drugs.

nonmaleficence: The principle that one should do no harm.

orishas: Spirits that resemble the Catholic saints and reflect one of the manifestations of Olodumare (God). These religious deities are said to represent human characteristics.

peyote: A spineless, dome-shaped cactus (*Lophophora williamsii*) native to Mexico and the southwest United States. The plant has buttonlike tubercles that are chewed fresh or dry as a narcotic, hallucinogenic drug by certain Native American peoples.

prakriti: The combination of the doshas at the time of conception that are unique to each individual.

Principle of Specificity of the Individual: States that any condition must be matched to the distinctive symptoms of the person.

promotores (male) or promotoras (female): Community members who promote health in their own communities.

qi: In traditional Chinese medicine, the vital life force that animates all things.

qigong: Translates to "energy work." A part of traditional Chinese medicine that involves movement, breathing, and meditation that is intended to improve the flow of qi through the body.

race: The concept of dividing people into populations or groups on the basis of visible traits and beliefs about common ancestry.

racism: The belief that some races are superior to others by nature.

reciprocity: A reciprocal condition or relationship.

reiki: A form of alternative medicine in which the healer uses his or her hands to channel healing energy.

respect: Ethical principle that addresses an individual's right to make determinations about his or her health and to live or die with the consequences.

ritual: A set of actions that usually are very structured and have a symbolic value or meaning.

Romany: A language derived from Sanskrit that is spoken by the Roma people.

Rumspringa: Amish practice characterized by adolescents being free to explore the world outside of the Amish culture.

Santeria: An African-based religion that combines the worship of traditional Yoruban deities with the worship of roman Catholic saints.

sexual identity: A person's physical, romantic, emotional, and/or spiritual attraction to another person.

shaman: A member of certain tribal societies who acts as a medium between the visible world and an invisible spirit world and who practices magic or sorcery for purposes of healing, prediction, and control over natural events.

shrine: A place of religious devotion or commemoration.

sorcerer: Black magician; wizard.

spirituality: The belief in a higher power, something beyond the human experience, and its intercession in healing.

susto: In the Hispanic culture, an illness thought to be caused by soul loss or fright.

sweat lodge: An important ritual used by some American Indians a sauna that is usually a domed or oblong hut.

t'ai chi ch'uan: Traditional Chinese medicine exercise designed to improve the flow of qi through the body and encourage balance and harmony.

talking circles: A method used by many American Indians to discuss a topic or what is present for them in their lives. The group members sit in a circle and make comments on the topic of discussion, following specified rules.

telemedicine: The use of telecommunications technology to provide, enhance, or expedite health care services, such as accessing off-site databases, linking clinics or physicians' offices to central hospitals, or transmitting x-rays or other diagnostic images for examination at another site.

timbang: Filipino belief in a range of "hot" and "cold" humoral balances in the body and food and dietary balances.

transcendental meditation: A technique that allows a practitioner to experience ever-finer levels of thought until the source of thought is experienced.

transgender: Individuals who live full- or part-time in the gender role opposite to the one in which they were physically born. They may be heterosexual or homosexual.

Tuskegee study: A study that the U.S. Public Health Service conducted from 1932 to 1972 on hundreds of black men who had syphilis.

value: Personal beliefs about what is true or appropriate behavior. Not all values are moral values.

veracity: An ethical principle that involves being truthful.

vitalistic: The theory or doctrine that life cannot be explained entirely as a physical and chemical phenomenon and that life is partially self-determining through one's energy or soul.

voodoo: A religion that originated in Africa and was influenced by Roman Catholics in which a supreme God rules deities, deified ancestors, and saints who communicate with believers in dreams, trances, and ritual possessions.

worldviews: The overall perspective from which one sees and interprets the world.

wuzho: A Roma belief of what is pure, which is a foundation of their health traditions.

yin and yang: The traditional Chinese medicine theory that everything is made up of two polar energies.

yoga: An ancient system of exercises and breathing techniques designed to encourage physical and spiritual well-being.

PHOTO CREDITS

INDEX

Italicized page locators indicate a figure; tables are noted with a *t*.